50% OFF Online TEAS Prep Course!

By Mometrix University

Dear Customer,

We consider it an honor and a privilege that you chose our TEAS Study Guide. As a way of showing our appreciation and to help us better serve you, we are offering **50% off our online TEAS Prep Course.** Many TEAS courses cost hundreds of dollars and don't deliver enough value. With our course, you get access to the best TEAS prep material, and **you only pay half price.**

We have structured our online course to perfectly complement your printed study guide. The TEAS Prep Course contains **over 60 lessons** that cover all the most important topics, **70 video reviews** that explain difficult concepts, over **1,800 practice questions** to ensure you feel prepared, over **500 digital flashcards** for studying on the go, and even an **audio mode,** so you can listen to lessons as you do other things.

Online TEAS Prep Course

Topics Covered:

- Reading
  - *Key Ideas and Details*
  - *Craft and Structure*
  - *Integration of Knowledge & Ideas*
- English & Language Usage
  - *Conventions of Standard English*
  - *Knowledge of Language*
  - *Vocabulary Acquisition*
- Science
  - *Human Anatomy & Physiology*
  - *Life & Physical Sciences*
  - *Scientific Reasoning*
- Math
  - *Numbers & Algebra*
  - *Measurement & Data*

Course Features:

- TEAS Study Guide
  - Get content that complements our best-selling study guide.
- 8 Full-Length Practice Tests
  - With over 1,800 practice questions, you can test yourself again and again.
- Mobile Friendly
  - If you need to study on the go, the course is easily accessible from your mobile device.
- TEAS Flashcards
  - Our course includes a flashcard mode consisting of over 500 content cards to help you study.
- Audio Mode
  - Every lesson in our course has an audio mode, allowing you to listen to the lessons.

To receive this discount, simply head to our website: mometrix.com/university/courses/teas and add the course to your cart. At the checkout page, enter the discount code: **teas50**

If you have any questions or concerns, please don't hesitate to contact us at universityhelp@mometrix.com.

Sincerely,

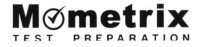

FREE Study Skills DVD Offer

Dear Customer,

Thank you for your purchase from Mometrix! We consider it an honor and a privilege that you have purchased our product and we want to ensure your satisfaction.

As a way of showing our appreciation and to help us better serve you, we have developed a Study Skills DVD that we would like to give you for <u>FREE</u>. This DVD covers our *best practices* for getting ready for your exam, from how to use our study materials to how to best prepare for the day of the test.

All that we ask is that you email us with feedback that would describe your experience so far with our product. Good, bad, or indifferent, we want to know what you think!

To get your FREE Study Skills DVD, email <u>freedvd@mometrix.com</u> with *FREE STUDY SKILLS DVD* in the subject line and the following information in the body of the email:

- The name of the product you purchased.
- Your product rating on a scale of 1-5, with 5 being the highest rating.
- Your feedback. It can be long, short, or anything in between. We just want to know your impressions and experience so far with our product. (Good feedback might include how our study material met your needs and ways we might be able to make it even better. You could highlight features that you found helpful or features that you think we should add.)
- Your full name and shipping address where you would like us to send your free DVD.

If you have any questions or concerns, please don't hesitate to contact me directly.

Thanks again!

Sincerely,

Jay Willis
Vice President
<u>jay.willis@mometrix.com</u>
1-800-673-8175

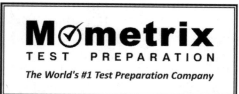

ATI TEAS®

Secrets Study Guide

TEAS® 6 Complete Study Manual for the 6th Edition Test of Essential Academic Skills

Full-Length Practice Tests

Step-by-Step Review
Video Tutorials

Written and edited by Mometrix Test Prep

Printed in the United States of America

This paper meets the requirements of ANSI/NISO Z39.48-1992 (Permanence of Paper).

Mometrix offers volume discount pricing to institutions. For more information or a price quote, please contact our sales department at sales@mometrix.com or 888-248-1219.

ATI TEAS® is a registered trademark of the Assessment Technologies Institute®, which was not involved in the production of, and does not endorse, this product.

Paperback
ISBN 13: 978-1-5167-4604-0
ISBN 10: 1-5167-4604-X

Dear Future Exam Success Story

First of all, **THANK YOU** for purchasing Mometrix study materials!

Second, congratulations! You are one of the few determined test-takers who are committed to doing whatever it takes to excel on your exam. **You have come to the right place.** We developed these study materials with one goal in mind: to deliver you the information you need in a format that's concise and easy to use.

In addition to optimizing your guide for the content of the test, we've outlined our recommended steps for breaking down the preparation process into small, attainable goals so you can make sure you stay on track.

We've also analyzed the entire test-taking process, identifying the most common pitfalls and showing how you can overcome them and be ready for any curveball the test throws you.

Standardized testing is one of the biggest obstacles on your road to success, which only increases the importance of doing well in the high-pressure, high-stakes environment of test day. Your results on this test could have a significant impact on your future, and this guide provides the information and practical advice to help you achieve your full potential on test day.

Your success is our success

We would love to hear from you! If you would like to share the story of your exam success or if you have any questions or comments in regard to our products, please contact us at **800-673-8175** or **support@mometrix.com**.

Thanks again for your business and we wish you continued success!

Sincerely,
The Mometrix Test Preparation Team

Need more help? Check out our flashcards at:
http://MometrixFlashcards.com/TEAS

TABLE OF CONTENTS

Introduction

Thank you for purchasing this resource! You have made the choice to prepare yourself for a test that could have a huge impact on your future, and this guide is designed to help you be fully ready for test day. Obviously, it's important to have a solid understanding of the test material, but you also need to be prepared for the unique environment and stressors of the test, so that you can perform to the best of your abilities.

For this purpose, the first section that appears in this guide is the **Secret Keys**. We've devoted countless hours to meticulously researching what works and what doesn't, and we've boiled down our findings to the five most impactful steps you can take to improve your performance on the test. We start at the beginning with study planning and move through the preparation process, all the way to the testing strategies that will help you get the most out of what you know when you're finally sitting in front of the test.

We recommend that you start preparing for your test as far in advance as possible. However, if you've bought this guide as a last-minute study resource and only have a few days before your test, we recommend that you skip over the first two Secret Keys since they address a long-term study plan.

If you struggle with **test anxiety**, we strongly encourage you to check out our recommendations for how you can overcome it. Test anxiety is a formidable foe, but it can be beaten, and we want to make sure you have the tools you need to defeat it.

Secret Key #1 – Plan Big, Study Small

There's a lot riding on your performance. If you want to ace this test, you're going to need to keep your skills sharp and the material fresh in your mind. You need a plan that lets you review everything you need to know while still fitting in your schedule. We'll break this strategy down into three categories.

Information Organization

Start with the information you already have: the official test outline. From this, you can make a complete list of all the concepts you need to cover before the test. Organize these concepts into groups that can be studied together, and create a list of any related vocabulary you need to learn so you can brush up on any difficult terms. You'll want to keep this vocabulary list handy once you actually start studying since you may need to add to it along the way.

Time Management

Once you have your set of study concepts, decide how to spread them out over the time you have left before the test. Break your study plan into small, clear goals so you have a manageable task for each day and know exactly what you're doing. Then just focus on one small step at a time. When you manage your time this way, you don't need to spend hours at a time studying. Studying a small block of content for a short period each day helps you retain information better and avoid stressing over how much you have left to do. You can relax knowing that you have a plan to cover everything in time. In order for this strategy to be effective though, you have to start studying early and stick to your schedule. Avoid the exhaustion and futility that comes from last-minute cramming!

Study Environment

The environment you study in has a big impact on your learning. Studying in a coffee shop, while probably more enjoyable, is not likely to be as fruitful as studying in a quiet room. It's important to keep distractions to a minimum. You're only planning to study for a short block of time, so make the most of it. Don't pause to check your phone or get up to find a snack. It's also important to **avoid multitasking**. Research has consistently shown that multitasking will make your studying dramatically less effective. Your study area should also be comfortable and well-lit so you don't have the distraction of straining your eyes or sitting on an uncomfortable chair.

The time of day you study is also important. You want to be rested and alert. Don't wait until just before bedtime. Study when you'll be most likely to comprehend and remember. Even better, if you know what time of day your test will be, set that time aside for study. That way your brain will be used to working on that subject at that specific time and you'll have a better chance of recalling information.

Finally, it can be helpful to team up with others who are studying for the same test. Your actual studying should be done in as isolated an environment as possible, but the work of organizing the information and setting up the study plan can be divided up. In between study sessions, you can discuss with your teammates the concepts that you're all studying and quiz each other on the details. Just be sure that your teammates are as serious about the test as you are. If you find that your study time is being replaced with social time, you might need to find a new team.

Secret Key #2 – Make Your Studying Count

You're devoting a lot of time and effort to preparing for this test, so you want to be absolutely certain it will pay off. This means doing more than just reading the content and hoping you can remember it on test day. It's important to make every minute of study count. There are two main areas you can focus on to make your studying count:

Retention

It doesn't matter how much time you study if you can't remember the material. You need to make sure you are retaining the concepts. To check your retention of the information you're learning, try recalling it at later times with minimal prompting. Try carrying around flashcards and glance at one or two from time to time or ask a friend who's also studying for the test to quiz you.

To enhance your retention, look for ways to put the information into practice so that you can apply it rather than simply recalling it. If you're using the information in practical ways, it will be much easier to remember. Similarly, it helps to solidify a concept in your mind if you're not only reading it to yourself but also explaining it to someone else. Ask a friend to let you teach them about a concept you're a little shaky on (or speak aloud to an imaginary audience if necessary). As you try to summarize, define, give examples, and answer your friend's questions, you'll understand the concepts better and they will stay with you longer. Finally, step back for a big picture view and ask yourself how each piece of information fits with the whole subject. When you link the different concepts together and see them working together as a whole, it's easier to remember the individual components.

Finally, practice showing your work on any multi-step problems, even if you're just studying. Writing out each step you take to solve a problem will help solidify the process in your mind, and you'll be more likely to remember it during the test.

Modality

Modality simply refers to the means or method by which you study. Choosing a study modality that fits your own individual learning style is crucial. No two people learn best in exactly the same way, so it's important to know your strengths and use them to your advantage.

For example, if you learn best by visualization, focus on visualizing a concept in your mind and draw an image or a diagram. Try color-coding your notes, illustrating them, or creating symbols that will trigger your mind to recall a learned concept. If you learn best by hearing or discussing information, find a study partner who learns the same way or read aloud to yourself. Think about how to put the information in your own words. Imagine that you are giving a lecture on the topic and record yourself so you can listen to it later.

For any learning style, flashcards can be helpful. Organize the information so you can take advantage of spare moments to review. Underline key words or phrases. Use different colors for different categories. Mnemonic devices (such as creating a short list in which every item starts with the same letter) can also help with retention. Find what works best for you and use it to store the information in your mind most effectively and easily.

Secret Key #3 – Practice the Right Way

Your success on test day depends not only on how many hours you put into preparing, but also on whether you prepared the right way. It's good to check along the way to see if your studying is paying off. One of the most effective ways to do this is by taking practice tests to evaluate your progress. Practice tests are useful because they show exactly where you need to improve. Every time you take a practice test, pay special attention to these three groups of questions:

- The questions you got wrong
- The questions you had to guess on, even if you guessed right
- The questions you found difficult or slow to work through

This will show you exactly what your weak areas are, and where you need to devote more study time. Ask yourself why each of these questions gave you trouble. Was it because you didn't understand the material? Was it because you didn't remember the vocabulary? Do you need more repetitions on this type of question to build speed and confidence? Dig into those questions and figure out how you can strengthen your weak areas as you go back to review the material.

Additionally, many practice tests have a section explaining the answer choices. It can be tempting to read the explanation and think that you now have a good understanding of the concept. However, an explanation likely only covers part of the question's broader context. Even if the explanation makes sense, **go back and investigate** every concept related to the question until you're positive you have a thorough understanding.

As you go along, keep in mind that the practice test is just that: practice. Memorizing these questions and answers will not be very helpful on the actual test because it is unlikely to have any of the same exact questions. If you only know the right answers to the sample questions, you won't be prepared for the real thing. **Study the concepts** until you understand them fully, and then you'll be able to answer any question that shows up on the test.

It's important to wait on the practice tests until you're ready. If you take a test on your first day of study, you may be overwhelmed by the amount of material covered and how much you need to learn. Work up to it gradually.

On test day, you'll need to be prepared for answering questions, managing your time, and using the test-taking strategies you've learned. It's a lot to balance, like a mental marathon that will have a big impact on your future. Like training for a marathon, you'll need to start slowly and work your way up. When test day arrives, you'll be ready.

Start with the strategies you've read in the first two Secret Keys—plan your course and study in the way that works best for you. If you have time, consider using multiple study resources to get different approaches to the same concepts. It can be helpful to see difficult concepts from more than one angle. Then find a good source for practice tests. Many times, the test website will suggest potential study resources or provide sample tests.

Practice Test Strategy

When you're ready to start taking practice tests, follow this strategy:

UNTIMED AND OPEN-BOOK PRACTICE

Take the first test with no time constraints and with your notes and study guide handy. Take your time and focus on applying the strategies you've learned.

TIMED AND OPEN-BOOK PRACTICE

Take the second practice test open-book as well, but set a timer and practice pacing yourself to finish in time.

TIMED AND CLOSED-BOOK PRACTICE

Take any other practice tests as if it were test day. Set a timer and put away your study materials. Sit at a table or desk in a quiet room, imagine yourself at the testing center, and answer questions as quickly and accurately as possible.

Keep repeating timed and closed-book tests on a regular basis until you run out of practice tests or it's time for the actual test. Your mind will be ready for the schedule and stress of test day, and you'll be able to focus on recalling the material you've learned.

Secret Key #4 – Pace Yourself

Once you're fully prepared for the material on the test, your biggest challenge on test day will be managing your time. Just knowing that the clock is ticking can make you panic even if you have plenty of time left. Work on pacing yourself so you can build confidence against the time constraints of the exam. Pacing is a difficult skill to master, especially in a high-pressure environment, so **practice is vital**.

Set time expectations for your pace based on how much time is available. For example, if a section has 60 questions and the time limit is 30 minutes, you know you have to average 30 seconds or less per question in order to answer them all. Although 30 seconds is the hard limit, set 25 seconds per question as your goal, so you reserve extra time to spend on harder questions. When you budget extra time for the harder questions, you no longer have any reason to stress when those questions take longer to answer.

Don't let this time expectation distract you from working through the test at a calm, steady pace, but keep it in mind so you don't spend too much time on any one question. Recognize that taking extra time on one question you don't understand may keep you from answering two that you do understand later in the test. If your time limit for a question is up and you're still not sure of the answer, mark it and move on, and come back to it later if the time and the test format allow. If the testing format doesn't allow you to return to earlier questions, just make an educated guess; then put it out of your mind and move on.

On the easier questions, be careful not to rush. It may seem wise to hurry through them so you have more time for the challenging ones, but it's not worth missing one if you know the concept and just didn't take the time to read the question fully. Work efficiently but make sure you understand the question and have looked at all of the answer choices, since more than one may seem right at first.

Even if you're paying attention to the time, you may find yourself a little behind at some point. You should speed up to get back on track, but do so wisely. Don't panic; just take a few seconds less on each question until you're caught up. Don't guess without thinking, but do look through the answer choices and eliminate any you know are wrong. If you can get down to two choices, it is often worthwhile to guess from those. Once you've chosen an answer, move on and don't dwell on any that you skipped or had to hurry through. If a question was taking too long, chances are it was one of the harder ones, so you weren't as likely to get it right anyway.

On the other hand, if you find yourself getting ahead of schedule, it may be beneficial to slow down a little. The more quickly you work, the more likely you are to make a careless mistake that will affect your score. You've budgeted time for each question, so don't be afraid to spend that time. Practice an efficient but careful pace to get the most out of the time you have.

Secret Key #5 – Have a Plan for Guessing

When you're taking the test, you may find yourself stuck on a question. Some of the answer choices seem better than others, but you don't see the one answer choice that is obviously correct. What do you do?

The scenario described above is very common, yet most test takers have not effectively prepared for it. Developing and practicing a plan for guessing may be one of the single most effective uses of your time as you get ready for the exam.

In developing your plan for guessing, there are three questions to address:

- When should you start the guessing process?
- How should you narrow down the choices?
- Which answer should you choose?

When to Start the Guessing Process

Unless your plan for guessing is to select C every time (which, despite its merits, is not what we recommend), you need to leave yourself enough time to apply your answer elimination strategies. Since you have a limited amount of time for each question, that means that if you're going to give yourself the best shot at guessing correctly, you have to decide quickly whether or not you will guess.

Of course, the best-case scenario is that you don't have to guess at all, so first, see if you can answer the question based on your knowledge of the subject and basic reasoning skills. Focus on the key words in the question and try to jog your memory of related topics. Give yourself a chance to bring the knowledge to mind, but once you realize that you don't have (or you can't access) the knowledge you need to answer the question, it's time to start the guessing process.

It's almost always better to start the guessing process too early than too late. It only takes a few seconds to remember something and answer the question from knowledge. Carefully eliminating wrong answer choices takes longer. Plus, going through the process of eliminating answer choices can actually help jog your memory.

Summary: Start the guessing process as soon as you decide that you can't answer the question based on your knowledge.

How to Narrow Down the Choices

The next chapter in this book (**Test-Taking Strategies**) includes a wide range of strategies for how to approach questions and how to look for answer choices to eliminate. You will definitely want to read those carefully, practice them, and figure out which ones work best for you. Here though, we're going to address a mindset rather than a particular strategy.

Your chances of guessing an answer correctly depend on how many options you are choosing from.

How many choices you have	How likely you are to guess correctly
5	20%
4	25%
3	33%
2	50%
1	100%

You can see from this chart just how valuable it is to be able to eliminate incorrect answers and make an educated guess, but there are two things that many test takers do that cause them to miss out on the benefits of guessing:

- Accidentally eliminating the correct answer
- Selecting an answer based on an impression

We'll look at the first one here, and the second one in the next section.

To avoid accidentally eliminating the correct answer, we recommend a thought exercise called **the $5 challenge**. In this challenge, you only eliminate an answer choice from contention if you are willing to bet $5 on it being wrong. Why $5? Five dollars is a small but not insignificant amount of money. It's an amount you could afford to lose but wouldn't want to throw away. And while losing $5 once might not hurt too much, doing it twenty times will set you back $100. In the same way, each small decision you make—eliminating a choice here, guessing on a question there—won't by itself impact your score very much, but when you put them all together, they can make a big difference. By holding each answer choice elimination decision to a higher standard, you can reduce the risk of accidentally eliminating the correct answer.

The $5 challenge can also be applied in a positive sense: If you are willing to bet $5 that an answer choice *is* correct, go ahead and mark it as correct.

Summary: Only eliminate an answer choice if you are willing to bet $5 that it is wrong.

Which Answer to Choose

You're taking the test. You've run into a hard question and decided you'll have to guess. You've eliminated all the answer choices you're willing to bet $5 on. Now you have to pick an answer. Why do we even need to talk about this? Why can't you just pick whichever one you feel like when the time comes?

The answer to these questions is that if you don't come into the test with a plan, you'll rely on your impression to select an answer choice, and if you do that, you risk falling into a trap. The test writers know that everyone who takes their test will be guessing on some of the questions, so they intentionally write wrong answer choices to seem plausible. You still have to pick an answer though, and if the wrong answer choices are designed to look right, how can you ever be sure that you're not falling for their trap? The best solution we've found to this dilemma is to take the decision out of your hands entirely. Here is the process we recommend:

Once you've eliminated any choices that you are confident (willing to bet $5) are wrong, select the first remaining choice as your answer.

Whether you choose to select the first remaining choice, the second, or the last, the important thing is that you use some preselected standard. Using this approach guarantees that you will not be enticed into selecting an answer choice that looks right, because you are not basing your decision on how the answer choices look.

This is not meant to make you question your knowledge. Instead, it is to help you recognize the difference between your knowledge and your impressions. There's a huge difference between thinking an answer is right because of what you know, and thinking an answer is right because it looks or sounds like it should be right.

Summary: To ensure that your selection is appropriately random, make a predetermined selection from among all answer choices you have not eliminated.

Test-Taking Strategies

This section contains a list of test-taking strategies that you may find helpful as you work through the test. By taking what you know and applying logical thought, you can maximize your chances of answering any question correctly!

It is very important to realize that every question is different and every person is different: no single strategy will work on every question, and no single strategy will work for every person. That's why we've included all of them here, so you can try them out and determine which ones work best for different types of questions and which ones work best for you.

Question Strategies

READ CAREFULLY

Read the question and answer choices carefully. Don't miss the question because you misread the terms. You have plenty of time to read each question thoroughly and make sure you understand what is being asked. Yet a happy medium must be attained, so don't waste too much time. You must read carefully, but efficiently.

CONTEXTUAL CLUES

Look for contextual clues. If the question includes a word you are not familiar with, look at the immediate context for some indication of what the word might mean. Contextual clues can often give you all the information you need to decipher the meaning of an unfamiliar word. Even if you can't determine the meaning, you may be able to narrow down the possibilities enough to make a solid guess at the answer to the question.

PREFIXES

If you're having trouble with a word in the question or answer choices, try dissecting it. Take advantage of every clue that the word might include. Prefixes and suffixes can be a huge help. Usually they allow you to determine a basic meaning. Pre- means before, post- means after, pro - is positive, de- is negative. From prefixes and suffixes, you can get an idea of the general meaning of the word and try to put it into context.

HEDGE WORDS

Watch out for critical hedge words, such as *likely, may, can, sometimes, often, almost, mostly, usually, generally, rarely*, and *sometimes*. Question writers insert these hedge phrases to cover every possibility. Often an answer choice will be wrong simply because it leaves no room for exception. Be on guard for answer choices that have definitive words such as *exactly* and *always*.

SWITCHBACK WORDS

Stay alert for *switchbacks*. These are the words and phrases frequently used to alert you to shifts in thought. The most common switchback words are *but, although*, and *however*. Others include *nevertheless, on the other hand, even though, while, in spite of, despite, regardless of*. Switchback words are important to catch because they can change the direction of the question or an answer choice.

FACE VALUE

When in doubt, use common sense. Accept the situation in the problem at face value. Don't read too much into it. These problems will not require you to make wild assumptions. If you have to go beyond creativity and warp time or space in order to have an answer choice fit the question, then you should move on and consider the other answer choices. These are normal problems rooted in reality. The applicable relationship or explanation may not be readily apparent, but it is there for you to figure out. Use your common sense to interpret anything that isn't clear.

Answer Choice Strategies

ANSWER SELECTION

The most thorough way to pick an answer choice is to identify and eliminate wrong answers until only one is left, then confirm it is the correct answer. Sometimes an answer choice may immediately seem right, but be careful. The test writers will usually put more than one reasonable answer choice on each question, so take a second to read all of them and make sure that the other choices are not equally obvious. As long as you have time left, it is better to read every answer choice than to pick the first one that looks right without checking the others.

ANSWER CHOICE FAMILIES

An answer choice family consists of two (in rare cases, three) answer choices that are very similar in construction and cannot all be true at the same time. If you see two answer choices that are direct opposites or parallels, one of them is usually the correct answer. For instance, if one answer choice says that quantity *x* increases and another either says that quantity *x* decreases (opposite) or says that quantity *y* increases (parallel), then those answer choices would fall into the same family. An answer choice that doesn't match the construction of the answer choice family is more likely to be incorrect. Most questions will not have answer choice families, but when they do appear, you should be prepared to recognize them.

ELIMINATE ANSWERS

Eliminate answer choices as soon as you realize they are wrong, but make sure you consider all possibilities. If you are eliminating answer choices and realize that the last one you are left with is also wrong, don't panic. Start over and consider each choice again. There may be something you missed the first time that you will realize on the second pass.

AVOID FACT TRAPS

Don't be distracted by an answer choice that is factually true but doesn't answer the question. You are looking for the choice that answers the question. Stay focused on what the question is asking for so you don't accidentally pick an answer that is true but incorrect. Always go back to the question and make sure the answer choice you've selected actually answers the question and is not merely a true statement.

EXTREME STATEMENTS

In general, you should avoid answers that put forth extreme actions as standard practice or proclaim controversial ideas as established fact. An answer choice that states the "process should be used in certain situations, if…" is much more likely to be correct than one that states the "process should be discontinued completely." The first is a calm rational statement and doesn't even make a definitive, uncompromising stance, using a hedge word *if* to provide wiggle room, whereas the second choice is a radical idea and far more extreme.

BENCHMARK

As you read through the answer choices and you come across one that seems to answer the question well, mentally select that answer choice. This is not your final answer, but it's the one that will help you evaluate the other answer choices. The one that you selected is your benchmark or standard for judging each of the other answer choices. Every other answer choice must be compared to your benchmark. That choice is correct until proven otherwise by another answer choice beating it. If you find a better answer, then that one becomes your new benchmark. Once you've decided that no other choice answers the question as well as your benchmark, you have your final answer.

PREDICT THE ANSWER

Before you even start looking at the answer choices, it is often best to try to predict the answer. When you come up with the answer on your own, it is easier to avoid distractions and traps because you will know exactly what to look for. The right answer choice is unlikely to be word-for-word what you came up with, but it should be a close match. Even if you are confident that you have the right answer, you should still take the time to read each option before moving on.

General Strategies

TOUGH QUESTIONS

If you are stumped on a problem or it appears too hard or too difficult, don't waste time. Move on! Remember though, if you can quickly check for obviously incorrect answer choices, your chances of guessing correctly are greatly improved. Before you completely give up, at least try to knock out a couple of possible answers. Eliminate what you can and then guess at the remaining answer choices before moving on.

CHECK YOUR WORK

Since you will probably not know every term listed and the answer to every question, it is important that you get credit for the ones that you do know. Don't miss any questions through careless mistakes. If at all possible, try to take a second to look back over your answer selection and make sure you've selected the correct answer choice and haven't made a costly careless mistake (such as marking an answer choice that you didn't mean to mark). This quick double check should more than pay for itself in caught mistakes for the time it costs.

PACE YOURSELF

It's easy to be overwhelmed when you're looking at a page full of questions; your mind is confused and full of random thoughts, and the clock is ticking down faster than you would like. Calm down and maintain the pace that you have set for yourself. Especially as you get down to the last few minutes of the test, don't let the small numbers on the clock make you panic. As long as you are on track by monitoring your pace, you are guaranteed to have time for each question.

DON'T RUSH

It is very easy to make errors when you are in a hurry. Maintaining a fast pace in answering questions is pointless if it makes you miss questions that you would have gotten right otherwise. Test writers like to include distracting information and wrong answers that seem right. Taking a little extra time to avoid careless mistakes can make all the difference in your test score. Find a pace that allows you to be confident in the answers that you select.

KEEP MOVING

Panicking will not help you pass the test, so do your best to stay calm and keep moving. Taking deep breaths and going through the answer elimination steps you practiced can help to break through a stress barrier and keep your pace.

Final Notes

The combination of a solid foundation of content knowledge and the confidence that comes from practicing your plan for applying that knowledge is the key to maximizing your performance on test day. As your foundation of content knowledge is built up and strengthened, you'll find that the strategies included in this chapter become more and more effective in helping you quickly sift through the distractions and traps of the test to isolate the correct answer.

Now it's time to move on to the test content chapters of this book, but be sure to keep your goal in mind. As you read, think about how you will be able to apply this information on the test. If you've already seen sample questions for the test and you have an idea of the question format and style, try to come up with questions of your own that you can answer based on what you're reading. This will give you valuable practice applying your knowledge in the same ways you can expect to on test day.

Good luck and good studying!

About the TEAS Test

ATI TEAS Secrets by Mometrix Test Preparation includes comprehensive review sections on each of the four TEAS test sections. Following those review sections are two complete TEAS practice tests, and a link to an additional **online interactive practice test**.

> **Online Interactive Practice Test**
> Visit mometrix.com/university/teas-bonus-practice-test

The TEAS is an important test, so it is essential that you adequately prepare for your test day. Be sure to set aside enough study time to be able to take each of the practice tests using only the amount of time that is specified. You are encouraged to minimize your external distractions in order to make the practice test conditions as similar to the real test conditions as possible.

Below is a breakdown of the four sections on the exam, including the subcategories, how many questions are in each section, and how much time will be allotted for you to complete that section. Each section of the test contains more questions for you to answer than will actually be scored. Those extra questions are being evaluated by the test makers for future use.

Content Areas	Time	Test Items	% of Test	Scored Items
Reading	**64 min**	**53**	**31%**	**47**
Key Ideas and Details				22
Craft and Structure				14
Integration of Knowledge and Ideas				11
Mathematics	**54 min**	**36**	**21%**	**32**
Number and Algebra				23
Measurement and Data				9
Science	**63 min**	**53**	**31%**	**47**
Human Anatomy and Physiology				32
Life and Physical Sciences				8
Scientific Reasoning				7
English and Language Usage	**28 min**	**28**	**17%**	**24**
Conventions of Standard English				9
Knowledge of Language				9
Vocabulary Acquisition				6
Total	**209 min**	**170**		**150**

Reading

Key Ideas and Details

SUMMARIZING A COMPLEX TEXT

SUMMARIZE

A helpful tool is the ability to **summarize** the information that you have read in a paragraph or passage format. This process is similar to creating an effective outline. First, a summary should accurately define the **main idea** of the passage though the summary does not need to explain this main idea in exhaustive detail. The summary should continue by laying out the most important **supporting details** or arguments from the passage. All of the significant supporting details should be included, and none of the details included should be irrelevant or insignificant. Also, the summary should accurately report all of these details. Too often, the desire for brevity in a summary leads to the sacrifice of clarity or accuracy. Summaries are often difficult to read because they omit all of the graceful language, digressions, and asides that distinguish great writing. However, an effective summary should contain much the same message as the original text.

PARAPHRASE

Paraphrasing is another method that the reader can use to aid in comprehension. When paraphrasing, one puts what they have read into their words by **rephrasing** what the author has written, or one "translates" all of what the author shared into their words by including as many details as they can.

IDENTIFYING THE LOGICAL CONCLUSION

Identifying a logical conclusion can help you determine whether you agree with the writer or not. Coming to this conclusion is much like making an inference: the approach requires you to combine the information given by the text with what you already know in order to make a **logical conclusion**. If the author intended the reader to draw a certain conclusion, then you can expect the author's argumentation and detail to be leading in that direction. One way to approach the task of drawing conclusions is to make brief **notes** of all the points made by the author. When the notes are arranged on paper, they may clarify the logical conclusion. Another way to approach conclusions is to consider whether the reasoning of the author raises any **pertinent questions**. Sometimes you will be able to draw several conclusions from a passage. On occasion these will be conclusions that were never imagined by the author. Therefore, be aware that these conclusions must be **supported** directly by the text.

DIRECTLY STATED INFORMATION

A reader should always be drawing conclusions from the text. Sometimes conclusions are implied from written information, and other times the information is **stated directly** within the passage. One should always aim to draw **conclusions** from information stated within a passage, rather than to draw them from mere implications. At times an author may provide some information and then describe a **counterargument**. Readers should be alert for direct statements that are subsequently rejected or weakened by the author. Furthermore, you should always read through the **entire passage** before drawing conclusions. Many readers are trained to expect the author's conclusions at either the beginning or the end of the passage, but many texts do not adhere to this format.

INFERENCES

Readers are often required to understand a text that claims and suggests ideas without stating them directly. An **inference** is a piece of information that is implied but not written outright by the author. For instance, consider the following sentence: *After the final out of the inning, the fans were filled with joy and rushed the field.* From this sentence, a reader can infer that the fans were watching a baseball game and their team won the game. Readers should take great care to avoid using information **beyond the provided passage** before making inferences. As you practice drawing inferences, you will find that they require concentration and attention.

> **Review Video: Inference**
> Visit mometrix.com/academy and enter code: 379203

Test-taking tip: While being tested on your ability to make correct inferences, you must look for **contextual clues**. An answer can be *true* but not *correct*. The contextual clues will help you find the answer that is the **best answer** out of the given choices. Be careful in your reading to understand the context in which a phrase is stated. When asked for the implied meaning of a statement made in the passage, you should immediately locate the statement and read the **context** in which the statement was made. Also, look for an answer choice that has a similar phrase to the statement in question.

IMPLICATIONS

Drawing conclusions from information implied within a passage requires confidence on the part of the reader. **Implications** are things that the author does not state directly, but readers can assume based on what the author does say. Consider the following passage: *I stepped outside and opened my umbrella. By the time I got to work, the cuffs of my pants were soaked.* The author never states that it is raining, but this fact is clearly implied. Conclusions based on implication must be well supported by the text. In order to draw a solid conclusion, readers should have multiple pieces of **evidence**. If readers have only one piece, they must be assured that there is no other possible explanation than their conclusion. A good reader will be able to draw many conclusions from information implied by the text which will be a great help in the exam.

TOPICS, MAIN IDEAS, AND SUPPORTING DETAILS

TOPICS AND MAIN IDEAS

One of the most important skills in reading comprehension is the identification of **topics** and **main ideas.** There is a subtle difference between these two features. The topic is the **subject** of a text (i.e., what the text is all about). The main idea, on the other hand, is the **most important point** being made by the author. The topic is usually expressed in a few words at the most while the main idea often needs a full sentence to be completely defined. As an example, a short passage might have the topic of penguins and the main idea could be written as: *Penguins are different from other birds in many ways.* In most nonfiction writing, the topic and the main idea will be stated directly and often appear in a sentence at the very **beginning** or **end** of the text. When being tested on an understanding of the author's topic, you may be able to **skim** the passage for the general idea, by reading only the first sentence of each paragraph. A body paragraph's first sentence is often—but not always—the main topic sentence which gives you a summary of the content in the paragraph.

However, there are cases in which the reader must figure out an **unstated** topic or main idea. In these instances, you must read every sentence of the text and try to come up with an overarching idea that is supported by each of those sentences.

> **Review Video: Topics and Main Ideas**
> Visit mometrix.com/academy and enter code: 407801

SUPPORTING DETAILS

Supporting details provide **evidence** and backing for the main point. In order to show that a main idea is correct, or valid, authors add details that prove their point. All texts contain details, but they are only classified as **supporting details** when they serve to reinforce some larger point. Supporting details are most commonly found in **informative** and **persuasive** texts. In some cases, they will be clearly indicated with terms like *for example* or *for instance*, or they will be enumerated with terms like *first*, *second*, and *last*. However, you need to be prepared for texts that do not contain those indicators. As a reader, you should consider whether the author's supporting details really back up his or her **main point**. Supporting details can be factual and correct, yet they may not be relevant to the author's point. Conversely, supporting details can seem pertinent, but they can be ineffective because they are based on opinion or assertions that cannot be proven.

> **Review Video: Supporting Details**
> Visit mometrix.com/academy and enter code: 396297

TOPIC AND SUMMARY SENTENCES

Topic and summary sentences are a convenient way to encapsulate the **main idea** of a text. In some textbooks and academic articles, the author will place a **topic** or **summary sentence** at the beginning of each section as a means of preparing the reader for what is to come. Research suggests that the brain is more receptive to new information when it has been prepared by the presentation of the main idea or some key words. The phenomenon is somewhat akin to the primer coat of paint that allows subsequent coats of paint to absorb more easily. A good topic sentence will be **clear** and not contain any **jargon**. When topic or summary sentences are not provided, good readers can jot down their own so that they can find their place in a text and refresh their memory.

FOLLOWING DIRECTIONS

Technical passages often require the reader to **follow a set of directions**. For many people, especially those who are tactile or visual learners, this can be a difficult process. It is important to approach a set of directions differently than other texts. First, it is a good idea to **scan** the directions to determine whether special equipment or preparations are needed. Sometimes in a recipe, for instance, the author fails to mention that the oven should be preheated first, and then halfway through the process, the cook is supposed to be baking. After briefly reading the directions, the reader should return to the first step. When following directions, it is appropriate to **complete each step** before moving on to the next. If this is not possible, it is useful at least to visualize each step before reading the next.

INFORMATION FROM PRINTED COMMUNICATION

MEMO

A memo (short for *memorandum*) is a common form of written communication. There is a standard format for these documents. It is typical for there to be a **heading** at the top indicating the author, date, and recipient. In some cases, this heading will also include the author's title and the name of his or her institution. Below this information will be the **body** of the memo. These documents are typically written by and for members of the same organization. They usually contain a plan of action, a request for information on a specific topic, or a response to such a request. Memos are considered to be official documents, and so are usually written in a **formal** style. Many memos are organized with numbers or bullet points, which make it easier for the reader to identify key ideas.

POSTED ANNOUNCEMENT

People post **announcements** for all sorts of occasions. Many people are familiar with notices for lost pets, yard sales, and landscaping services. In order to be effective, these announcements need to *contain all of the information* the reader requires to act on the message. For instance, a lost pet announcement needs to include a good description of the animal and a contact number for the owner. A yard sale notice should include the address, date, and hours of the sale, as well as a brief description of the products that will be available there. When composing an announcement, it is important to consider the perspective of the **audience**—what will they need to know in order to respond to the message? Although a posted announcement can have color and decoration to attract the eye of the passerby, it must also convey the necessary information clearly.

CLASSIFIED ADVERTISEMENT

Classified advertisements, or **ads**, are used to sell or buy goods, to attract business, to make romantic connections, and to do countless other things. They are an inexpensive, and sometimes free, way to make a brief *pitch*. Classified ads used to be found only in newspapers or special advertising circulars, but there are now online listings as well. The style of these ads has remained basically the same. An ad usually begins with a word or phrase indicating what is being **sold** or **sought**. Then, the listing will give a brief **description** of the product or service. Because space is limited and costly in newspapers, classified ads there will often contain abbreviations for common attributes. For instance, two common abbreviations are *bk* for *black*, and *obo* for *or best offer*. Classified ads will then usually conclude by listing the **price** (or the amount the seeker is willing to pay), followed by **contact information** like a telephone number or email address.

SCALE READINGS OF STANDARD MEASUREMENT INSTRUMENTS

The scales used on **standard measurement instruments** are fairly easy to read with a little practice. Take the **ruler** as an example. A typical ruler has different units along each long edge. One side measures inches, and the other measures centimeters. The units are specified close to the zero reading for the ruler. Note that the ruler does not begin measuring from its outermost edge. The zero reading is a black line a tiny distance inside of the edge. On the inches side, each inch is indicated with a long black line and a number. Each half-inch is noted with a slightly shorter line. Quarter-inches are noted with still shorter lines, eighth-inches are noted with even shorter lines, and sixteenth-inches are noted with the shortest lines of all. On the centimeter side, the second-largest black lines indicate half-centimeters, and the smaller lines indicate tenths of centimeters, otherwise known as millimeters.

LEGEND OR KEY OF A MAP

Almost all maps contain a **key**, or **legend**, that defines the **symbols** used on the map for various landmarks. This key is usually placed in a corner of the map. It should contain listings for all of the important symbols on the map. Of course, these symbols will vary depending on the nature of the map. A road map uses different colored lines to indicate roads, highways, and interstates. A legend might also show different dots and squares that are used to indicate towns of various sizes. The legend may contain information about the map's **scale**, though this may be elsewhere on the map. Many legends will contain special symbols, such as a picnic table indicating a campground.

EVENTS IN A SEQUENCE

Readers must be able to identify a text's **sequence**, or the order in which things happen. Often, when the sequence is very important to the author, the text is indicated with signal words like *first*, *then*, *next*, and *last*. However, a sequence can be merely implied and must be noted by the reader. Consider the sentence: *He walked through the garden and gave water and fertilizer to the plants.* Clearly, the man did not walk through the garden before he collected water and fertilizer for the plants. So, the implied sequence is that he first collected water, then he collected fertilizer, next he walked through the garden, and last he gave water or fertilizer as necessary to the plants. Texts do not always proceed in an **orderly** sequence from first to last. Sometimes they begin at the end and start over at the beginning. As a reader, you can enhance your understanding of the passage by taking brief **notes** to clarify the sequence.

> **Review Video: Sequence**
> Visit mometrix.com/academy and enter code: 489027

Craft and Structure

FACT AND OPINION

Readers must always be conscious of the distinction between **fact** and **opinion**. A fact can be subjected to analysis and can be either **proved or disproved**. An opinion, on the other hand, is the author's **personal thoughts or feelings** which may not be alterable by research or evidence. If the author writes that the distance from New York to Boston is about two hundred miles, then he or she is stating a fact. If the author writes that New York is too crowded, then he or she is giving an opinion because there is no objective standard for overpopulation.

An opinion may be indicated by words like *believe*, *think*, or *feel*. Readers must be aware that an **opinion** may be supported by **facts**. For instance, the author might give the population density of New York as evidence of an overcrowded population. An opinion supported by fact tends to be more convincing. On the other hand, when authors support their opinions with other opinions, readers should not be persuaded by the argument to any degree.

> **Review Video: How to Tell the Difference Between Facts and Opinions**
> Visit mometrix.com/academy and enter code: 717670

BIASES AND STEREOTYPES

Every author has a point-of-view, but authors demonstrate a **bias** when they ignore reasonable counterarguments or distort opposing viewpoints. A bias is evident whenever the author is **unfair** or **inaccurate** in his or her presentation. Bias may be intentional or unintentional, and readers should be skeptical of the author's argument. Remember that a biased author may still be correct; however, the author will be correct in spite of his or her bias, not because of the bias. A **stereotype** is like a bias, yet a stereotype is applied specifically to a **group** or **place**. Stereotyping is considered to be particularly abhorrent because the practice promotes negative generalizations about people. Readers should be very cautious of authors who stereotype in their writing. These faulty assumptions typically reveal the author's ignorance and lack of curiosity.

> **Review Video: Bias and Stereotype**
> Visit mometrix.com/academy and enter code: 644829

STRUCTURE OF TEXTS

PROBLEM-SOLUTION TEXT STRUCTURE

Some nonfiction texts are organized to present a **problem** followed by a **solution**. For this type of text, the problem is often explained before the solution is offered. In some cases, as when the problem is well known, the solution may be introduced briefly at the beginning. Other passages may focus on the solution, and the problem will be referenced only occasionally. Some texts will outline *multiple solutions* to a problem, leaving readers to choose among them. If the author has an interest or an allegiance to one solution, he or she may fail to mention or describe accurately some of the other solutions. Readers should be careful of the author's **agenda** when reading a problem-solution text. Only by understanding the author's perspective and interests can one develop a proper judgment of the proposed solution.

DESCRIPTIVE TEXT

In a sense, almost all writing is descriptive, insofar as an author seeks to describe *events, ideas, or people* to the reader. Some texts, however, are primarily concerned with **description**. A descriptive text focuses on a particular subject and attempts to depict the subject in a way that will be clear to readers. Descriptive texts contain many **adjectives** and **adverbs** (i.e., words that give shades of meaning and create a more detailed mental picture for the reader). A descriptive text fails when it is unclear to the reader. A descriptive text will certainly be informative, and the passage may be persuasive and entertaining as well.

> **Review Video: Descriptive Texts**
> Visit mometrix.com/academy and enter code: 174903

COMPARISON AND CONTRAST

Authors will use different stylistic and writing devices to make their meaning clear for readers. One of those devices is **comparison and contrast**. As mentioned previously, when an author describes the ways in which two things are **alike**, he or she is comparing them. When the author describes the ways in which two things are **different**, he or she is contrasting them. The "compare and contrast" essay is one of the most common forms in nonfiction. These passages are often signaled with certain words: a comparison may have indicating terms such as *both, same, like, too,* and *as well*; while a contrast may have terms like *but, however, on the other hand, instead,* and *yet*. Of course, comparisons and contrasts may be implicit without using any such signaling language. A single sentence may both compare and contrast. Consider the sentence *Brian and Sheila love ice cream, but Brian prefers vanilla and Sheila prefers strawberry*. In one sentence, the author has described both a similarity (love of ice cream) and a difference (favorite flavor).

> **Review Video: Compare and Contrast**
> Visit mometrix.com/academy and enter code: 171799

CAUSE AND EFFECT

One of the most common text structures is **cause and effect**. A cause is an **act** or **event** that makes something happen, and an effect is the thing that happens as a **result** of the cause. A cause-and-effect relationship is not always explicit, but there are some terms in English that signal causes, such as *since, because,* and *due to*. Furthermore, terms that signal effects include *consequently, therefore, this lead(s) to*. As an example, consider this sentence: *Because the sky was clear, Ron did not bring an umbrella*. The cause is the clear sky, and the effect is that Ron did not bring an umbrella. However, readers may find that sometimes the cause-and-effect relationship will not be clearly noted. For instance, the sentence *He was late and missed the meeting* does not contain any signaling words, but the sentence still contains a cause (he was late) and an effect (he missed the meeting).

> **Review Video: Rhetorical Strategy of Cause-and-Effect Analysis**
> Visit mometrix.com/academy and enter code: 725944

TYPES OF PASSAGES

NARRATIVE PASSAGE

A **narrative** passage is a story that can be fiction or nonfiction. However, there are a few elements that a text must have in order to be classified as a narrative. First, the text must have a **plot** (i.e., a series of events). Narratives often proceed in a clear sequence, but this is not a requirement. If the narrative is good, then these events will be interesting to readers. Second, a narrative has **characters**. These characters could be people, animals, or even inanimate objects—so long as they participate in the plot. Third, a narrative passage often contains **figurative language** which is meant to stimulate the imagination of readers by making comparisons and observations. For instance, a *metaphor*, a common piece of figurative language, is a description of one thing in terms of another. *The moon was a frosty snowball* is an example of a metaphor. In the literal sense this is obviously untrue, but the comparison suggests a certain mood for the reader.

EXPOSITORY PASSAGE

An **expository** passage aims to **inform** and enlighten readers. The passage is nonfiction and usually centers around a simple, easily defined topic. Since the goal of exposition is to teach, such a passage should be as clear as possible. Often, an expository passage contains helpful organizing words, like *first, next, for example*, and *therefore*. These words keep the reader **oriented** in the text. Although expository passages do not need to feature colorful language and artful writing, they are often more effective with these features. For a reader, the challenge of expository passages is to maintain steady attention. Expository passages are not always about subjects that will naturally interest a reader, so the writer is often more concerned with **clarity** and **comprehensibility** than with engaging the reader. By reading actively, you will ensure a good habit of focus when reading an expository passage.

TECHNICAL PASSAGE

A **technical** passage is written to *describe* a complex object or process. Technical writing is common in medical and technological fields, in which complex ideas of mathematics, science, and engineering need to be explained *simply* and *clearly*. To ease comprehension, a technical passage usually proceeds in a very logical order. Technical passages often have clear headings and subheadings, which are used to keep the reader oriented in the text. Additionally, you will find that these passages divide sections up with numbers or letters. Many technical passages look more like an outline than a piece of prose. The amount of **jargon** or difficult vocabulary will vary in a technical passage depending on the intended audience. As much as possible, technical passages try to avoid language that the reader will have to research in order to understand the message, yet readers will find that jargon cannot always be avoided.

PERSUASIVE PASSAGE

A **persuasive** passage is meant to change the mind of readers and lead them into **agreement** with the author. The persuasive intent may be very obvious or quite difficult to discern. In some cases, a persuasive passage will be indistinguishable from one that is informative. Both passages make an assertion and offer supporting details. However, a persuasive passage is more likely to appeal to the reader's **emotions** and to make claims based on **opinion**. Persuasive passages may not describe alternate positions, but when they do, they often display significant **bias**. Readers may find that a persuasive passage is giving the author's viewpoint, or the passage may adopt a seemingly objective tone. A persuasive passage is successful if it can make a convincing argument and win the trust of the reader.

WORD MEANING FROM CONTEXT

One of the benefits of reading is the expansion of one's vocabulary. In order to obtain this benefit, however, one needs to know how to identify the definition of a **word from its context**. This means defining a word based on the **words around it** and the way it is **used in a sentence**. Consider the following sentence: *The elderly scholar spent his evenings hunched over arcane texts that few other people even knew existed.* The adjective *arcane* is uncommon, but you can obtain significant information about it based on its use in the sentence. The fact that few other people know of their existence allows you to assume that "arcane texts" must be rare and be of interest to few people. Also, the texts are being read by an elderly scholar. So, you can assume that they focus on difficult academic subjects. Sometimes, words can be defined by **what they are not**. Consider the following sentence: *Ron's fealty to his parents was not shared by Karen, who disobeyed their every command.*

Someone who disobeys is not demonstrating *fealty*. So, you can infer that the word means something like *obedience* or *respect*.

FIGURATIVE LANGUAGE

There are many types of language devices that authors use to convey their meaning in a descriptive way. Understanding these concepts will help you understand what you read. These types of devices are called **figurative language** – language that goes beyond the literal meaning of a word or phrase. **Descriptive language** that evokes imagery in the reader's mind is one type of figurative language. **Exaggeration** is another type of figurative language. Also, when you compare two things, you are using figurative language. **Similes** and **metaphors** are ways of comparing things, and both are types of figurative language commonly found in poetry. An example of figurative language (a simile in this case): *The child howled like a coyote when her mother told her to pick up the toys*. In this example, the child's howling is compared to that of a coyote and helps the reader understand the sound being made by the child.

METAPHOR

A **metaphor** is a type of figurative language in which the writer equates one thing with a different thing. For instance: *The bird was an arrow arcing through the sky*. In this sentence, the arrow is serving as a metaphor for the bird. The point of a metaphor is to encourage the reader to consider the item being described in a *different way*. Let's continue with this metaphor for a bird: you are asked to envision the bird's flight as being similar to the arc of an arrow. So, you imagine the flight to be swift and bending. Metaphors are a way for the author to describe an item *without being direct and obvious*. This literary device is a lyrical and suggestive way of providing information. Note that the reference for a metaphor will not always be mentioned explicitly by the author. Consider the following description of a forest in winter: *Swaying skeletons reached for the sky and groaned as the wind blew through them.* In this example, the author is using *skeletons* as a metaphor for leafless trees. This metaphor creates a spooky tone while inspiring the reader's imagination.

> **Review Video: Metaphor**
> Visit mometrix.com/academy and enter code: 133295

SIMILE

A **simile** is a figurative expression that is similar to a metaphor, yet the expression requires the use of the distancing words *like* or *as*. Some examples: *The sun was like an orange, eager as a beaver*, and *nimble as a mountain goat*. Because a simile includes *like* or *as,* the device creates a space between the description and the thing being described. If an author says that *a house was like a shoebox*, then the tone is different than the author saying that the house *was* a shoebox. In a simile, authors explicitly indicate that the description is **not** the same thing as the thing being described. In a metaphor, there is no such distinction. The decision of which device to use will be made based on the authors' intended **tone**.

> **Review Video: Simile**
> Visit mometrix.com/academy and enter code: 642949

PERSONIFICATION

Another type of figurative language is **personification**. This is the description of a nonhuman thing as if the item were **human**. Literally, the word means the process of making something into a person. The general intent of personification is to describe things in a manner that will be comprehensible to readers. When an author states that a tree *groans* in the wind, he or she does not mean that the tree is emitting a low, pained sound from a mouth. Instead, the author means that the tree is making a noise similar to a human groan. Of course, this personification establishes a tone of sadness or suffering. A different tone would be established if the author said that the tree was *swaying* or *dancing*.

> **Review Video: Personification**
> Visit mometrix.com/academy and enter code: 260066

DENOTATIVE AND CONNOTATIVE MEANING OF WORDS

The **denotative** meaning of a word is the literal meaning of the word. The **connotative** meaning goes beyond the denotative meaning to include the **emotional reaction** that a word may invoke. The connotative meaning often takes the denotative meaning a step further due to associations which the reader makes with the denotative meaning. Readers can differentiate between the denotative and connotative meanings by first recognizing how authors use each meaning. Most nonfiction, for example, is fact-based and authors do not use flowery, figurative language. The reader can assume that the writer is using the denotative meaning of words. In fiction, the author may use the connotative meaning. Readers can determine whether the author is using the denotative or connotative meaning of a word by implementing **context clues**.

> **Review Video: Denotation and Connotation**
> Visit mometrix.com/academy and enter code: 310092

DICTIONARY ENTRY

Dictionaries can be used to find a word's meaning, to check spelling, and to find out how to say or pronounce a word. **Dictionary entries** are in alphabetical order. **Guide words** are the two words at the top of each page. One word is the first word listed on the page and the other word is the last word listed on the page. Using these guide words will help you use the dictionaries more effectively. You may notice that many words have more than one definition. These different definitions are numbered. Also, some words can be used as different **parts of speech**. The definitions for each part of speech are separated. A simple entry might look like this:

WELL: (adverb) 1. in a good way | (noun) 1. a hole drilled into the earth

The correct definition of a word depends on how the word is used in a sentence. To know that you are using the word correctly, you can try to replace the dictionary's definitions for the word in the passage. Then, choose the definition that seems to be the best fit.

PURPOSE

Usually, identifying the **purpose** of an author is easier than identifying his or her position. In most cases, the author has no interest in hiding his or her purpose. A text that is meant to entertain, for instance, should be written to please the reader. Most narratives, or stories, are written to entertain, though they may also inform or persuade. Informative texts are easy to identify, while the most difficult purpose of a text to identify is persuasion because the author has an interest in making this purpose *hard to detect*. When a reader discovers that the author is trying to persuade, he or she should be skeptical of the argument. For this reason, persuasive texts often try to establish an entertaining tone and hope to amuse the reader into agreement. On the other hand, an informative tone may be implemented to create an appearance of authority and objectivity.

> **Review Video: Purpose**
> Visit mometrix.com/academy and enter code: 511819

An author's purpose is evident often in the **organization** of the text (e.g., section headings in bold font points to an informative text). However, you may not have such organization available to you in your exam. Instead, if the author makes his or her main idea clear from the beginning, then the likely purpose of the text is to **inform**. If the author begins by making a claim and provides various arguments to support that claim, then the purpose is probably to **persuade**. If the author tells a story or seems to want the attention of the reader more than to push a particular point or deliver information, then his or her purpose is most likely to **entertain**. As a reader, you must judge authors on how well they accomplish their purpose. In other words, you need to consider the type of passage (e.g., technical, persuasive, etc.) that the author has written and whether the author has followed the requirements of the passage type.

PERSUASIVE WRITING

In a persuasive essay, the author is attempting to change the reader's mind or **convince** him or her of something that he or she did not believe previously. There are several identifying characteristics of **persuasive writing**. One is **opinion presented as fact**. When authors attempt to persuade readers, they often present their opinions as if they were fact. Readers must be on guard for statements that sound factual but which cannot be subjected to research, observation, or experiment. Another characteristic of persuasive writing is **emotional language**. An author will often try to play on the emotions of readers by appealing to their sympathy or sense of morality. When an author uses colorful or evocative language with the intent of arousing the reader's passions, then the author may be attempting to persuade. Finally, in many cases, a persuasive text will give an **unfair explanation of opposing positions**, if these positions are mentioned at all.

INFORMATIVE TEXTS

An informative text is written to **educate** and **enlighten** readers. Informative texts are almost always nonfiction and are rarely structured as a story. The intention of an informative text is to deliver information in the most *comprehensible* way. So, look for the structure of the text to be very clear. In an informative text, the **thesis statement** is one or sometimes two sentences that normally appear at the end of the first paragraph. The author may use some colorful language, but he or she is likely to put more emphasis on **clarity** and **precision**. Informative essays do not typically appeal to the emotions. They often contain *facts* and *figures* and rarely include the opinion of the author; however, readers should remain aware of the possibility for a bias as those facts are presented. Sometimes a persuasive essay can resemble an informative essay, especially if the author maintains an even tone and presents his or her views as if they were established fact.

Review Video: Informative Text
Visit mometrix.com/academy and enter code: 924964

ENTERTAINING TEXTS

The success or failure of an author's intent to **entertain** is determined by those who read the author's work. Entertaining texts may be either fiction or nonfiction, and they may describe real or imagined people, places, and events. Entertaining texts are often narratives or poems. A text that is written to entertain is likely to contain **colorful language** that engages the imagination and the emotions. Such writing often features a great deal of figurative language, which typically enlivens the subject matter with images and analogies.

Though an entertaining text is not usually written to persuade or inform, authors may accomplish both of these tasks in their work. An entertaining text may *appeal to the reader's emotions* and cause him or her to think differently about a particular subject. In any case, entertaining texts tend to showcase the personality of the author more than other types of writing.

EXPRESSION OF FEELINGS

When an author intends to **express feelings,** he or she may use **expressive and bold language**. An author may write with emotion for any number of reasons. Sometimes, authors will express feelings because they are describing a personal situation of great pain or happiness. In other situations, authors will attempt to persuade the reader and will use emotion to stir up the passions. This kind of expression is easy to identify when the writer uses phrases like *I felt* and *I sense*. However, readers may find that the author will simply describe feelings without introducing them. As a reader, you must know the importance of recognizing when an author is expressing emotion and not to become overwhelmed by sympathy or passion. Readers should maintain some **detachment** so that they can still evaluate the strength of the author's argument or the quality of the writing.

IDENTIFYING AN AUTHOR'S POSITION

In order to be an effective reader, one must pay attention to the author's **position** and purpose. Even those texts that seem objective and impartial, like textbooks, have a position and **bias**. Readers need to take these positions into account when considering the author's message. When an author uses emotional language or clearly favors one side of an argument, his or her position is clear. However, the author's position may be evident not only in what he or she writes, but also in what he or she doesn't write. In a normal setting, a reader would want to review some other texts on the same topic in order to develop a view of the author's position. If this was not possible, then you would want to acquire some *background* about the author. However, since you are in the middle of an exam and the only source of information is the text, you should look for *language and argumentation that seems to indicate a particular stance* on the subject.

TEXT FEATURES

HEADINGS AND SUBHEADINGS

Many informative texts, especially textbooks, use **headings** and **subheadings** for organization. Headings and subheadings are printed in larger and bolder fonts. Sometimes, they are in a different color than the main body of the book. Headings may be larger than subheadings. Also, headings and subheadings are not always complete sentences. A heading gives the **topic** that will be addressed in the paragraphs below. Headings are meant to alert you about what is coming next. Subheadings give the **topics of smaller sections**. For example, the heading of a section in a science textbook might be *AMPHIBIANS*. Within that section, you may have subheadings for *Frogs*, *Salamanders*, and *Newts*. Pay close attention to headings and subheadings. They make it easy to go back and find specific details in a book.

FOOTNOTES AND ENDNOTES

Footnotes and endnotes can also be used in word processing programs. A **footnote** is text that is listed at the *bottom of a page* which lists where facts and figures within that document page were obtained. An **endnote** is similar to a footnote, but differs in the fact that it is listed at the *end of paragraphs and chapters* of a document, instead of the bottom of each page of the document.

BOLD TEXT AND UNDERLINING

Authors will often incorporate text features like bold text and underlining to communicate meaning to the reader. When text is made **bold**, it is often because the author wants to emphasize the point that is being made. Bold text indicates **importance**. Also, many textbooks place key terms in bold. This not only draws the reader's attention, but also makes it easy to find these terms when reviewing before a test. **Underlining** serves a similar purpose. It is often used to suggest **emphasis**. However, underlining is also used on occasion beneath the **titles** of books, magazines, and works of art. This was more common when people used typewriters, which weren't able to create italics. Now that word processing software is nearly universal, italics are generally used for longer works.

ITALICS

Italics, like bold text and underlines, are used to **emphasize** important words, phrases, and sentences in a text. However, italics have other uses as well. A word is placed in italics when it is being discussed *as* a word; that is, when it is being **defined** or its use in a sentence is being **described**. For instance, it is appropriate to use italics when saying that *esoteric* is an unusual adjective. Italics are also used for the titles of long or large works, like books, magazines, long operas, and epic poems. Shorter works are typically placed within **quotation marks**. A reader should note how an author uses italics, as this is a marker of *style and tone*. Some authors use them frequently, creating a tone of high emotion, while others are more restrained in their use, suggesting calm and reason.

INDEX

Normally, a nonfiction book will have an **index** at the end. The index is for you to find *information about specific topics*. An index lists the topics in alphabetical order (i.e., a, b, c, d...). The names of people are listed by last name. For example, *Adams, John* would come before *Washington, George*. To the right of a topic, the page numbers are listed for that topic. When a topic is spread over several pages, the index will connect these pages with a dash. For example, the topic is said to be on pages 35 to 42 and again on 53. The topic will be labeled as 35–42, 53. Some topics will have **subtopics**. These subtopics are listed below the main topic, indented slightly, and placed in alphabetical order. This is common for subjects that are covered over several pages in the book. For example, you have a book about Elizabethan drama; William Shakespeare is an important topic. Beneath Shakespeare's name in the index, you may find listings for *death of, dramatic works of, life of*, etc. These specific sub-topics help you narrow your search.

TABLE OF CONTENTS

Most books, magazines, and journals have a **table of contents** at the beginning. The table of contents lists the different **subjects** or **chapter titles** with a page number. This information allows you to find what you need with ease. Normally, the table of contents is found a page or two after the title page in a book or in the first few pages of a magazine. In a book, the table of contents will have the chapters listed on the left side. The page number for each chapter comes on the right side. Many books have a **preface** (i.e., a note that explains the background of the book) or introduction. The preface and introduction come with Roman numerals. The chapters are listed in order from the beginning to the end.

Integration of Knowledge and Ideas

PRIMARY SOURCES AND INTERNET SOURCES

PRIMARY SOURCES

When conducting research, it is important to depend on reputable **primary sources**. A primary source is the **documentary evidence** closest to the subject being studied. For instance, the primary sources for an essay about penguins would be photographs and recordings of the birds, as well as accounts of people who have studied penguins in person. A **secondary source** would be a review of a movie about penguins or a book outlining the observations made by others. A primary source should be credible and, if it is on a subject that is still being explored, recent. One way to assess the credibility of a work is to see how often it is mentioned in other books and articles on the same subject. Just by reading the works cited and bibliographies of other books, one can get a sense of what the reliable sources authorities in the field are.

INTERNET SOURCES

The Internet was once considered a poor place to find sources for an essay or article, but its credibility has improved greatly over the years. Still, students need to exercise caution when performing research online. The best sources are those affiliated with **established institutions**, such as *universities, public libraries, and think tanks*. Most newspapers are available online, and many of them allow the public to browse their archives. Magazines frequently offer similar services. When obtaining information from an unknown website, however, one must exercise considerably more caution. A website can be considered trustworthy if it is referenced by other sites that are known to be reputable. Also, credible sites tend to be properly maintained and frequently updated. A site is easier to trust when the author provides some information about himself, including some credentials that indicate expertise in the subject matter.

MAKING PREDICTIONS AND DRAWING CONCLUSIONS

PREDICTIONS

A prediction is a **guess** about what will happen next. Readers constantly make predictions based on what they have read and what they already know. Consider the following sentence: *Staring at the computer screen in shock, Kim blindly reached over for the brimming glass of water on the shelf to her side.* The sentence suggests that Kim is agitated, and that she is not looking at the glass that she is going to pick up. So, a reader might **predict** that Kim is going to knock over the glass. Of course, not every prediction will be accurate: perhaps Kim will pick the glass up cleanly. Nevertheless, the author has certainly created the expectation that the water might be spilled. Predictions are always subject to revision as the reader acquires more information.

> **Review Video: Predictions**
> Visit mometrix.com/academy and enter code: 437248

FORESHADOWING

Foreshadowing uses hints in a narrative to let the audience **anticipate** future events in the plot. Foreshadowing can be indicated by a number of literary devices and figures of speech, as well as through dialogue between characters.

DRAWING CONCLUSIONS

In addition to inference and prediction, readers must often **draw conclusions** about the information they have read. When asked for a *conclusion* that may be drawn, look for critical "hedge" phrases, such as *likely, may, can, will often,* among many others. When you are being tested on this knowledge, remember the question that writers insert into these hedge phrases to cover every possibility. Often an answer will be wrong simply because there is no room for exception. Extreme positive or negative answers (such as always or never) are usually not correct. The reader should not use any outside knowledge that is not gathered from the passage to answer the related questions. Correct answers can be derived *straight from the passage.*

THEMES IN PRINT AND OTHER SOURCES

Themes are seldom expressed directly in a text and can be difficult to identify. A **theme** is *an issue, an idea, or a question raised by the text.* For instance, a theme of *Cinderella* (the Charles Perrault version) is perseverance as the title character serves her step-sisters and step-mother, and the prince seeks to find the girl with the missing slipper. A passage may have many themes, and you, as a dedicated reader, must take care to identify only themes that you are asked to find. One common characteristic of themes is that they raise more questions than they answer. In a good piece of fiction, authors are trying to elevate the reader's perspective and encourage him or her to consider the themes in a deeper way. In the process of reading, one can identify themes by constantly *asking about the general issues that the text is addressing.* A good way to evaluate an author's approach to a theme is to begin reading with a question in mind (e.g., How does this text approach the theme of love?) and to look for evidence in the text that addresses that question.

> **Review Video: Theme**
> Visit mometrix.com/academy and enter code: 732074

SIMILAR THEMES ACROSS CULTURES

A brief study of world literature suggests that writers from vastly different cultures address **similar themes**. For instance, works like the *Odyssey* and *Hamlet* both consider the individual's battle for self-control and independence. In most cultures, authors address themes of *personal growth and the struggle for maturity.* Another universal theme is the *conflict between the individual and society.* Works that are as culturally disparate as *Native Son,* the *Aeneid,* and *1984* dramatize how people struggle to maintain their personalities and dignity in large (sometimes) oppressive groups. Finally, many cultures have versions of the *hero's or heroine's journey* in which an adventurous person must overcome many obstacles in order to gain greater knowledge, power, and perspective. Some famous works that treat this theme are the *Epic of Gilgamesh,* Dante's *Divine Comedy,* and Cervantes' *Don Quixote.*

DIFFERENCES IN ADDRESSING THEMES IN VARIOUS CULTURES AND GENRES

Authors from different **genres** and **cultures** may address similar themes, but they do so in different ways. For instance, poets are likely to address subject matter indirectly through the use of *images and allusions.* In a play, the author is more likely to dramatize themes by using characters to express opposing viewpoints; this disparity is known as a *dialectical approach.* In a passage, the author does not need to express themes directly; indeed, they can be expressed through *events and actions.* In some regional literatures, such as Greece or England, authors use more irony: their works have characters that express views and make decisions that are clearly disapproved of by the author. In Latin America, there is a great tradition of using supernatural events to illustrate themes about real life. Chinese and Japanese authors frequently use well-established regional forms (e.g., haiku poetry in Japan) to organize their treatment of universal themes.

EVALUATING AN ARGUMENT

Argumentative and persuasive passages take a **stand** on a debatable issue, seek to explore all sides of the issue, and find the best possible solution. Argumentative and persuasive passages should not be combative or abusive. The word *argument* may remind you of two or more people shouting at each other and walking away in anger. However, an argumentative or persuasive passage should be a *calm and reasonable presentation of an author's ideas* for others to consider. When an author writes reasonable arguments, his or her goal is not to win or have the last word. Instead, authors want to reveal current understanding of the question at hand and suggest a **solution** to a problem. The purpose of argument and persuasion in a free society is to reach the best solution.

EVIDENCE

The term **text evidence** refers to information that supports a **main point** or **minor points** and can help lead the reader to a conclusion. Information used as text evidence is precise, descriptive, and factual. A main point is often followed by **supporting details** that provide evidence to back up a claim. For example, a passage may include the claim that winter occurs during opposite months in the Northern and Southern hemispheres. Text evidence based on this claim may include countries where winter occurs in opposite months along with reasons that winter occurs at different times of the year in separate hemispheres (due to the tilt of the Earth as it rotates around the sun).

> **Review Video: Text Evidence**
> Visit mometrix.com/academy and enter code: 486236

Evidence needs to be provided that supports the thesis and additional arguments. Most arguments must be supported by facts or statistics. A **fact** is something that is *known with certainty* and has been verified by several independent individuals. **Examples** and **illustrations** add an emotional component to arguments. With this component, you persuade readers in ways that facts and statistics cannot. The emotional component is effective when used with objective information that can be confirmed.

CREDIBILITY

The text used to support an argument can be the argument's downfall if the text is not credible. A text is **credible**, or believable, when the author is knowledgeable and objective, or unbiased. The author's **motivations** for writing the text play a critical role in determining the credibility of the text and must be evaluated when assessing that credibility. Reports written about the ozone layer by an environmental scientist and a hairdresser will have different levels of credibility.

APPEAL TO EMOTION

Sometimes, authors will **appeal to the reader's emotion** in an attempt to *persuade or to distract the reader from the weakness of the argument*. For instance, the author may try to inspire the **pity** of the reader by delivering a heart-rending story. An author also might use the **bandwagon** approach, in which he suggests that his opinion is correct because it is held by the majority. Some authors resort to **name-calling**, in which insults and harsh words are delivered to the opponent in an attempt to distract. In advertising, a common appeal is the **celebrity testimonial**, in which a famous person endorses a product. Of course, the fact that a famous person likes something should not really mean anything to the reader. These and other emotional appeals are usually evidence of poor reasoning and a weak argument.

> **Review Video: Appeal to Emotion**
> Visit mometrix.com/academy and enter code: 163442

COUNTERARGUMENTS

When authors give both sides to the argument, they build trust with their readers. As a reader, you should start with an undecided or neutral position. If an author presents only his or her side to the argument, then you will need to be concerned at best.

Building common ground with neutral or opposed readers can be appealing to skeptical readers. Sharing values with undecided readers can allow people to switch positions without giving up what they feel is important. For people who may oppose a position, they need to feel that they can change their minds without betraying who they are as a person. This *appeal to having an open mind* can be a powerful tool in arguing a position without antagonizing other views. Objections can be countered on a point-by-point basis or in a summary paragraph. Be mindful of how an author points out flaws in **counterarguments**. If they are unfair to the other side of the argument, then you should lose trust with the author.

DATA FROM DIFFERENT SOURCES AND IN DIFFERENT FORMATS

JOURNAL ARTICLES

Although published journal articles listed in library databases have been reviewed and edited to be acceptable for publication, you should still evaluate them by six criteria.

1. **Source**: Articles by experts in their subjects, published in scholarly journals, are more *reliable*. They also contain *references* to more publications on the same topic. Try to start your search with a database that includes searching by article type (e.g., reviews, clinical trials, editorials, and research articles).
2. **Length**: The citation states an article's number of pages, an indication of its research *utility*.
3. **Authority**: Research sources should be authoritative, written by *experts* affiliated with academic institutions.
4. **Date**: Many research fields are constantly changing, so research must be as *current* as possible. In areas with new research breakthroughs, some articles are not up-to-date.
5. **Audience**: If an author wrote an article for professional colleagues, it will include subject-specific language and *terminology*.
6. **Usefulness**: Evaluate whether an article is *relevant* to one's own research topic.

LINE GRAPH

A line graph is a type of graph that is typically used for *measuring trends over time*. The graph is set up along a vertical and a horizontal **axis**. The variables being measured are listed along the left side and the bottom side of the axes. Points are then plotted along the graph as they correspond with their values for each variable. For instance, imagine a line graph measuring a person's income for each month of the year. If the person earned $1500 in January, there should be a point directly above January (perpendicular to the horizontal axis) and directly to the right of $1500 (perpendicular to the vertical axis). Once all of the lines are plotted, they are connected with a line from left to right. This line provides a nice visual illustration of the general **trends**. For instance, using the earlier example, if the line sloped up, then one would see that the person's income had increased over the course of the year.

BAR GRAPH

The bar graph is one of the most common visual representations of information. **Bar graphs** are used to illustrate sets of numerical **data**. The graph has a vertical axis (along which numbers are listed) and a horizontal axis (along which categories, words, or some other indicators are placed). One example of a bar graph is a depiction of the respective heights of famous basketball players: the vertical axis would contain numbers ranging from five to eight feet, and the horizontal axis would contain the names of the players. The length of the bar above the player's name would illustrate his height, and the top of the bar would stop perpendicular to the height listed along the left side. In this representation, one would see that Yao Ming is taller than Michael Jordan because Yao's bar would be higher.

PIE CHART

A pie chart, also known as a circle graph, is useful for depicting how a single unit or category is divided. The standard pie chart is a circle with designated wedges. Each wedge is **proportional** in size to a part of the whole. For instance, consider a pie chart representing a student's budget. If the student spends half of his or her money on rent, then the pie chart will represent that amount with a line through the center of the pie. If she spends a quarter of her money on food, there will be a line extending from the edge of the circle to the center at a right angle to the line depicting rent. This illustration would make it clear that the student spends twice the amount of money on rent as she does on food.

A pie chart is effective at showing how a single entity is *divided into parts*. They are not effective at demonstrating the relationships between parts of different wholes. For example, an unhelpful use of a pie chart would be to compare the respective amounts of state and federal spending devoted to infrastructure since these values are only meaningful in the context of the entire budget.

RESEARCH ASSISTANCE

Today's **library media specialists** are important figures in contemporary learning communities, which now consist of administrators, teachers, and parents; and international, national, state, regional, and local communities. Such communities transcend the borders of disciplinary field, occupation, age, time, and place. They are connected by shared needs, interests, and rapidly increasing technologies in telecommunications. Library media specialists and student-centered library media programs aim to aid students in attaining and improving their **information literacy**. As such, library media specialists and library media programs have the objective of helping every student to creatively and actively find, evaluate, and use information toward the ends of fulfilling their own curiosities and imaginations by pursuing reading and research activities and of exercising and developing their own critical thinking abilities.

INFORMATION SPECIALIST

In fulfilling the function of an **information specialist**, library media specialists bring their skills for finding and evaluating information in a variety of formats as resources for learners and educators. They bring an awareness of various issues related to information to the attention of students, teachers, administrators, and other involved parties. Library media specialists also serve to model for students the **strategies** they can learn to find, access, and evaluate information inside and outside of the library media centers. The environment of the library media center has experienced a critical impact from the development of technology. Accordingly, the library media specialist not only attains mastery over current advanced electronic resources, but she or he must also continually sustain attention focused on how information—both in more traditional forms and in the newest technological forms—is used ethically, as well as its quality and its character.

ORGANIZING AND SYNTHESIZING DATA

ORGANIZING INFORMATION

Organizing information effectively is an important part of research. The data must be organized in a useful manner so that it can be effectively used. Three basic ways to organize information are:

1. **Spatial Organization** – This is useful as it lets the user "see" the information, to fix it in *space*. This has benefits for those individuals who are visually adept at processing information.
2. **Chronological Organization** – This is the most common presentation of information. This method places information in the *sequence* with which it occurs. Chronological organization is very useful in explaining a process that occurs in a step-by-step pattern.
3. **Logical Organization** – This includes presenting material in a logical *pattern* that makes intuitive sense. Some patterns that are frequently used are illustrated, definition, compare/contrast, cause/effect, problem/solution, and division/classification.

LOGICAL ORGANIZATION

There are six major types of logical organization that are frequently used:

1. **Illustrations** may be used to support the thesis. Examples are the most common form of this organization.
2. **Definitions** say what something is or is not. A helpful question for this type of organization is, "What are the characteristics of the topic?"
3. Dividing or **classifying** information into separate items according to their similarities is a common and effective organizing method.
4. **Comparing** (focusing on the similarities of things) and **contrasting** (highlighting the differences between things) are excellent tools to use with certain kinds of information.
5. **Cause and effect** is a simple tool to logically understand relationships between things. A phenomenon may be traced to its causes for organizing a subject logically.
6. **Problem and solution** is a simple and effective manner of logically organizing material. It is very commonly used and lucidly presents information.

SYNTHESIS OF RESEARCH

When you must generate questions about what the data that you have collected, you realize whether you understand it and whether you can answer your own questions. You can learn to ask yourself questions which require that you **synthesize** content from different portions of the data, such as asking questions about the data's important information.

Understanding how to **summarize** what you have collected allows you to discern what is important in the data, and to be able to express the important content in your own words. When you learn to summarize your data, you are better able to identify the main ideas of the research, and to connect these main ideas. Then, you will be better able to generate central ideas from your research. Also, you will be able to avoid irrelevant information and to remember what you have researched.

Mathematics

Numbers and Operations

Numbers are the basic building blocks of mathematics. Specific features of numbers are identified by the following terms:

Integer – any positive or negative whole number, including zero. Integers do not include fractions $\left(\frac{1}{3}\right)$, decimals (0.56), or mixed numbers $\left(7\frac{3}{4}\right)$.

Prime number – any whole number greater than 1 that has only two factors, itself and 1; that is, a number that can be divided evenly only by 1 and itself.

Composite number – any whole number greater than 1 that has more than two different factors; in other words, any whole number that is not a prime number. For example: The composite number 8 has the factors of 1, 2, 4, and 8.

Even number – any integer that can be divided by 2 without leaving a remainder. For example: 2, 4, 6, 8, and so on.

Odd number – any integer that cannot be divided evenly by 2. For example: 3, 5, 7, 9, and so on.

Decimal number – any number that uses a decimal point to show the part of the number that is less than one. Example: 1.234.

Decimal point – a symbol used to separate the ones place from the tenths place in decimals or dollars from cents in currency.

Decimal place – the position of a number to the right of the decimal point. In the decimal 0.123, the 1 is in the first place to the right of the decimal point, indicating tenths; the 2 is in the second place, indicating hundredths; and the 3 is in the third place, indicating thousandths.

The **decimal**, or base 10, system is a number system that uses ten different digits (0, 1, 2, 3, 4, 5, 6, 7, 8, 9). An example of a number system that uses something other than ten digits is the **binary**, or base 2, number system, used by computers, which uses only the numbers 0 and 1. It is thought that the decimal system originated because people had only their 10 fingers for counting.

Rational numbers include all integers, decimals, and fractions. Any terminating or repeating decimal number is a rational number.

Irrational numbers cannot be written as fractions or decimals because the number of decimal places is infinite and there is no recurring pattern of digits within the number. For example, pi (π) begins with 3.141592 and continues without terminating or repeating, so pi is an irrational number.

Real numbers are the set of all rational and irrational numbers.

> **Review Video: Numbers and Their Classifications**
> Visit mometrix.com/academy and enter code: 461071

PLACE VALUE

Write the place value of each digit in the following number: 14,059.826

1: ten thousands
4: thousands
0: hundreds
5: tens
9: ones
8: tenths
2: hundredths
6: thousandths

WRITING NUMBERS IN WORD FORM

EXAMPLE 1

Write each number in words.

29: twenty-nine
478: four hundred seventy-eight
9,435: nine thousand four hundred thirty-five
98,542: ninety-eight thousand five hundred forty-two
302, 876: three hundred two thousand eight hundred seventy-six

EXAMPLE 2

Write each decimal in words.

0.06: six hundredths
0.6: six tenths
6.0: six
0.009: nine thousandths
0.113: one hundred thirteen thousandths
0.901: nine hundred one thousandths

FRACTIONS

A **fraction** is a number that is expressed as one integer written above another integer, with a dividing line between them $\left(\frac{x}{y}\right)$. It represents the **quotient** of the two numbers: x divided by y. It can also be thought of as x out of y equal parts.

The top number of a fraction is called the **numerator**, and it represents the number of parts under consideration. The 1 in $\frac{1}{4}$ means that 1 part out of the whole is being considered in the calculation. The bottom number of a fraction is called the **denominator**, and it represents the total number of equal parts. The 4 in $\frac{1}{4}$ means that the whole consists of 4 equal parts. A fraction cannot have a denominator of zero; this is referred to as *undefined*.

Fractions can be manipulated, without changing the value of the fraction, by multiplying or dividing (but not adding or subtracting) both the numerator and denominator by the same number. If you divide both numbers by a common factor, you are **reducing** or simplifying the fraction. Two fractions that have the same value, but are expressed differently are known as **equivalent**

fractions. For example, $\frac{2}{10}, \frac{3}{15}, \frac{4}{20}$, and $\frac{5}{25}$ are all equivalent fractions. They can also all be reduced or simplified to $\frac{1}{5}$.

PROPER FRACTIONS AND MIXED NUMBERS

A fraction whose denominator is greater than its numerator is known as a **proper fraction**, while a fraction whose numerator is greater than its denominator is known as an **improper fraction**. Proper fractions have values *less than one* and improper fractions have values *greater than one*.

A **mixed number** is a number that contains both an integer and a fraction. Any improper fraction can be rewritten as a mixed number. Example: $\frac{8}{3} = \frac{6}{3} + \frac{2}{3} = 2 + \frac{2}{3} = 2\frac{2}{3}$. Similarly, any mixed number can be rewritten as an improper fraction. Example: $1\frac{3}{5} = 1 + \frac{3}{5} = \frac{5}{5} + \frac{3}{5} = \frac{8}{5}$.

> **Review Video: <u>Fractions</u>**
> Visit mometrix.com/academy and enter code: 262335

DECIMALS

DECIMAL ILLUSTRATION

Use a model to represent the decimal: 0.24. Write 0.24 as a fraction.

The decimal 0.24 is twenty-four hundredths. One possible model to represent this fraction is to draw 100 pennies, since each penny is worth one hundredth of a dollar. Draw one hundred circles to represent one hundred pennies. Shade 24 of the pennies to represent the decimal twenty-four hundredths.

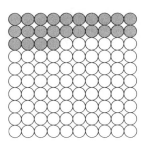

To write the decimal as a fraction, write a fraction: $\frac{\#\ shaded\ spaces}{\#\ total\ spaces}$. The number of shaded spaces is 24, and the total number of spaces is 100, so as a fraction 0.24 equals $\frac{24}{100}$. This fraction can then be reduced to $\frac{6}{25}$.

PERCENTAGES

Percentages can be thought of as fractions that are based on a whole of 100; that is, one whole is equal to 100%. The word **percent** means *per hundred*. Fractions can be expressed as percentages by finding equivalent fractions with a denomination of 100. Example: $\frac{7}{10} = \frac{70}{100} = 70\%$; $\frac{1}{4} = \frac{25}{100} = 25\%$.

To express a percentage as a fraction, divide the percentage number by 100 and reduce the fraction to its simplest possible terms. Example: $60\% = \frac{60}{100} = \frac{3}{5}$; $96\% = \frac{96}{100} = \frac{24}{25}$.

Review Video: Percentages
Visit mometrix.com/academy and enter code: 141911

CONVERTING PERCENTAGES, FRACTIONS, AND DECIMALS

Converting decimals to percentages and percentages to decimals is as simple as moving the decimal point. To *convert from a decimal to a percentage*, move the decimal point **two places to the right**. To *convert from a percentage to a decimal*, move it **two places to the left**. Example: 0.23 = 23%; 5.34 = 534%; 0.007 = 0.7%; 700% = 7.00; 86% = 0.86; 0.15% = 0.0015.

It may be helpful to remember that the percentage number will always be larger than the equivalent decimal number.

Review Video: Converting Decimals to Fractions and Percentages
Visit mometrix.com/academy and enter code: 986765

EXAMPLE 1

Write 15% as a fraction and as a decimal.

To convert a percentage to a fraction, follow these steps:

1. Write the percentage over 100. 15% can be written as $\frac{15}{100}$.
2. Fractions should be written in simplest form, which means that the numbers in the numerator and denominator should be reduced if possible. Both 15 and 100 can be divided by 5.
3. Therefore, $\frac{15 \div 5}{100 \div 5} = \frac{3}{20}$.

To convert a percentage to a decimal, simply remove the percent sign and move the decimal point two places to the left:

$$15\% \rightarrow 15. \rightarrow 0.15$$

EXAMPLE 2

Write 24.36% as a fraction and as a decimal.

24.36% written as a fraction is $\frac{24.36}{100}$, or $\frac{2436}{10,000}$, which reduces to $\frac{609}{2500}$.

24.36% written as a decimal is 0.2436.

Review Video: Converting Percentages to Decimals and Fractions
Visit mometrix.com/academy and enter code: 287297

EXAMPLE 3

Write $\frac{4}{5}$ as a decimal and as a percentage.

One way to convert a fraction to a decimal is to divide the numerator by the denominator:

$$\frac{4}{5} = 4 \div 5 = 0.80 = 0.8$$

Alternatively, the fraction can be manipulated to make the denominator a multiple of ten. Once the denominator is a multiple of ten, write the numerator as a decimal with as many decimal places as there are zeros in the denominator:

$$\frac{4}{5} = \frac{4 \times 2}{5 \times 2} = \frac{8}{10} = 0.8$$

Converting a decimal to a percentage may be done in much the same way as the method shown above, except that the denominator must be changed specifically to 100:

$$\frac{4 \times 20}{5 \times 20} = \frac{80}{100} = 80\%$$

EXAMPLE 4

Write $3\frac{2}{5}$ as a decimal and as a percentage.

The mixed number $3\frac{2}{5}$ has a whole number and a fractional part. The fractional part $\frac{2}{5}$ can be written as a decimal by dividing 5 into 2, which gives 0.4. Adding the whole to the part gives 3.4. Alternatively, note that $3\frac{2}{5} = 3\frac{4}{10} = 3.4$.

To change a decimal to a percentage, multiply it by 100%, or equivalently move the decimal point two places to the right and add a percent sign:

$$3.4 \times 100\% = 340\%$$

Notice that this percentage is greater than 100%. This makes sense because the original mixed number $3\frac{2}{5}$ is greater than 1.

> **Review Video: Converting Fractions to Percentages and Decimals**
> Visit mometrix.com/academy and enter code: 306233

OPERATIONS

There are four basic mathematical operations:

Addition increases the value of one quantity by the value of another quantity. Example: $2 + 4 = 6$; $8 + 9 = 17$. The result is called the **sum**. With addition, the order does not matter. $4 + 2 = 2 + 4$.

Subtraction is the opposite operation to addition; it decreases the value of one quantity by the value of another quantity. Example: $6 - 4 = 2$; $17 - 8 = 9$. The result is called the **difference**. Note that with subtraction, the order does matter. $6 - 4 \neq 4 - 6$.

Multiplication can be thought of as repeated addition. One number tells how many times to add the other number to itself. Example: 3×2 (three times two) $= 2 + 2 + 2 = 6$. With multiplication, the order does not matter. $2 \times 3 = 3 \times 2$ or $3 + 3 = 2 + 2 + 2$.

Division is the opposite operation to multiplication; one number tells us how many parts to divide the other number into. Example: $20 \div 4 = 5$; if 20 is split into 4 equal parts, each part is 5. With division, the order of the numbers does matter. $20 \div 4 \neq 4 \div 20$.

ORDER OF OPERATIONS

Order of Operations is a set of rules that dictates the order in which we must perform each operation in an expression so that we will evaluate it accurately. If we have an expression that includes multiple different operations, **Order of Operations** tells us which operations to do first. The most common mnemonic for Order of Operations is **PEMDAS**, or "Please Excuse My Dear Aunt Sally." PEMDAS stands for Parentheses, Exponents, Multiplication, Division, Addition, and Subtraction. It is important to understand that multiplication and division have equal precedence, as do addition and subtraction, so those pairs of operations are simply worked from left to right in order.

Example: Evaluate the expression $5 + 20 \div 4 \times (2 + 3) - 6$ using the correct order of operations.

- P: Perform the operations inside the parentheses: $(2 + 3) = 5$
- E: Simplify the exponents. (Not required on the ATI TEAS).
  - The equation now looks like this: $5 + 20 \div 4 \times 5 - 6$
- MD: Perform multiplication and division from left to right: $20 \div 4 = 5$; then $5 \times 5 = 25$
  - The equation now looks like this: $5 + 25 - 6$
- AS: Perform addition and subtraction from left to right: $5 + 25 = 30$; then $30 - 6 = 24$

> **Review Video: Order of Operations**
> Visit mometrix.com/academy and enter code: 259675

PARENTHESES

Parentheses are used to designate which operations should be done first when there are multiple operations. Example: $4 - (2 + 1) = 1$; the parentheses tell us that we must add 2 and 1, and then subtract the sum from 4, rather than subtracting 2 from 4 and then adding 1 (this would give us an answer of 3).

EXPONENTS

An exponent is a superscript number placed next to another number at the top right. It indicates how many times the base number is to be multiplied by itself. **Exponents** provide a shorthand way to write what would be a longer mathematical expression. Example: $a^2 = a \times a$; $2^4 = 2 \times 2 \times 2 \times 2$. A number with an exponent of 2 is said to be **squared**, while a number with an exponent of 3 is said to be **cubed**. The value of a number raised to an exponent is called its power. So, 8^4 is read as "8 to the 4th power," or "8 raised to the power of 4." A negative exponent is the same as the **reciprocal** of a positive exponent. Example: $a^{-2} = \frac{1}{a^2}$.

ABSOLUTE VALUE

A precursor to working with negative numbers is understanding what **absolute values** are. A number's absolute value is simply the distance away from zero a number is on the number line. The absolute value of a number is always positive and is written $|x|$.

EXAMPLE

Show that $|3| = |-3|$.

The absolute value of 3, written as $|3|$, is 3 because the distance between 0 and 3 on a number line is three units. Likewise, the absolute value of –3, written as $|-3|$, is 3 because the distance between 0 and –3 on a number line is three units. So, $|3| = |-3|$.

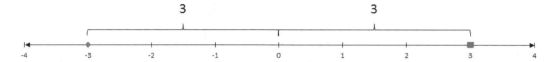

OPERATIONS WITH POSITIVE AND NEGATIVE NUMBERS

ADDITION

When adding signed numbers, if the signs are the same simply add the absolute values of the addends and apply the original sign to the sum. For example, $(+4) + (+8) = +12$ and $(-4) + (-8) = -12$. When the original signs are different, take the absolute values of the addends and subtract the smaller value from the larger value, then apply the original sign of the larger value to the difference. For instance, $(+4) + (-8) = -4$ and $(-4) + (+8) = +4$.

SUBTRACTION

For subtracting signed numbers, change the sign of the number after the minus symbol and then follow the same rules used for addition. For example, $(+4) - (+8) = (+4) + (-8) = -4$.

MULTIPLICATION

If the signs are the same the product is positive when multiplying signed numbers. For example, $(+4) \times (+8) = +32$ and $(-4) \times (-8) = +32$. If the signs are opposite, the product is negative. For example, $(+4) \times (-8) = -32$ and $(-4) \times (+8) = -32$. When more than two factors are multiplied together, the sign of the product is determined by how many negative factors are present. If there are an odd number of negative factors then the product is negative, whereas an even number of negative factors indicates a positive product. For instance, $(+4) \times (-8) \times (-2) = +64$ and $(-4) \times (-8) \times (-2) = -64$.

DIVISION

The rules for dividing signed numbers are similar to multiplying signed numbers. If the dividend and divisor have the same sign, the quotient is positive. If the dividend and divisor have opposite signs, the quotient is negative. For example, $(-4) \div (+8) = -0.5$.

OPERATIONS WITH DECIMALS

ADDING AND SUBTRACTING DECIMALS

When adding and subtracting decimals, the decimal points must always be aligned. Adding decimals is just like adding regular whole numbers. Example: $4.5 + 2 = 6.5$.

If the problem-solver does not properly align the decimal points, an incorrect answer of 4.7 may result. An easy way to add decimals is to align all of the decimal points in a vertical column visually. This will allow one to see exactly where the decimal should be placed in the final answer. Begin adding from right to left. Add each column in turn, making sure to carry the number to the left if a column adds up to more than 9. The same rules apply to the subtraction of decimals.

> **Review Video: Adding and Subtracting Decimals**
> Visit mometrix.com/academy and enter code: 381101

MULTIPLYING DECIMALS

A simple multiplication problem has two components: a **multiplicand** and a **multiplier**. When multiplying decimals, work as though the numbers were whole rather than decimals. Once the final product is calculated, count the number of places to the right of the decimal in both the multiplicand and the multiplier. Then, count that number of places from the right of the product and place the decimal in that position.

For example, 12.3 × 2.56 has three places to the right of the respective decimals. Multiply 123 × 256 to get 31488. Now, beginning on the right, count three places to the left and insert the decimal. The final product will be 31.488.

> **Review Video: Multiplying Decimals**
> Visit mometrix.com/academy and enter code: 731574

DIVIDING DECIMALS

Every division problem has a **divisor** and a **dividend**. The dividend is the number that is being divided. In the problem 14 ÷ 7, 14 is the dividend and 7 is the divisor. In a division problem with decimals, the divisor must be converted into a whole number. Begin by moving the decimal in the divisor to the right until a whole number is created. Next, move the decimal in the dividend the same number of spaces to the right. For example, 4.9 into 24.5 would become 49 into 245. The decimal was moved one space to the right to create a whole number in the divisor, and then the same was done for the dividend. Once the whole numbers are created, the problem is carried out normally: 245 ÷ 49 = 5.

> **Review Video: Dividing Decimals**
> Visit mometrix.com/academy and enter code: 560690

OPERATIONS WITH FRACTIONS

ADDING AND SUBTRACTING FRACTIONS

If two fractions have a common denominator, they can be added or subtracted simply by adding or subtracting the two numerators and retaining the same denominator. Example: $\frac{1}{2} + \frac{1}{4} = \frac{2}{4} + \frac{1}{4} = \frac{3}{4}$. If the two fractions do not already have the same denominator, one or both of them must be manipulated to achieve a common denominator before they can be added or subtracted.

MULTIPLYING FRACTIONS

Two fractions can be multiplied by multiplying the two numerators to find the new numerator and the two denominators to find the new denominator. Example: $\frac{1}{3} \times \frac{2}{3} = \frac{1 \times 2}{3 \times 3} = \frac{2}{9}$.

DIVIDING FRACTIONS

Two fractions can be divided by flipping the numerator and denominator of the second fraction and then proceeding as though it were a multiplication. Example: $\frac{2}{3} \div \frac{3}{4} = \frac{2}{3} \times \frac{4}{3} = \frac{8}{9}$.

THE NUMBER LINE

A number line is a graph to see the distance between numbers. Basically, this graph shows the relationship between numbers. So, a number line may have a point for zero and may show negative numbers on the left side of the line. Also, any positive numbers are placed on the right side of the line.

EXAMPLE

Name each point on the number line below:

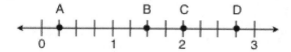

Use the dashed lines on the number line to identify each point. Each dashed line between two whole numbers is $\frac{1}{4}$. The line halfway between two numbers is $\frac{1}{2}$.

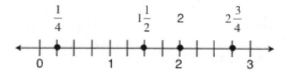

> **Review Video: Numbers and Their Classifications**
> Visit mometrix.com/academy and enter code: 461071

RATIONAL NUMBERS FROM LEAST TO GREATEST

EXAMPLE

Order the following rational numbers from least to greatest: 0.55, 17%, $\sqrt{25}$, $\frac{64}{4}$, $\frac{25}{50}$, 3.

Recall that the term **rational** simply means that the number can be expressed as a ratio or fraction. The set of rational numbers includes integers and decimals. Notice that each of the numbers in the problem can be written as a decimal or integer:

$$17\% = 0.17$$
$$\sqrt{25} = 5$$
$$\frac{64}{4} = 16$$
$$\frac{25}{50} = \frac{1}{2} = 0.5$$

So, the answer is 17%, $\frac{25}{50}$, 0.55, 3, $\sqrt{25}$, $\frac{64}{4}$.

RATIONAL NUMBERS FROM GREATEST TO LEAST

EXAMPLE

Order the following rational numbers from greatest to least: 0.3, 27%, $\sqrt{100}$, $\frac{72}{9}$, $\frac{1}{9}$. 4.5

Recall that the term **rational** simply means that the number can be expressed as a ratio or fraction. The set of rational numbers includes integers and decimals. Notice that each of the numbers in the problem can be written as a decimal or integer:

$$27\% = 0.27$$
$$\sqrt{100} = 10$$
$$\frac{72}{9} = 8$$
$$\frac{1}{9} \approx 0.11$$

So, the answer is $\sqrt{100}, \frac{72}{9}, 4.5, 0.3, 27\%, \frac{1}{9}$.

COMMON DENOMINATORS WITH FRACTIONS

When two fractions are manipulated so that they have the same denominator, this is known as finding a **common denominator**. The number chosen to be that common denominator should be the **least common multiple** of the two original denominators. Example: $\frac{3}{4}$ and $\frac{5}{6}$; the least common multiple of 4 and 6 is 12. Manipulating to achieve the common denominator: $\frac{3}{4} = \frac{9}{12}; \frac{5}{6} = \frac{10}{12}$.

FACTORS AND GREATEST COMMON FACTOR

Factors are numbers that are multiplied together to obtain a **product**. For example, in the equation $2 \times 3 = 6$, the numbers 2 and 3 are factors. A **prime number** has only two factors (1 and itself), but other numbers can have many factors.

A **common factor** is a number that divides exactly into two or more other numbers. For example, the factors of 12 are 1, 2, 3, 4, 6, and 12, while the factors of 15 are 1, 3, 5, and 15. The common factors of 12 and 15 are 1 and 3.

A **prime factor** is also a prime number. Therefore, the prime factors of 12 are 2 and 3. For 15, the prime factors are 3 and 5.

Review Video: Factors
Visit mometrix.com/academy and enter code: 920086

The **greatest common factor** (GCF) is the largest number that is a factor of two or more numbers. For example, the factors of 15 are 1, 3, 5, and 15; the factors of 35 are 1, 5, 7, and 35. Therefore, the greatest common factor of 15 and 35 is 5.

MULTIPLES AND LEAST COMMON MULTIPLE

The least common multiple (**LCM**) is the smallest number that is a multiple of two or more numbers. For example, the multiples of 3 include 3, 6, 9, 12, 15, etc.; the multiples of 5 include 5, 10, 15, 20, etc. Therefore, the least common multiple of 3 and 5 is 15.

Review Video: Multiples
Visit mometrix.com/academy and enter code: 626738

SOLVE EQUATIONS IN ONE VARIABLE

MANIPULATING EQUATIONS

Sometimes you will have variables missing in equations. So, you need to find the missing variable. To do this, you need to remember one important thing: *whatever you do to one side of an equation, you need to do to the other side*. If you subtract 100 from one side of an equation, you need to subtract 100 from the other side of the equation. This will allow you to change the form of the equation to find missing values.

EXAMPLE

Ray earns $10 an hour. This can be given with the expression $10x$, where x is equal to the number of hours that Ray works. This is the independent variable. The independent variable is the amount that can change. The money that Ray earns is in y hours. So, you would write the equation: $10x = y$. The variable y is the dependent variable. This depends on x and cannot be changed. Now, let's say that Ray makes $360. How many hours did he work to make $360?

$$10x = 360$$

Now, you want to know how many hours that Ray worked. So, you want to get x by itself. To do that, you can divide both sides of the equation by 10.

$$\frac{10x}{10} = \frac{360}{10}$$

So, you have: $x = 36$. Now, you know that Ray worked 36 hours to make $360.

SOLVING ONE VARIABLE LINEAR EQUATIONS

Another way to write an equation is $ax + b = 0$ where $a \neq 0$. This is known as a **one-variable linear equation**. A solution to an equation is called a **root**.

Example: $5x + 10 = 0$

If we solve for x, the solution is $x = -2$. In other words, the root of the equation is –2.

The first step is to subtract 10 from both sides. This gives $5x = -10$.

Next, divide both sides by the **coefficient** of the variable. For this example, that is 5. So, you should have $x = -2$. You can make sure that you have the correct answer by placing –2 back into the original equation. So, the equation now looks like this: $(5)(-2) + 10 = -10 + 10 = 0$.

EXAMPLE 1

Solve for x in the following equation:

$$\frac{45\%}{12\%} = \frac{15\%}{x}$$

First, cross multiply; then solve for x:

$$45x = 12 \times 15 = 180$$

$$x = \frac{180}{45} = 4\%$$

Alternatively, notice that $\frac{45\% \div 3}{12\% \div 3} = \frac{15\%}{4\%}$, so $x = 4\%$.

EXAMPLE 2

Solve for x in the following equation:

$$\frac{0.50}{2} = \frac{1.50}{x}$$

First, cross multiply; then, solve for x:

$$0.5x = 1.5 \times 2 = 3$$

$$x = \frac{3}{0.5} = 3 \times 2 = 6$$

Alternatively, notice that $\frac{0.50 \times 3}{2 \times 3} = \frac{1.50}{6}$, so $x = 6$.

EXAMPLE 3

Solve for x in the following equation:

$$\frac{40}{8} = \frac{x}{24}$$

First, cross multiply; then, solve for x:

$$8x = 40 \times 24 = 960$$

$$x = \frac{960}{8} = 120$$

Alternatively, notice that $\frac{40 \times 3}{8 \times 3} = \frac{120}{24}$, so $x = 120$.

SUBTRACTION WITH REGROUPING

EXAMPLE 1

Demonstrate how to subtract 189 from 525 using regrouping.

First, set up the subtraction problem:

$$\begin{array}{r} 525 \\ -\ 189 \\ \hline \end{array}$$

Notice that the numbers in the ones and tens columns of 525 are smaller than the numbers in the ones and tens columns of 189. This means you will need to use regrouping to perform subtraction.

$$\begin{array}{ccc} 5 & 2 & 5 \\ -\ 1 & 8 & 9 \\ \hline \end{array}$$

To subtract 9 from 5 in the ones column you will need to borrow from the 2 in the tens columns:

```
      5    1   15
  –   1    8    9
                6
```

Next, to subtract 8 from 1 in the tens column you will need to borrow from the 5 in the hundreds column:

```
      4   11   15
  –   1    8    9
            3    6
```

Last, subtract the 1 from the 4 in the hundreds column:

```
      4   11   15
  –   1    8    9
      3    3    6
```

EXAMPLE 2

Demonstrate how to subtract 477 from 620 using regrouping.

First, set up the subtraction problem:

```
    620
  – 477
```

Notice that the numbers in the ones and tens columns of 620 are smaller than the numbers in the ones and tens columns of 477. This means you will need to use regrouping to perform subtraction.

```
      6    2    0
  –   4    7    7
```

To subtract 7 from 0 in the ones column you will need to borrow from the 2 in the tens column.

```
      6    1   10
  –   4    7    7
                3
```

Next, to subtract 7 from the 1 that's still in the tens column you will need to borrow from the 6 in the hundreds column.

```
      5   11   10
  –   4    7    7
            4    3
```

Lastly, subtract 4 from the 5 remaining in the hundreds column to get:

```
      5   11   10
  –   4    7    7
      1    4    3
```

REAL WORLD ONE OR MULTI-STEP PROBLEMS WITH RATIONAL NUMBERS

EXAMPLE 1

A patient's age is thirteen more than half of 60. How old is the patient?

The words *more than* indicate addition, and *of* indicates multiplication. The expression can be written as $\frac{1}{2} \times 60 + 13$, so the patient's age is $\frac{1}{2} \times 60 + 13 = 30 + 13 = 43$. The patient is 43 years old.

EXAMPLE 2

A patient was given pain medicine at a dosage of 0.22 grams. The patient's dosage was then increased to 0.80 grams. By how much was the patient's dosage increased?

The first step is to determine what operation (addition, subtraction, multiplication, or division) the problem requires. Notice the key words and phrases *by how much* and *increased*. This indicates that you are looking for the amount of change or the difference between the two amounts. This difference is found by subtracting the smaller amount from the larger amount. Remember to line up the decimal when subtracting:

$$
\begin{array}{r}
0.80 \\
- 0.22 \\
\hline
0.58
\end{array}
$$

EXAMPLE 3

At a hospital, $\frac{3}{4}$ of the 100 beds are occupied today. Yesterday, $\frac{4}{5}$ of the 100 beds were occupied. On which day were more of the hospital beds occupied and by how much more?

First, find the number of beds that were occupied each day. To do so, multiply the fraction of beds occupied by the number of beds available:

Number of beds occupied today $= \frac{3}{4} \times 100 = 75$.

Number of beds occupied yesterday $= \frac{4}{5} \times 100 = 80$.

The difference in the number of beds occupied is $80 - 75 = 5$ beds.

Therefore, 5 more beds were occupied yesterday than today.

EXAMPLE 4

At a hospital, 40% of the nurses work in labor and delivery. If 20 nurses work in labor and delivery, how many nurses work at the hospital?

To answer this problem, first think about the number of nurses that work at the hospital. Will it be more or less than the number of nurses who work in a specific department such as labor and delivery? More nurses work at the hospital, so the number you find to answer this question will be greater than 20.

40% of the nurses are labor and delivery nurses. The word *of* indicates multiplication, and the words *is* and *are* indicate equivalence. Translating the problem into a mathematical sentence gives

$40\% \times n = 20$, where n represents the total number of nurses. Solving for n gives $n = \frac{20}{40\%} = \frac{20}{0.40} = 50$. Fifty nurses work at the hospital.

EXAMPLE 5

A patient was given blood pressure medicine at a dosage of 2 grams. The patient's dosage was then decreased to 0.45 grams. By how much was the patient's dosage decreased?

The decrease is represented by the difference between the two amounts. Remember to line up the decimal point before subtracting:

$$\begin{array}{r} 2.00 \\ - \quad 0.45 \\ \hline 1.55 \end{array}$$

EXAMPLE 6

Two weeks ago, $\frac{2}{3}$ of the 60 patients at a hospital were male. Last week, $\frac{3}{6}$ of the 80 patients were male. During which week were there more male patients?

First, you need to find the number of male patients that were in the hospital each week. You are given this amount in terms of fractions. To find the number of male patients, multiply the fraction of male patients by the number of patients in the hospital.

Number of male patients = fraction of male patients × total number of patients.

Number of male patients two weeks ago $= \frac{2}{3} \times 60 = \frac{120}{3} = 40$.

Number of male patients last week $= \frac{3}{6} \times 80 = \frac{1}{2} \times 80 = \frac{80}{2} = 40$.

The number of male patients was the same both weeks.

EXAMPLE 7

Jane ate lunch at a local restaurant. She ordered a $4.99 appetizer, a $12.50 entrée, and a $1.25 soda. If she wants to tip her server 20%, how much money will she spend in all?

To find total amount, first find the sum of the items she ordered from the menu and then add 20% of this sum to the total:

$$\$4.99 + \$12.50 + \$1.25 = \$18.74$$

$$\$18.74 \times 20\% = \$18.74 \times 0.2 = \$3.748 \approx \$3.75$$

$$\text{Total} = \$18.74 + \$3.75 = \$22.49$$

Another way to find this sum is to multiply the cost of the meal by 120%:

$$\$18.74 \times 120\% = \$18.74 \times 1.2 = \$22.488 \approx \$22.49$$

REAL WORLD PROBLEMS WITH PERCENTAGES

A percentage problem can be presented three main ways: (1) Find what percentage of some number another number is. Example: What percentage of 40 is 8? (2) Find what number is some percentage of a given number. Example: What number is 20% of 40? (3) Find what number another number is a given percentage of. Example: What number is 8 20% of?

The three components in all of these cases are the same: a **whole** (W), a **part** (P), and a **percentage** (%). These are related by the equation: $P = W \times \%$. This is the form of the equation you would use to solve problems of type (2). To solve types (1) and (3), you would use these two forms:

$$\% = \frac{P}{W} \text{ and } W = \frac{P}{\%}$$

The thing that frequently makes percentage problems difficult is that they are most often also word problems, so a large part of solving them is figuring out which quantities are what. Example: In a school cafeteria, 7 students choose pizza, 9 choose hamburgers, and 4 choose tacos. Find the percentage that chooses tacos. To find the whole, you must first add all of the parts: $7 + 9 + 4 = 20$. The percentage can then be found by dividing the part by the whole $\left(\% = \frac{P}{W}\right)$: $\frac{4}{20} = \frac{20}{100} = 20\%$.

> **Review Video: <u>Word Problems and Percentages</u>**
> Visit mometrix.com/academy and enter code: 715536

EXAMPLE 1

What is 30% of 120?

The word *of* indicates multiplication, so 30% of 120 is found by multiplying 120 by 30%. Change 30% to a fraction or decimal, then multiply:

$$30\% = \frac{30}{100} = 0.3$$

$$120 \times 0.3 = 36$$

EXAMPLE 2

What is 150% of 20?

The word *of* indicates multiplication, so 150% of 20 is found by multiplying 20 by 150%. Change 150% to a fraction or decimal, then multiply:

$$150\% = \frac{150}{100} = 1.5$$

$$20 \times 1.5 = 30$$

Notice that 30 is greater than the original number of 20. This makes sense because you are finding a number that is more than 100% of the original number.

EXAMPLE 3

What is 14.5% of 96?

Change 14.5% to a decimal and multiply:

$$0.145 \times 96 = 13.92$$

Notice that 13.92 is much smaller than the original number of 96. This makes sense because you are finding a small percentage of the original number.

EXAMPLE 4

According to a hospital survey, 82% of nurses were highly satisfied at their job. Of 145 nurses, how many were highly satisfied?

Write 82% of 145 as an equation:

$$0.82 \times 145 = 118.9$$

Because you can't have 0.9 of a person, the answer is, "About 119 nurses are highly satisfied with their jobs."

EXAMPLE 5

During a shift, a new nurse spent five hours of her time observing procedures, three hours working in the oncology department, and four hours doing paperwork. During the next shift, she spent four hours observing procedures, six hours in the oncology department, and two hours doing paperwork. What was the percent change for each task between the two shifts?

The three tasks are observing procedures, working in the oncology department, and doing paperwork. To find the amount of change, compare the first amount with the second amount for each task. Then, write this difference as a percentage compared to the initial amount.

Amount of change for observing procedures: 5 hr − 4 hr = 1 hr.

The percent of change is $\frac{\text{amount of change}}{\text{original amount}} \times 100\%$. $\frac{1 \text{ hour}}{5 \text{ hours}} \times 100\% = 20\%$. The nurse spent 20% less time observing procedures on her second shift than on her first.

Amount of change for working in the oncology department: 6 hr − 3 hr = 3 hr.

The percent of change is $\frac{\text{amount of change}}{\text{original amount}} \times 100\%$. $\frac{3 \text{ hours}}{3 \text{ hours}} \times 100\% = 100\%$. The nurse spent 100% more time (or twice as much time) working in the oncology department during her second shift than she did in her first.

Amount of change for doing paperwork: 4 hr − 2 hr = 2 hr.

The percent of change is $\frac{\text{amount of change}}{\text{original amount}} \times 100\%$. $\frac{2 \text{ hours}}{4 \text{ hours}} \times 100\% = 50\%$. The nurse spent 50% less time (or half as much time) working on paperwork during her second shift than she did in her first.

EXAMPLE 6

A patient was given 40 mg of a certain medicine. Later, the patient's dosage was increased to 45 mg. What was the percent increase in his medication?

To find the percent increase, first compare the original and increased amounts. The original amount was 40 mg, and the increased amount is 45 mg, so the dosage of medication was increased by 5 mg (45 – 40 = 5). Note, however, that the question asks not by how much the dosage increased but by what percentage it increased. Percent increase $= \frac{\text{new amount} - \text{original amount}}{\text{original amount}} \times 100\%$.

$$\frac{45 \text{ mg} - 40 \text{ mg}}{40 \text{ mg}} \times 100\% = \frac{5}{40} \times 100\% = 0.125 \times 100\% = 12.5\%$$

The percent increase is 12.5%.

EXAMPLE 7

A patient was given 100 mg of a certain medicine. The patient's dosage was later decreased to 88 mg. What was the percent decrease?

The medication was decreased by 12 mg (100 mg − 88 mg = 12 mg). To find by what percent the medication was decreased, this change must be written as a percentage when compared to the original amount.

In other words, $\frac{\text{original amount} - \text{new amount}}{\text{original amount}} \times 100\% = \text{percent decrease}$

$$\frac{12 \text{ mg}}{100 \text{ mg}} \times 100\% = 0.12 \times 100\% = 12\%$$

The percent decrease is 12%.

EXAMPLE 8

A patient complaining of fatigue and weight gain was diagnosed with hypothyroidism and was prescribed 125 mcg of medication. Three months later, her symptoms had improved, and her thyroid stimulation hormone (TSH) level was found to be 0.5 mIU/L. The doctor reduced the patient's thyroid medication dosage to 100 mcg, after which the patient's TSH level was found to be 1.5 mIU/L, which is within the normal range. By what percentage did the doctor reduce the patient's thyroid medication?

In this problem you must determine which information is necessary to answer the question. The question asks by what percentage the doctor reduced the patient's thyroid medication dosage. Find the two dosage amounts and perform subtraction to find their difference. The first dosage amount is 125 mcg. The second dosage amount is 100 mcg. Therefore, the difference is 125 mcg − 100 mcg = 25 mcg. The percentage reduction can then be calculated as $\frac{\text{change}}{\text{original}} = \frac{25 \text{ mcg}}{125 \text{ mcg}} = \frac{1}{5} = 20\%$.

EXAMPLE 9

In a performance review, an employee received a score of 70 for efficiency and 90 for meeting project deadlines. Six months later, the employee received a score of 65 for efficiency and 96 for meeting project deadlines. What was the percent change for each score on the performance review?

To find the percent change, compare the first amount with the second amount for each score; then, write this difference as a percentage of the initial amount.

Percent change for efficiency score:

$$70 - 65 = 5; \quad \frac{5}{70} \approx 7.1\%$$

The employee's efficiency decreased by about 7.1%.

Percent change for meeting project deadlines score:

$$96 - 90 = 6; \quad \frac{6}{90} \approx 6.7\%$$

The employee increased his ability to meet project deadlines by about 6.7%.

ROUNDING AND ESTIMATION

Rounding is reducing the number of non-zero digits in a number while trying to keep the value similar to what it was before. The result will be less accurate, but will be in a simpler form, and will be easier to use. Numbers can be **rounded** to the nearest ten, hundred, thousand, etc.

EXAMPLE 1

Round each number:

1. Round each number to the nearest ten: 11, 47, 118
2. Round each number to the nearest hundred: 78, 980, 248
3. Round each number to the nearest thousand: 302, 1274, 3756

Answer

1. Remember, when rounding to the nearest ten, anything ending in 5 or greater rounds up. So, 11 rounds to 10, 47 rounds to 50, and 118 rounds to 120.
2. Remember, when rounding to the nearest hundred, anything ending in 50 or greater rounds up. So, 78 rounds to 100, 980 rounds to 1000, and 248 rounds to 200.
3. Remember, when rounding to the nearest thousand, anything ending in 500 or greater rounds up. So, 302 rounds to 0, 1274 rounds to 1000, and 3756 rounds to 4000.

When you are asked to estimate the solution a problem, you will need to provide only an approximate figure or **estimation** for your answer. In this situation, you will need to round each number in the calculation to the level indicated (nearest hundred, nearest thousand, etc.) or to a level that makes sense for the numbers involved. When estimating a sum **all numbers must be rounded to the same level**. You cannot round one number to the nearest thousand while rounding another to the nearest hundred.

EXAMPLE 2

Estimate the solution to 345,932 + 96,369 *by rounding each number to the nearest ten thousand.*

Start by rounding each number to the nearest ten thousand: 345,932 becomes 350,000, and 96,369 becomes 100,000.

Then, add the rounded numbers: 350,000 + 100,000 = 450,000. So, the answer is approximately 450,000.

The exact answer would be 345,932 + 96,369 = 442,301. So, the estimate of 450,000 is a similar value to the exact answer.

EXAMPLE 3

A patient's heart beat 422 times over the course of six minutes. About how many times did the patient's heart beat during each minute?

The words *about how many* indicate that you need to estimate the solution. In this case, look at the numbers you are given. 422 can be rounded down to 420, which is easily divisible by 6. A good estimate is 420 ÷ 6 = 70 beats per minute. More accurately, the patient's average heart rate was just over 70 beats per minute since his heart actually beat a little more than 420 times in six minutes.

PROPORTIONS AND RATIOS

PROPORTIONS

A proportion is a relationship between two quantities that dictates how one changes when the other changes. A **direct proportion** describes a relationship in which a quantity increases by a set amount for every increase in the other quantity, or decreases by that same amount for every decrease in the other quantity. Example: Assuming a constant driving speed, the time required for a car trip increases as the distance of the trip increases. The distance to be traveled and the time required to travel are directly proportional.

Inverse proportion is a relationship in which an increase in one quantity is accompanied by a decrease in the other, or vice versa. Example: the time required for a car trip decreases as the speed increases, and increases as the speed decreases, so the time required is inversely proportional to the speed of the car.

RATIOS

A ratio is a comparison of two quantities in a particular order. Example: If there are 14 computers in a lab, and the class has 20 students, there is a student to computer **ratio** of 20 to 14, commonly written as 20:14. Ratios are normally reduced to their smallest whole number representation, so 20:14 would be reduced to 10:7 by dividing both sides by 2.

> **Review Video: Word Problems with Ratios**
> Visit mometrix.com/academy and enter code: 104804

REAL WORLD PROBLEMS WITH PROPORTIONS AND RATIOS

EXAMPLE 1

A patient receives 100 mg of a medication every two hours. How much medication does the patient receive on average in five hours?

Using proportional reasoning, since five hours is 2.5 times as long as two hours, the patient will receive two and a half times as much medication: 2.5×100 mg $= 250$ mg, in five hours.

To compute the answer methodically, create two ratios for medication over time—one for the given values, and one that includes the missing value:

$$\frac{\text{medication}}{\text{time}} = \frac{100 \text{ mg}}{2 \text{ hr}} = \frac{x \text{ mg}}{5 \text{ hr}}$$

Cross multiply, and then solve for x:

$$2x = 100 \times 5 = 500$$

$$x = \frac{500}{2} = 250$$

Therefore, the patient receives 250 mg every five hours.

EXAMPLE 2

At a hospital, for every 20 female patients there are 15 male patients. This same patient ratio happens to exist at another hospital. If there are 100 female patients at the second hospital, how many male patients are there?

One way to find the number of male patients is to set up and solve a proportion.

$$\frac{\text{number of female patients}}{\text{number of male patients}} = \frac{20}{15} = \frac{100}{x}$$

Cross multiply and then solve for x:

$$20x = 15 \times 100 = 1500$$

$$x = \frac{1500}{20} = 75$$

Alternatively, notice that: $\frac{20 \times 5}{15 \times 5} = \frac{100}{75}$, so $x = 75$.

EXAMPLE 3

In a hospital emergency room, there are 4 nurses for every 12 patients. What is the ratio of nurses to patients? If the nurse-to-patient ratio remains constant, how many nurses must be present to care for 24 patients?

The ratio of nurses to patients can be written as 4 to 12, 4:12, or $\frac{4}{12}$. Because four and twelve have a common factor of four, the ratio should be reduced to 1:3, which means that there is one nurse present for every three patients. If this ratio remains constant, there must be eight nurses present to care for 24 patients.

EXAMPLE 4

In an intensive care unit, the nurse-to-patient ratio is 1:2. If seven nurses are on duty, how many patients are currently in the ICU?

Use proportional reasoning or set up a proportion to solve. Because there are twice as many patients as nurses, there must be fourteen patients when seven nurses are on duty. Setting up and solving a proportion gives the same result:

$$\frac{\text{number of nurses}}{\text{number of patients}} = \frac{1}{2} = \frac{7}{x}$$

Cross multiply, then solve for x:

$$x = 7 \times 2 = 14$$

CONSTANT OF PROPORTIONALITY

When two quantities have a proportional relationship, there exists a **constant of proportionality** between the quantities; the product of this constant and one of the quantities is equal to the other quantity. For example, if one lemon costs $0.25, two lemons cost $0.50, and three lemons cost $0.75, there is a proportional relationship between the total cost of lemons and the number of lemons purchased. The constant of proportionality is the **unit price**, namely $0.25/lemon. Notice that the total price of lemons, t, can be found by multiplying the unit price of lemons, p, and the number of lemons, n: $t = pn$.

SLOPE

On a graph with two points, (x_1, y_1) and (x_2, y_2), the **slope** m is found with the formula $m = \frac{y_2 - y_1}{x_2 - x_1}$; where $x_1 \neq x_2$. If the value of the slope is **positive**, the line has an *upward direction* from left to right. If the value of the slope is **negative**, the line has a *downward direction* from left to right.

UNIT RATE AS THE SLOPE

A new book goes on sale. In the first month, 5,000 copies of the book are sold. Over time, the book maintains its popularity. The data for the number of copies sold is in the table below.

# of Months on Sale	1	2	3	4	5
# of Copies Sold (Thousands)	5	10	15	20	25

So, the number of copies that are sold and the time that the book is on sale have a proportional relationship. In this example, an equation can be used to show the data: $y = 5x$, where x is the number of months that the book is on sale, and y is the number of copies sold. The slope is $\frac{rise}{run} = \frac{5}{1}$, which can be reduced to 5.

WORK/UNIT RATE

Unit rate expresses a quantity of one thing in terms of one unit of another. For example, if you travel 30 miles every two hours, a **unit rate** expresses this comparison in terms of one hour: in one hour you travel 15 miles, so your unit rate is 15 miles per hour. Other examples are how much one ounce of food costs (price per ounce), or figuring out how much one egg costs out of the dozen (price per 1 egg, instead of price per 12 eggs). The denominator of a unit rate is always 1.

Unit rates are used to compare different options to solve problems. For example, to make sure you get the best deal when deciding which kind of soda to buy, you can find the unit rate of each. If soda #1 costs $1.50 for a 1-liter bottle, and soda #2 costs $2.75 for a 2-liter bottle, it would be a better deal to buy soda #2, because its unit rate is only $1.375 per liter, which is cheaper than soda #1.

Unit rates can also help determine the length of time a given event will take. For example, if you can paint 2 rooms in 4.5 hours, you can determine how long it will take you to paint 5 rooms by solving for the unit rate per room and then multiplying by 5:

$$\text{unit rate} = \frac{4.5 \text{ hr}}{2 \text{ rooms}} = 2.25 \frac{\text{hr}}{\text{room}}$$

$$5 \times \text{unit rate} = 5 \times 2.25 = 11.25 \text{ hr}$$

EXAMPLE 1

Janice made $40 during the first 5 hours she spent babysitting. She will continue to earn money at this rate until she finishes babysitting in 3 more hours. Find how much money Janice earned babysitting and how much she earns per hour.

The total Janice will earn can be found by setting up a proportion comparing money earned to babysitting hours. Since she earned $40 for 5 hours and since the rate is constant, she will earn a proportional amount in 8 hours: $\frac{40}{5} = \frac{x}{8}$. Cross multiplying yields $5x = 8 \times 40 = 320$, and division by 5 shows that $x = \frac{320}{5} = 64$. Janice made a total of $64.

The hourly rate can be found by taking her total amount earned and dividing it by the number of hours worked. Since $\frac{64}{8} = 8$, Janice makes \$8 per hour.

EXAMPLE 2

The McDonalds are taking a family road trip, driving 300 miles to their cabin. It took them 2 hours to drive the first 120 miles. They will drive at the same speed all the way to their cabin. Find the speed at which the McDonalds are driving and how much longer it will take them to get to their cabin.

The McDonalds' speed can be found by dividing the distance traveled by the time it took to travel:

$$\text{Speed} = \frac{120 \text{ mi}}{2 \text{ hr}} = 60 \text{ mph}$$

To determine the amount of time it will take for them to drive the rest of the way, first find how many miles they have left: $300 - 120 = 180$ mi. Divide the remaining distance by the rate of travel to find the remaining travel time:

$$\text{Time} = \frac{180 \text{ mi}}{60 \text{ mph}} = 3 \text{ hr}$$

EXAMPLE 3

It takes Andy 10 minutes to read 6 pages of his book. He has already read 150 pages in his book that is 210 pages long. Find how long it takes Andy to read 1 page and also find how long it will take him to finish his book if he continues to read at the same speed.

Andy's reading time per page can be found by dividing the time it takes him to read 6 pages by 6:

$$Rate = \frac{10}{6} = \frac{5}{3} = 1\frac{2}{3} \text{ min} = 1 \text{ min}, 40 \text{ sec per page}$$

The time it will take Andy to finish the book can be found by first figuring out how many pages he has left to read, and then multiplying this number by his reading time per page:

$$210 - 150 = 60 \text{ pages}$$

$$60 \times \frac{5}{3} = \frac{300}{3} = 100 \text{ min} = 1 \text{ hr}, 40 \text{ min}$$

TRANSLATING WORD PROBLEMS

To write an **expression**, you must first put **variables** with the unknown values in the problem. Then, **translate** the words and phrases into expressions that have numbers and symbols.

INEQUALITIES

= **is**, was, were, will be, equals, is equal to, yields, is the same as, amounts to, becomes

> **is** greater than, **is** more than

≥ **is** greater than or equal to, is at least, is no less than

< **is** less than, **is** fewer than

≤ **is** less than or equal to, is at most, is no more than

To write out an **inequality**, you may need to translate a sentence into an inequality. This translation is putting the words into symbols. When translating, choose a variable to stand for the unknown value. Then, change the words or phrases into symbols. For example, the sum of 2 and a number is at most 12. So, you would write: $2 + b \leq 12$.

<u>EXAMPLE</u>

A farm sells vegetables and dairy products. One third of the sales from dairy products plus half of the sales from vegetables should be greater than the monthly payment (P) for the farm.

Let *d* stand for the sales from dairy products. Let *v* stand for the sales from vegetables. One third of the sales from dairy products is the expression $\frac{d}{3}$. One half of the sales from vegetables is the expression $\frac{v}{2}$. The sum of these expressions should be greater than the monthly payment for the farm. An inequality for this is $\frac{d}{3} + \frac{v}{2} > P$.

RATIONAL EXPRESSIONS

John and Luke play basketball every week. John shoots free throws while Luke shoots three-point shots. John can make 5 more shots per minute than Luke. On one day, John made 30 free throws in the same time that it took Luke to make 20 three-point shots. How fast are Luke and John making shots?

First, determine what you know and what values you can set as equal to each other. You know how many shots each player made in an unknown time period and their rate relative to the other player. The values that can be set as equal are the times it took each player to make their shots. Even though you don't know the value for the time, you know it's the same for both players. When you have a quantity and a rate, dividing the quantity by the rate gives you the time. So divide each player's number of made shots by their rate and set those values equal. Luke made 20 shots at a rate of *x* shots per minute: $\frac{20}{x}$. John made 30 shots at a rate of *x* + 5 shots per minute (he made 5 shots per minute more than Luke): $\frac{30}{x+5}$. Set these two values equal to one another because they both represent the amount of time it took to make the shots:

$$\frac{30}{x+5} = \frac{20}{x}$$

Cross multiply the proportion: $30x = 20(x + 5)$

Distribute the 20 across the parentheses: $30x = 20x + 100$

Subtract 20*x* from both sides of the equation, and you are left with: $10x = 100$

Divide both sides by 10: $x = \frac{100}{10} = 10$

Luke's speed was 10 three-point shots per minute, so John's speed was 15 free throws per minute.

Review Video: <u>Rational Expressions</u>
Visit mometrix.com/academy and enter code: 415183

POLYNOMIAL EXPRESSIONS

Fred buys some CDs for $12 each. He also buys two DVDs. The total that Fred spent is $60. Write an equation that shows the connection between the number of CDs and the average cost of a DVD.

Let c stand for the number of CDs that Fred buys. Also, let D stand for the cost of each DVD that Fred buys. The expression $12c$ gives the cost of the CDs, and the expression $2D$ gives the cost of the DVDs. So the equation $12c + 2D = 60$ represents the situation described.

GRAPHING AND SOLVING INEQUALITIES

Solving inequalities can be done with the same rules as for solving equations. However, when multiplying or dividing by a negative number, the direction of the **inequality sign** must be flipped or **reversed**.

EXAMPLE 1

Simplify the inequality $7x > 5$.

To solve for x, divide both sides by 7:

$$x > \frac{5}{7}$$

EXAMPLE 2

Graph the inequality $10 > -2x + 4$.

In order to graph the inequality $10 > -2x + 4$, you need to solve for x. The opposite of addition is subtraction. So, subtract 4 from both sides. This gives you $6 > -2x$. Next, the opposite of multiplication is division. So, divide both sides by -2. Don't forget to flip the inequality symbol because you are dividing by a negative number. Now, you have $-3 < x$. You can rewrite this as $x > -3$.

To graph an inequality, you make a **number line**. Then, put a circle around the value that is being compared to x. If you are graphing a *greater than* or *less than* inequality, the circle remains open. This represents all of the values up to, but not including, -3. If the inequality is *greater than or equal to* or *less than or equal to*, you draw a closed circle around the value. This would represent all of the values up to, and including, the number. Finally, look over the values that the solution stands for. Then, shade the number line in the needed direction. This example calls for graphing all of the values greater than -3. This is all of the numbers to the right of -3, so you would then shade this area on the number line.

SIMPLIFY

EXAMPLE 1

Simplify the following expression:

$$\frac{\frac{2}{5}}{\frac{4}{7}}$$

Dividing a fraction by a fraction may appear tricky, but it's not if you write out your steps carefully. Follow these steps to divide a fraction by a fraction.

Step 1: Rewrite the problem as a multiplication problem. Dividing by a fraction is the same as multiplying by its **reciprocal**, also known as its **multiplicative inverse**. The product of a number and its reciprocal is 1. Because $\frac{4}{7}$ times $\frac{7}{4}$ is 1, these numbers are reciprocals. Note that reciprocals can be found by simply interchanging the numerators and denominators. So, rewriting the problem as a multiplication problem gives $\frac{2}{5} \times \frac{7}{4}$.

Step 2: Perform multiplication of the fractions by multiplying the numerators by each other and the denominators by each other. In other words, multiply across the top and then multiply across the bottom.

$$\frac{2}{5} \times \frac{7}{4} = \frac{2 \times 7}{5 \times 4} = \frac{14}{20}$$

Step 3: Make sure the fraction is reduced to lowest terms. Both 14 and 20 can be divided by 2.

$$\frac{14}{20} = \frac{14 \div 2}{20 \div 2} = \frac{7}{10}$$

The answer is $\frac{7}{10}$.

EXAMPLE 2

Simplify the following expression:

$$\frac{1}{4} + \frac{3}{6}$$

Fractions with common denominators can be easily added or subtracted. Recall that the denominator is the bottom number in the fraction and that the numerator is the top number in the fraction.

The denominators of $\frac{1}{4}$ and $\frac{3}{6}$ are 4 and 6, respectively. The lowest common denominator of 4 and 6 is 12 because 12 is the least common multiple of 4 (multiples 4, 8, 12, 16, ...) and 6 (multiples 6, 12, 18, 24, ...). Convert each fraction to its equivalent with the newly found common denominator of 12.

$\frac{1 \times 3}{4 \times 3} = \frac{3}{12}; \frac{3 \times 2}{6 \times 2} = \frac{6}{12}$.

Now that the fractions have the same denominator, you can add them.

$\frac{3}{12} + \frac{6}{12} = \frac{9}{12}$.

Be sure to write your answer in lowest terms. Both 9 and 12 can be divided by 3, so the answer is $\frac{3}{4}$.

EXAMPLE 3

Simplify the following expression:

$$\frac{7}{8} - \frac{8}{16}$$

Fractions with common denominators can be easily added or subtracted. Recall that the denominator is the bottom number in the fraction and that the numerator is the top number in the fraction.

The denominators of $\frac{7}{8}$ and $\frac{8}{16}$ are 8 and 16, respectively. The lowest common denominator of 8 and 16 is 16 because 16 is the least common multiple of 8 (multiples 8, 16, 24 ...) and 16 (multiples 16, 32, 48, ...). Convert each fraction to its equivalent with the newly found common denominator of 16.

$$\frac{7 \times 2}{8 \times 2} = \frac{14}{16} \qquad \frac{8 \times 1}{16 \times 1} = \frac{8}{16}$$

Now that the fractions have the same denominator, you can subtract them.

$$\frac{14}{16} - \frac{8}{16} = \frac{6}{16}$$

Be sure to write your answer in lowest terms. Both 6 and 16 can be divided by 2, so the answer is $\frac{3}{8}$.

EXAMPLE 4

Simplify the following expression:

$$\frac{1}{2} + \left(3\left(\frac{3}{4}\right) - 2\right) + 4$$

When simplifying expressions, first perform operations within groups. Within the set of parentheses are multiplication and subtraction operations. Perform the multiplication first to get $\frac{1}{2} + \left(\frac{9}{4} - 2\right) + 4$. Then, subtract two to obtain $\frac{1}{2} + \frac{1}{4} + 4$. Finally, perform addition from left to right: $\frac{1}{2} + \frac{1}{4} + 4 = \frac{2}{4} + \frac{1}{4} + \frac{16}{4} = \frac{19}{4}$.

EXAMPLE 5

Simplify the following expression:

$$0.22 + 0.5 - (5.5 + 3.3 \div 3)$$

First, evaluate the terms in the parentheses $(5.5 + 3.3 \div 3)$ using order of operations. $3.3 \div 3 = 1.1$, and $5.5 + 1.1 = 6.6$.

Next, rewrite the problem: $0.22 + 0.5 - 6.6$.

Finally, add and subtract from left to right: $0.22 + 0.5 = 0.72$; $0.72 - 6.6 = -5.88$. The answer is -5.88.

EXAMPLE 6

Simplify the following expression:

$$\frac{3}{2} + (4(0.5) - 0.75) + 2$$

First change the fraction to a decimal:

$$1.5 + (4(0.5) - 0.75) + 2$$

$$1.5 + (2 - 0.75) + 2$$

Then perform addition from left to right:

$$1.5 + 1.25 + 2 = 4.75$$

EXAMPLE 7

Simplify the following expression:

$$1.45 + 1.5 + (6 - 9 \div 2) + 45$$

First, evaluate the terms in the parentheses using proper order of operations.

$$1.45 + 1.5 + (6 - 4.5) + 45$$

$$1.45 + 1.5 + 1.5 + 45$$

Finally, add from left to right.

$$1.45 + 1.5 + 1.5 + 45 = 49.45$$

Data Interpretation

STATISTICS

Statistics is the branch of mathematics that deals with collecting, recording, interpreting, illustrating, and analyzing large amounts of **data**. The following terms are often used in the discussion of data and **statistics**:

- **Data** – the collective name for pieces of *information* (singular is datum).
- **Quantitative data** – measurements (such as length, mass, and speed) that provide information about *quantities* in numbers
- **Qualitative data** – information (such as colors, scents, tastes, and shapes) that *cannot be measured* using numbers
- **Discrete data** – information that can be expressed only by a *specific value*, such as whole or half numbers. For example, since people can be counted only in whole numbers, a population count would be discrete data.
- **Continuous data** – information (such as time and temperature) that can be expressed by *any value within a given range*
- **Primary data** – information that has been *collected* directly from a survey, investigation, or experiment, such as a questionnaire or the recording of daily temperatures. Primary data that has not yet been organized or analyzed is called raw data.
- **Secondary data** – information that has been collected, sorted, and *processed* by the researcher
- **Ordinal data** – information that *can be placed in numerical order*, such as age or weight
- **Nominal data** – information that *cannot be placed in numerical order*, such as names or places.

DISPLAYING DATA

A **bar graph** is a graph that uses bars to compare data, as if each bar were a ruler being used to measure the data. The graph includes a **scale** that identifies the units being measured.

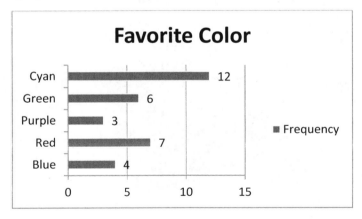

A **line graph** is a graph that connects points to show how data increases or decreases over time. The time line is the **horizontal axis**. The connecting lines between data points on the graph are a way to more clearly show how the data changes.

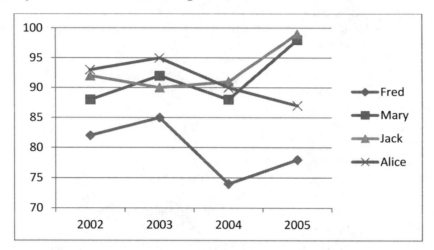

A **pictograph** is a graph that uses pictures or symbols to show data. The pictograph will have a **key** to identify what each symbol represents. Generally, each symbol stands for one or more objects.

A **pie chart** or circle graph is a diagram used to compare parts of a whole. The full pie represents the whole, and it is divided into sectors that each represent something that is a part of the whole. Each sector or slice of the pie is either labeled to indicate what it represents, or explained on a key associated with the chart. The size of each slice is determined by the *percentage of the whole* that the associated quantity represents. Numerically, the angle measurement of each sector can be computed by solving the proportion: $x/360 = \text{part/whole}$.

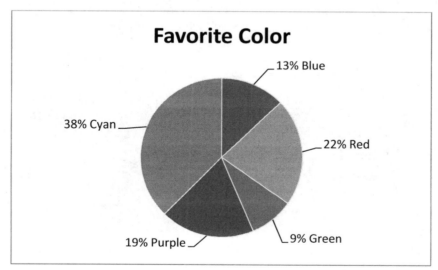

A **histogram** is a special type of bar graph where the data are grouped in **intervals** (for example 20–29, 30–39, 40–49, etc.). The **frequency**, or number of times a value occurs in each interval, is indicated by the height of the bar. The intervals do not have to be the same amount but usually are (all data in ranges of 10 or all in ranges of 5, for example). The smaller the intervals, the more detailed the information.

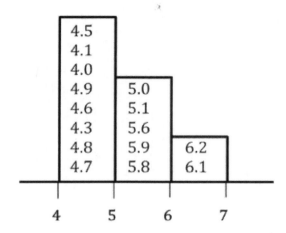

A **stem-and-leaf plot** can outline groups of data that fall into a range of values. Each piece of data is split into two parts: the first, or left, part is called the stem. The second, or right, part is called the leaf. Each **stem** is listed in a column from smallest to largest. Each **leaf** that has the common stem is listed in that stem's row from smallest to largest.

For example, in a set of two-digit numbers, the digit in the tens place is the stem. So, the digit in the ones place is the leaf. With a stem-and-leaf plot, you can see which subset of numbers (10s, 20s, 30s, etc.) is the largest. This information can be found by looking at a histogram. However, a stem and leaf plot also lets you look closer and see which values fall in that range. Using all of the test scores from the line graph, we can put together a stem and leaf plot:

Test Scores								
7	4	8						
8	2	5	7	8	8			
9	0	0	1	2	2	3	5	8	9

Again, a stem-and-leaf plot is similar to histograms and frequency plots. However, a stem-and-leaf plot keeps all of the original data. In this example, you can see that almost half of the students scored in the 80s. Also, all of the data has been maintained. These plots can be used for larger numbers as well. However, they work better for *small sets of data*.

Scatter plots are useful for knowing the types of functions that are given with the data. Also, they are helpful for finding the simple regression. A **simple regression** is a regression that uses an independent variable.

A **regression** is a chart that is used to predict future events. Linear scatter plots may be positive or negative. Many nonlinear scatter plots are exponential or quadratic. Below are some common types of scatter plots:

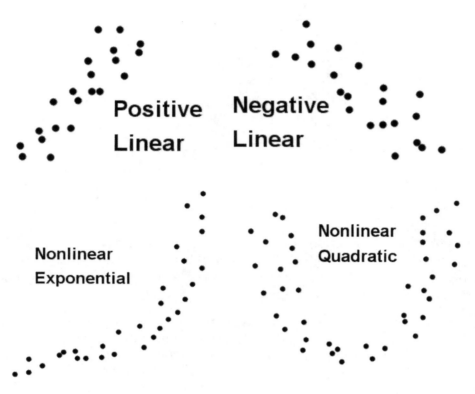

INTERPRETATION OF GRAPHS

EXAMPLE 1

The following graph shows the ages of five patients a nurse is caring for in the hospital:

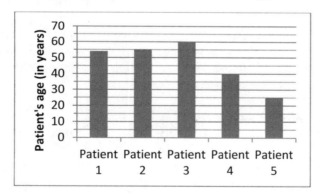

Use this graph to determine the age range of the patients for which the nurse is caring.

Use the graph to find the age of each patient: Patient 1 is 54 years old; Patient 2 is 55 years old; Patient 3 is 60 years old; Patient 4 is 40 years old; and Patient 5 is 25 years old. The age range is the age of the oldest patient minus the age of the youngest patient. In other words, 60 – 25 = 35. The age range is 35 years.

EXAMPLE 2

Below is a line graph representing the heart rate of a patient during the day. Use the graph to answer the questions that follow.

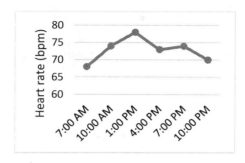

The patient's minimum measured heart rate occurred at what time? The patient's maximum measured heart rate occurred at what time? At what times during the day did the patient have the same measured heart rate? What trends, if any, can you find about the patient's heart rate throughout the day?

The patient's minimum measured heart rate occurred at the lowest data point on the graph, which is 68 bpm at 7:00 AM. The patient's maximum measured heart rate occurred at the highest data point on the graph, which is 78 bpm at 1:00 PM. The patient had the same measured heart rate of 74 bpm at 10:00 AM and 7:00 PM. The patient's heart rate increased through the morning to early afternoon, and generally declined as the afternoon progressed.

CONSISTENCY BETWEEN STUDIES

EXAMPLE

*In a drug study containing 100 patients, a new cholesterol drug was found to decrease low-density lipoprotein (LDL) levels in 25% of the patients. In a second study containing 50 patients, the same drug administered at the same dosage was found to decrease LDL levels in 50% of the patients. Are the results of these two studies **consistent** with one another?*

Even though in both studies 25 people (25% of 100 is 25 and 50% of 50 is 25) showed improvements in their LDL levels, the results of the studies are inconsistent. The results of the second study indicate that the drug has a much higher efficacy (desired result) than the results of the first study. Because 50 out of 150 total patients showed improvement on the medication, one could argue that the drug is effective in one third (or approximately 33%) of patients. However, one should be wary of the reliability of results when they're not **reproducible** from one study to the next and when the **sample size** is low.

DATA ORGANIZATION

EXAMPLE

A nurse found the heart rates of eleven different patients to be 76, 80, 90, 86, 70, 76, 72, 88, 88, 68, and 88 beats per minute. Organize this information in a table.

There are several ways to organize data in a table. The table below is an example.

Patient Number	1	2	3	4	5	6	7	8	9	10	11
Heart Rate (bpm)	76	80	90	86	70	76	72	88	88	68	88

When making a table, be sure to label the columns and rows appropriately.

INDEPENDENT AND DEPENDENT VARIABLES

A **variable** is a symbol, usually an alphabetic character, designating a *value that may change* within the scope of a given problem. Variables can be described as either independent or dependent variables. An **independent variable** is an input into a system that may take on values freely. **Dependent variables** are those that change as a consequence of changes in other values in the equation.

EXAMPLE 1

Ray earns $10 an hour at his job. Write an equation for his earnings as a function of time spent working. How long does Ray have to work in order to earn $360?

The number of dollars that Ray earns is dependent on the number of hours he works, so earnings will be represented by the dependent variable y and hours worked will be represented by the independent variable x. He earns 10 dollars per hour worked, so his earning can be calculated as $y = 10x$.

To calculate the number of hours Ray must work in order to earn $360, plug in 360 for y and solve for x:

$$360 = 10x$$

$$x = \frac{360}{10} = 36$$

So Ray must work 36 hours in order to earn $360.

EXAMPLE 2

A patient told a doctor she feels fine after running one mile but that her knee starts hurting after running two miles. Her knee throbs after running three miles and swells after running four. Identify the independent and dependent variables with regard to the distance she runs and her level of pain.

An independent variable is one that does not depend on any other variables in the situation. In this case, the distance the patient runs would be considered the independent variable. The dependent variable would be her level of pain because it depends on how far she runs.

BIVARIATE DATA

Bivariate data is data *from two different variables*. The prefix *bi-* means *two*. In a **scatter plot**, each value in the set of data is put on a grid. This is similar to the Cartesian plane where each axis represents one of the two variables.

When you look at the pattern made by the points on the grid, you may know if there is a relationship between the two variables. Also, you may know what that relationship is and if it exists.

The variables may be directly proportionate, inversely proportionate, or show no proportion. Also, you may be able to see if the data is linear. If the data is linear, you can find an equation to show the two variables. The following scatter plot shows the relationship between preference for brand "A" and the age of the consumers surveyed.

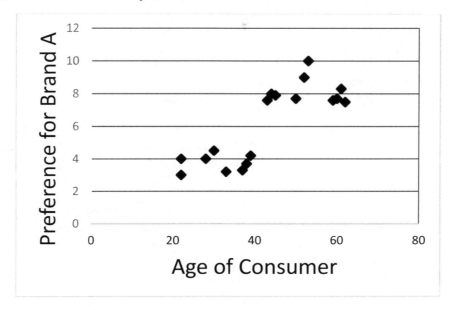

MEASURES OF CENTRAL TENDENCY

MEAN

The mean is the *average of the data points*; that is, it is the sum of the data points divided by the number of data points. Mathematically, the mean of a set of data points $\{x_1, x_2, x_3, \ldots x_n\}$ can be written as $\bar{X} = \sum \frac{X}{N}$. For instance, for the data set (1, 3, 6, 8, 100, 800), the mean is

$$\frac{1 + 3 + 6 + 8 + 100 + 800}{6} = 153$$

The mean is most useful when data is approximately normal and does not include extreme **outliers** (data values that are unusually high or unusually low compared to the rest of the data values). In the above example, the data shows much **variation**. Thus, the mean is not the best measure of central tendency to use, when interpreting the data. With this data set, the **median** will give a more complete picture of the distribution.

MEDIAN

The median is the value *in the middle of the data set*, in the sense that 50% of the data points lie above the median and 50% of the data points lie below. The median can be determined by simply putting the data points in order, and selecting the data point in the middle. If there is an even number of data points, then the median is the average of the middle two data points. For instance, for the data set {1, 3, 6, 8, 100, 800}, the median is $\frac{6+8}{2} = 7$.

For distributions with widely varying data points, especially those with large outliers, the median is a more appropriate measure of **central tendency**, and thus gives a better idea of a "typical" data point. Notice in the data set above, the mean is 153, while the median is 7.

MODE

The mode is the value that *appears most often in the data set*. For instance, for the data set {2, 6, 4, 9, 4, 5, 7, 6, 4, 1, 5, 6, 7, 5, 6}, the mode is 6: the number 6 appears four times in the data set, while the next most frequent values, 4 and 5, appear only three times each. It is possible for a data set to have more than one mode: in the data set {11, 14, 17, 16, 11, 17, 12, 14, 17, 14, 13}, 14 and 17 are both modes, appearing three times each. In the extreme case of a uniform distribution—a distribution in which all values appear with equal probability—all values in the data set are modes. However, if no value appears more than once in a data set, the set has no mode.

The mode is useful to get a general sense of the *shape of the distribution*; it shows where the peaks of the distribution are. More information is necessary to get a more detailed description of the full shape.

RANGE

The range of a distribution is the *difference between the highest and lowest values in the distribution*. For example, in the data set (1, 3, 5, 7, 9, 11), the highest and lowest values are 11 and 1, respectively. The range then would be calculated as 11 – 1 = 10.

SHAPE OF DATA DISTRIBUTION

SYMMETRY AND SKEWNESS

Symmetry is a characteristic of the shape of the plotted data. Specifically, it refers to how well the data on one side of the median *mirrors* the data on the other side.

A **skewed** data set is one that has a distinctly longer or fatter tail on one side of the peak or the other. A data set that is *skewed left* has more of its values to the left of the peak, while a set that is *skewed right* has more of its values to the right of the peak. When actually looking at the graph, these names may seem counterintuitive since, in a left-skewed data set, the bulk of the values seem to be on the right side of the graph, and vice versa. However, if the graph is viewed strictly in relation to the peak, the direction of skewness makes more sense.

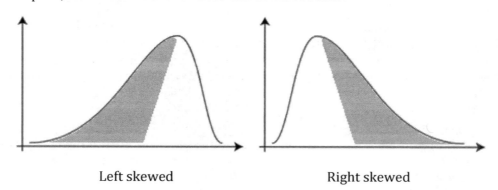

Left skewed   Right skewed

UNIMODAL VS. BIMODAL

If a distribution has a single peak, it would be considered **unimodal**. If it has two discernible peaks it would be considered **bimodal**. Bimodal distributions may be an indication that the set of data being considered is actually the combination of two sets of data with significant differences.

UNIFORMITY

A uniform distribution is a distribution in which there is *no distinct peak or variation* in the data. No values or ranges are particularly more common than any other values or ranges.

Measurement

POLYGONS

Quadrilateral: A closed two-dimensional geometric figure composed of exactly four straight sides. The sum of the interior angles of any quadrilateral is 360°.

Parallelogram: A quadrilateral that has exactly two pairs of opposite **parallel** sides. The sides that are parallel are also **congruent**. The opposite interior angles are always congruent, and the consecutive interior angles are **supplementary**. The **diagonals** of a parallelogram bisect each other. Each diagonal divides the parallelogram into two congruent triangles.

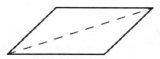

Trapezoid: Traditionally, a quadrilateral that has exactly one pair of parallel sides. Some math texts define trapezoid as a quadrilateral that has at least one pair of parallel sides. Because there are no rules governing the second pair of sides, there are no rules that apply to the properties of the diagonals of a trapezoid.

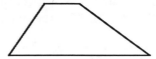

Rectangles, rhombuses, and squares are all special forms of parallelograms.

Rectangle: A parallelogram with four right angles. All rectangles are parallelograms, but not all parallelograms are rectangles. The diagonals of a rectangle are congruent.

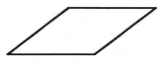

Rhombus: A parallelogram with four congruent sides. All rhombuses are parallelograms, but not all parallelograms are rhombuses. The diagonals of a rhombus are **perpendicular** to each other.

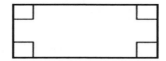

Square: A parallelogram with four right angles and four congruent sides. All squares are also parallelograms, rhombuses, and rectangles. The diagonals of a square are congruent and perpendicular to each other.

A quadrilateral whose diagonals bisect each other is a **parallelogram**. A quadrilateral whose opposite sides are parallel (2 pairs of parallel sides) is a parallelogram.

A quadrilateral whose diagonals are perpendicular bisectors is a **rhombus**. A quadrilateral whose opposite sides (both pairs) are parallel and congruent is a rhombus.

A parallelogram that has a right angle is a **rectangle**. (Consecutive angles of a parallelogram are supplementary. Therefore, if there is one right angle in a parallelogram, there are four right angles in that parallelogram.)

A rhombus that has a right angle is a **square**. Because the rhombus is a special form of a parallelogram, the rules about the angles of a parallelogram also apply to the rhombus.

> **Review Video: <u>Polygons</u>**
> Visit mometrix.com/academy and enter code: 271869

CIRCLE

The **center** is the single point inside the circle that is **equidistant** from every point on the circle. (Point O in the diagram below.)

The **radius** is a line segment that joins the center of the circle and any one point on the circle. All radii of a circle are equal. (Segments OX, OY, and OZ in the diagram below.)

The **diameter** is a line segment that passes through the center of the circle and has both endpoints on the circle. The length of the diameter is exactly *twice the length of the radius*. (Segment XZ in the diagram below.)

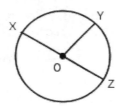

An **arc** is a portion of a circle. Specifically, an arc is the set of points between and including two points on a circle. An arc does not contain any points inside the circle. When a segment is drawn from the endpoints of an arc to the center of the circle, a **sector** is formed.

A **central angle** is an angle whose **vertex** is the center of a circle and whose legs intercept an arc of the circle. Angle XOY in the diagram above is a central angle. A **minor arc** is an arc that has a measure less than 180°. The measure of a central angle is equal to the measure of the minor arc it intercepts. A **major arc** is an arc having a measure of at least 180°. The measure of the major arc can be found by subtracting the measure of the central angle from 360°.

A **semicircle** is an arc whose endpoints are the endpoints of the diameter of a circle. A semicircle is exactly half of a circle.

A **chord** is a line segment that has both endpoints on a circle. In the diagram below, $\overline{EB}$ is a chord.

Secant: A line that passes through a circle and contains a chord of that circle. In the diagram below, $\overleftrightarrow{EB}$ is a secant and contains chord $\overline{EB}$.

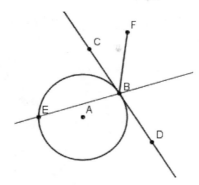

An **inscribed angle** is an angle whose vertex lies on a circle and whose legs contain chords of that circle. The portion of the circle intercepted by the legs of the angle is called the **intercepted arc**. The measure of the intercepted arc is exactly twice the measure of the inscribed angle. In the diagram below, angle ABC is an inscribed angle. $\widehat{AC} = 2(\text{m}\angle ABC)$.

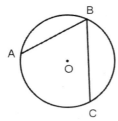

The **arc length** is the length of that portion of the circumference between two points on the circle. The formula for arc length is $s = \frac{\pi r \theta}{180°}$ where s is the arc length, r is the length of the radius, and θ is the angular measure of the arc in degrees, or $s = r\theta$, where θ is the angular measure of the arc in radians (2π radians = 360 degrees).

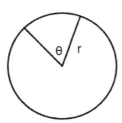

A **sector** is the portion of a circle formed by two radii and their intercepted arc. While the arc length is exclusively the points that are also on the circumference of the circle, the sector is the entire area bounded by the arc and the two radii.

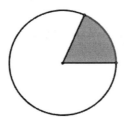

The **area** of a sector of a circle is found by the formula $A = \frac{\theta r^2}{2}$, where A is the area, θ is the measure of the central angle in radians, and r is the radius. To find the area when the central angle is in degrees, use the formula, $A = \frac{\theta \pi r^2}{360}$, where θ is the measure of the central angle in degrees and r is the radius.

PERIMETER FORMULAS

TRIANGLE

The **perimeter** of any triangle is found by summing the three side lengths; $P = a + b + c$. For an **equilateral triangle**, this is the same as $P = 3s$, where s is any side length, since all three sides are the same length.

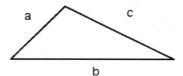

SQUARE

The perimeter of a square is found by using the formula $P = 4s$, where s is the length of one side. Because all four sides are equal in a square, it is faster to multiply the length of one side by 4 than to add the same number four times. You could use the formulas for rectangles and get the same answer.

RECTANGLE

The perimeter of a rectangle is found by the formula $P = 2l + 2w$ or $P = 2(l + w)$, where l is the length, and w is the width. It may be easier to add the length and width first and then double the result, as in the second formula.

PARALLELOGRAM

The perimeter of a parallelogram is found by the formula $P = 2a + 2b$ or $P = 2(a + b)$, where a and b are the lengths of the two sides.

TRAPEZOID

The perimeter of a trapezoid is found by the formula $P = a + b_1 + c + b_2$, where $a, b_1, c,$ and b_2 are the four sides of the trapezoid.

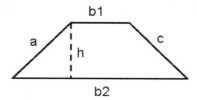

CIRCLE

The perimeter (**circumference**) of a circle is found by the formula $C = 2\pi r$, where r is the radius. Again, remember to convert the diameter if you are given that measure rather than the radius.

AREA FORMULAS

TRIANGLE

The **area** of any triangle can be found by taking half the product of one side length (base or *b*) and the perpendicular distance from that side to the opposite vertex (height or *h*). In equation form, $A = \frac{1}{2}bh$.

SQUARE

The area of a square is found by using the formula $A = s^2$, where and *s* is the length of one side.

RECTANGLE

The area of a rectangle is found by the formula $A = lw$, where *A* is the area of the rectangle, *l* is the length (usually considered to be the longer side) and *w* is the width (usually considered to be the shorter side). The numbers for *l* and *w* are interchangeable.

PARALLELOGRAM

The area of a parallelogram is found by the formula $A = bh$, where *b* is the length of the base and *h* is the height. Note that the base and height correspond to the length and width in a rectangle, so this formula would apply to rectangles as well. Do not confuse the height of a parallelogram with the length of the second side. The two are only the same measure in the case of a rectangle.

TRAPEZOID

The area of a trapezoid is found by the formula $A = \frac{1}{2}h(b_1 + b_2)$, where *h* is the height (segment joining and perpendicular to the parallel bases), and b_1 and b_2 are the two parallel sides (bases). Do not use one of the other two sides as the height unless that side is also perpendicular to the parallel bases.

CIRCLE

The area of a circle is found by the formula $A = \pi r^2$, where *r* is the length of the radius. If the diameter of the circle is given, remember to divide it in half to get the length of the radius before proceeding.

> **Review Video: How to Find the Area and Perimeter**
> Visit mometrix.com/academy and enter code: 471797

SURFACE AREA AND VOLUME FORMULAS

The surface area of a solid object is the *area of all sides or exterior surfaces*. For objects such as prisms and pyramids, a further distinction is made between **base surface area** (B) and **lateral surface area** (LA). For a prism, the total surface area (SA) is $SA = LA + 2B$. For a pyramid or cone, the total surface area is $SA = LA + B$.

PRISMS

The **surface area** of any prism is the sum of the areas of both bases and all sides. It can be calculated as $SA = 2B + Ph$, where *P* is the perimeter of the base. The **volume** of any prism is found with the formula $V = Bh$, where B is the area of the base and h is the height. The perpendicular distance between the bases is the height.

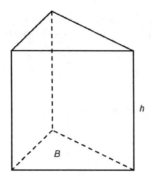

SPHERE

The **surface area** of a sphere can be found by the formula $A = 4\pi r^2$, where r is the radius. The **volume** of a sphere can be found with the formula $V = \frac{4}{3}\pi r^3$, where r is the radius. Both quantities are generally given in terms of π.

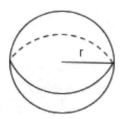

EXAMPLE

Dwight has a beach ball with a radius of 9 inches. He is planning to wrap the ball with wrapping paper. How many square feet of wrapping paper are needed to cover the surface of the ball?

The surface area of a sphere may be calculated using the formula $SA = 4\pi r^2$. Substituting 9 for r gives $SA = 4\pi(9)^2$, which simplifies to $SA \approx 1017.36$. So the surface area of the ball is approximately 1017.36 square inches. There are twelve inches in a foot. So, there are $12^2 = 144$ square inches in a square foot. To convert this measurement to square feet, the following proportion may be written and solved for x: $\frac{1}{144} = \frac{x}{1017.36}$. So $x \approx 7.07$, meaning it will take approximately 7.07 square feet of wrapping paper to cover the surface of the ball.

CUBE

The **volume** of a cube can be found with the formula $V = s^3$, where s is the length of a side.

The **surface area** of a cube is calculated as $SA = 6s^2$, where SA is the total surface area and s is the length of a side. These formulas are the same as the ones used for the volume and surface area of a rectangular prism. However, these are simple formulas because the three numbers (i.e., length, width, and height) are the same.

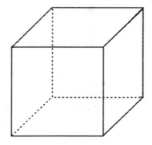

RECTANGULAR PRISM

The **surface area** can be calculated as $SA = 2lw + 2hl + 2wh$ or $SA = 2(lw + hl + wh)$. The **volume** of a rectangular prism can be found with the formula $V = lwh$, where V is the volume, l is the length, w is the width, and h is the height.

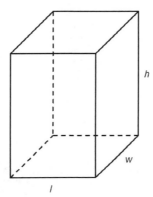

CYLINDER

The **surface area** of a cylinder can be found by the formula $SA = 2\pi r^2 + 2\pi rh$. The first term is the base area multiplied by two, and the second term is the perimeter of the base multiplied by the height. The **volume** of a cylinder can be found with the formula $V = \pi r^2 h$, where r is the radius and h is the height.

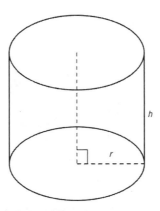

Review Video: How to Calculate the Volume of 3D Objects
Visit mometrix.com/academy and enter code: 163343

COORDINATE PLANE

When algebraic functions and equations are shown graphically, they are usually shown on a **Cartesian coordinate plane**. The Cartesian coordinate plane consists of two number lines placed perpendicular to each other, and intersecting at the **zero point**, also known as the **origin**. The horizontal number line is known as the **x-axis**, with positive values to the right of the origin and negative values to the left of the origin. The vertical number line is known as the **y-axis**, with positive values above the origin and negative values below the origin. Any point on the plane can be identified by an ordered pair in the form (*x,y*), called **coordinates**. The *x*-value of the coordinate is called the **abscissa**, and the *y*-value of the coordinate is called the **ordinate**. The two number lines divide the plane into four **quadrants**: I, II, III, and IV.

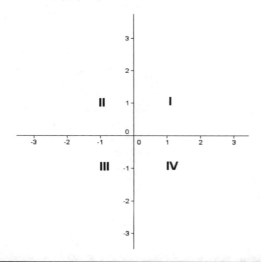

Review Video: <u>Cartesian Coordinate Plane and Graphing</u>
Visit mometrix.com/academy and enter code: 115173

EXAMPLE

Plot the following points on the coordinate plane:

A. (−4, −2)   B. (−1, 3)   C. (2, 2)   D. (3, −1)

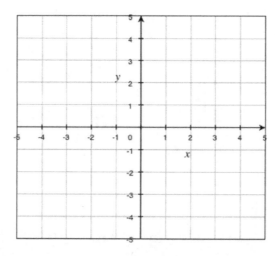

ANSWER

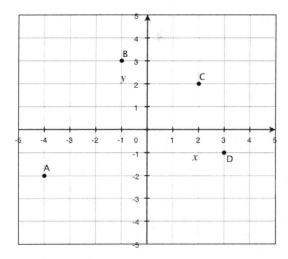

ACTUAL DRAWINGS AND SCALE DRAWINGS

A map has a key for measurements to compare real distances with a **scale distance**.

EXAMPLE

The key on one map says that 2 inches on the map is 12 real miles. Find the distance of a route that is 5 inches long on the map.

A **proportion** is needed to show the map measurements and real distances. First, write a ratio that has the information in the key. The map measurement can be in the numerator, and the real distance can be in the denominator.

$$\frac{2 \text{ inches}}{12 \text{ miles}}$$

Next, write a ratio with the known map distance and the unknown real distance. The unknown number for miles can be represented with the letter m.

$$\frac{5 \text{ inches}}{m \text{ miles}}$$

Then, write out the ratios in a proportion and solve it for m.

$$\frac{2 \text{ inches}}{12 \text{ miles}} = \frac{5 \text{ inches}}{m \text{ miles}}$$

Now, you have $2m = 60$. So, you are left with $m = 30$. Thus, the route is 30 miles long.

MEASUREMENT CONVERSION

When going from a larger unit to a smaller unit, multiply the number of the known amount by the **equivalent amount**. When going from a smaller unit to a larger unit, divide the number of the known amount by the equivalent amount.

Also, you can set up conversion fractions. In these fractions, one fraction is the **conversion factor**. The other fraction has the unknown amount in the numerator. So, the known value is placed in the denominator. Sometimes the second fraction has the known value from the problem in the numerator, and the unknown in the denominator. Multiply the two fractions to get the converted measurement.

CONVERSION UNITS

METRIC CONVERSIONS

1000 mcg (microgram)	1 mg
1000 mg (milligram)	1 g
1000 g (gram)	1 kg
1000 kg (kilogram)	1 metric ton
1000 mL (milliliter)	1 L
1000 um (micrometer)	1 mm
1000 mm (millimeter)	1 m
100 cm (centimeter)	1 m
1000 m (meter)	1 km

U.S. AND METRIC EQUIVALENTS

Unit	U.S. equivalent	Metric equivalent
Inch	1 inch	2.54 centimeters
Foot	12 inches	0.305 meters
Yard	3 feet	0.914 meters
Mile	5280 feet	1.609 kilometers

CAPACITY MEASUREMENTS

Unit	U.S. equivalent	Metric equivalent
Ounce	8 drams	29.573 milliliters
Cup	8 ounces	0.237 liter
Pint	16 ounces	0.473 liter
Quart	2 pints	0.946 liter
Gallon	4 quarts	3.785 liters

WEIGHT MEASUREMENTS

Unit	U.S. equivalent	Metric equivalent
Ounce	16 drams	28.35 grams
Pound	16 ounces	453.6 grams
Ton	2,000 pounds	907.2 kilograms

> **Review Video: Converting Kilograms to Pounds**
> Visit mometrix.com/academy and enter code: 241463

NURSING MEASUREMENTS

Unit	English equivalent	Metric equivalent
1 tsp	1 fluid dram	5 milliliters
3 tsp	4 fluid drams	15 or 16 milliliters
2 tbsp	1 fluid ounce	30 milliliters
1 glass	8 fluid ounces	240 milliliters

MEASUREMENT CONVERSION PRACTICE PROBLEMS

EXAMPLE 1

a. Convert 1.4 meters to centimeters.
b. Convert 218 centimeters to meters.

EXAMPLE 2

a. Convert 42 inches to feet.
b. Convert 15 feet to yards.

EXAMPLE 3

a. How many pounds are in 15 kilograms?
b. How many pounds are in 80 ounces?

EXAMPLE 4

a. How many kilometers are in 2 miles?
b. How many centimeters are in 5 feet?

EXAMPLE 5

a. How many gallons are in 15.14 liters?
b. How many liters are in 8 quarts?

EXAMPLE 6

a. How many grams are in 13.2 pounds?
b. How many pints are in 9 gallons?

MEASUREMENT CONVERSION SOLUTIONS

EXAMPLE 1

Write ratios with the conversion factor $\frac{100 \text{ cm}}{1 \text{ m}}$. Use proportions to convert the given units.

a. $\frac{100 \text{ cm}}{1 \text{ m}} = \frac{x \text{ cm}}{1.4 \text{ m}}$. Cross multiply to get $x = 140$. So, 1.4 m is the same as 140 cm.

b. $\frac{100 \text{ cm}}{1 \text{ m}} = \frac{218 \text{ cm}}{x \text{ m}}$. Cross multiply to get $100x = 218$, or $x = 2.18$. So, 218 cm is the same as 2.18 m.

EXAMPLE 2

Write ratios with the conversion factors $\frac{12 \text{ in}}{1 \text{ ft}}$ and $\frac{3 \text{ ft}}{1 \text{ yd}}$. Use proportions to convert the given units.

a. $\frac{12 \text{ in}}{1 \text{ ft}} = \frac{42 \text{ in}}{x \text{ ft}}$. Cross multiply to get $12x = 42$, or $x = 3.5$. So, 42 inches is the same as 3.5 feet.

b. $\frac{3 \text{ ft}}{1 \text{ yd}} = \frac{15 \text{ ft}}{x \text{ yd}}$. Cross multiply to get $3x = 15$, or $x = 5$. So, 15 feet is the same as 5 yards.

EXAMPLE 3

a. 15 kilograms $\times \frac{2.2 \text{ pounds}}{1 \text{ kilogram}} = 33$ pounds

b. 80 ounces $\times \frac{1 \text{ pound}}{16 \text{ ounces}} = 5$ pounds

EXAMPLE 4

a. 2 miles $\times \frac{1.609 \text{ kilometers}}{1 \text{ mile}} = 3.218$ kilometers

b. 5 feet $\times \frac{12 \text{ inches}}{1 \text{ foot}} \times \frac{2.54 \text{ centimeters}}{1 \text{ inch}} = 152.4$ centimeters

EXAMPLE 5

a. 15.14 liters $\times \frac{1 \text{ gallon}}{3.785 \text{ liters}} = 4$ gallons

b. 8 quarts $\times \frac{1 \text{ gallon}}{4 \text{ quarts}} \times \frac{3.785 \text{ liters}}{1 \text{ gallon}} = 7.57$ liters

EXAMPLE 6

a. 13.2 pounds $\times \frac{1 \text{ kilogram}}{2.2 \text{ pounds}} \times \frac{1000 \text{ grams}}{1 \text{ kilogram}} = 6000$ grams

b. 9 gallons $\times \frac{4 \text{ quarts}}{1 \text{ gallon}} \times \frac{2 \text{ pints}}{1 \text{ quarts}} = 72$ pints

Science

General Anatomy and Physiology

Cell

The cell is the basic *organizational unit* of all living things. Each piece within a cell has a function that helps organisms grow and survive. There are many different types of cells, but cells are unique to each type of organism. The one thing that all cells have in common is a **membrane**, which is comparable to a semi-permeable plastic bag. The membrane is composed of **phospholipids**. There are also some **transport holes**, which are proteins that help certain molecules and ions move in and out of the cell. The cell is filled with a fluid called **cytoplasm** or cytosol.

Within the cell are a variety of **organelles**, groups of complex molecules that help a cell survive, each with its own unique membrane that has a different chemical makeup from the cell membrane. The larger the cell, the more organelles it will need to live.

Cell Structural Organization

All organisms, whether plants, animals, fungi, protists, or bacteria, exhibit structural organization on the cellular and organism level. All cells contain **DNA** and **RNA** and can synthesize proteins. Cells are the basic structural units of all organisms. All organisms have a highly organized cellular structure. Each cell consists of **nucleic acids**, **cytoplasm**, and a **cell membrane**. Specialized organelles such as **mitochondria** and **chloroplasts** have specific functions within the cell. In single-celled organisms, that single cell contains all of the components necessary for life. In multicellular organisms, cells can become specialized. Different types of cells can have different functions. Life begins as a single cell whether by **asexual** or **sexual reproduction**. Cells are grouped together in **tissues**. Tissues are grouped together in **organs**. Organs are grouped together in **systems**. An **organism** is a complete individual.

Defining Characteristics of Eukaryotic Cells

Cells can be classified into two main groups based on the presence or absence of a nucleus. In fact, the terms **eukaryote** and **prokaryote** mean "true kernel" and "before the kernel," respectively. The nucleus is a membrane-bound structure that encloses nearly all the genetic material of a eukaryotic cell. Eukaryotic DNA molecules wrap around associated proteins to form linear chromosomes, and the genes within them are regulated by molecules within the nucleoplasm. For this reason, the nucleus is deemed the "control center" of the cell. Eukaryotic cells are also defined by the presence of other membrane-bound organelles, including mitochondria, endoplasmic reticulum, Golgi bodies, peroxisomes, and (in animal cells) lysosomes. Ribosomes and the cytoskeleton are not enclosed by membranes and are found in both prokaryotic and eukaryotic cells. These types of cells also differ in the way that they divide. While prokaryotes reproduce by a simple process called binary fission, eukaryotes undergo a more involved method of division called mitosis. During mitosis, duplicated chromosomes are lined up along the cell's equator and split at the centromere to form two identical daughter nuclei.

> **Review Video: Eukaryotic and Prokaryotic**
> Visit mometrix.com/academy and enter code: 231438

CELL STRUCTURE

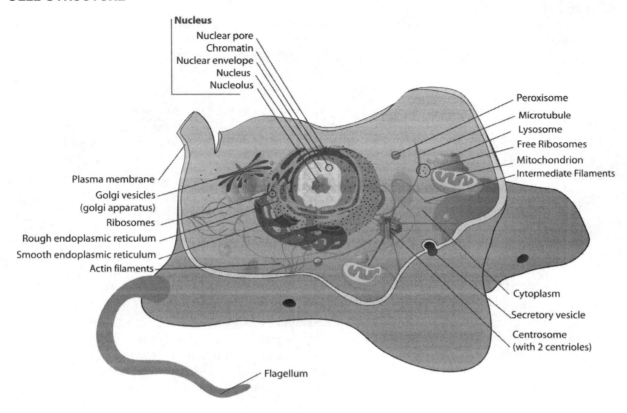

Ribosomes: Ribosomes are involved in *synthesizing proteins from amino acids*. They are numerous, making up about one quarter of the cell. Some cells contain thousands of ribosomes. Some are mobile and some are embedded in the rough **endoplasmic reticulum**.

Golgi complex (Golgi apparatus): This is involved in *synthesizing materials* such as proteins that are transported out of the cell. It is located near the nucleus and consists of layers of **membranes**.

Vacuoles: These are sacs used for *storage, digestion, and waste removal*. There is one large vacuole in plant cells. Animal cells have small, sometimes numerous vacuoles.

Vesicle: This is a small organelle within a cell. It has a membrane and performs varying functions, including *moving materials within a cell*.

Cytoskeleton: This consists of **microtubules** that help *shape and support the cell*.

Microtubules: These are part of the **cytoskeleton** and help *support the cell*. They are made of protein.

Cytosol: This is the *liquid material in the cell*. It is mostly water, but also contains some floating molecules.

Cytoplasm: This is a general term that refers to cytosol and the substructures (organelles) found *within the plasma membrane*, but not within the nucleus.

Cell membrane (plasma membrane): This defines the cell by acting as a *barrier*. It helps keeps cytoplasm in and substances located outside the cell out. It also determines what is allowed to enter and exit the cell.

Endoplasmic reticulum: The two types of endoplasmic reticulum are **rough** (has ribosomes on the surface) and **smooth** (does not have ribosomes on the surface). It is a tubular network that comprises the *transport system of a cell*. It is fused to the nuclear membrane and extends through the cytoplasm to the cell membrane.

Mitochondrion (pl. mitochondria): These cell structures vary in terms of size and quantity. Some cells may have one mitochondrion, while others have thousands. This structure performs various functions such as *generating ATP*, and is also involved in *cell growth and death*. Mitochondria contain their own DNA that is separate from that contained in the nucleus.

GOLGI APPARATUS: GENERAL STRUCTURE AND ROLE IN PACKAGING AND SECRETION

The **Golgi apparatus** consists of a series of curved, flattened sacs called cisternae. The cis face (the stack that is nearest to the ER) receives vesicles sent by the RER that contain immature proteins. The vesicles fuse with the membrane and release the proteins into the Golgi. The proteins then move from stack to stack, budding off a new vesicle which fuses with the next cisterna layer each time. During their travels, the proteins are modified by an assortment of Golgi enzymes. Proteins that were glycosylated in the ER may have some of their sugar residues removed, or more may be added. Sulfate and phosphate groups may be added as well. These "tags" influence the structure and function of the protein, and also aid in the sorting and delivery of these proteins to their destinations. The proteins are packaged into vesicles that bud from the trans face (or exit face) of the Golgi. Some of these proteins are secreted from the cell through exocytosis, while others become part of the cell membrane. Still others serve as hydrolytic enzymes inside lysosomes.

LYSOSOMES: MEMBRANE-BOUND VESICLES CONTAINING HYDROLYTIC ENZYMES

Lysosomes are organelles that function in the breakdown of various substances. They bud from the Golgi apparatus, and enclose hydrolytic enzymes that would damage the cell if not separated from the cytosol. These enzymes are active at a low pH of around 5, so hydrogen ions are pumped into the lysosome to maintain the acidic environment. Lysosomes play a vital role in cell homeostasis by dismantling various substrates and nonfunctioning intracellular components, and recycling them in a process called autophagy. Many of the substances destined for degradation are contained in a double-membrane vesicle called an autophagosome. Lysosomes can fuse with these (and with other vesicles created by endocytosis) releasing their enzymes and digesting the contents. Other substances can be transported into the lysosome directly by crossing the membrane. If enough lysosomes are damaged, the cell undergoes apoptosis, and in cases of severe damage, necrosis. Mutations of the hydrolases within the lysosomes are associated with a number of lysosomal storage diseases, including Tay Sachs.

CYTOSKELETON

GENERAL FUNCTION IN CELL SUPPORT AND MOVEMENT

The **cytoskeleton** is a membraneless structure found in all cell types, and it is made of various types of protein fibers. In eukaryotes, the cytoskeleton has three major components: microfilaments, intermediate fibers, and microtubules. While the cytoskeleton is known for its role in cell shape and structure, it is also involved in the movement of materials within the cell, and movement of the cell itself. The cytoskeleton is dynamic and can extend and retract, allowing cells to maintain their shape, or change shape as needed. The network of protein fibers stabilizes most of the organelles, and also provides a "railway" for motor proteins to use to direct vesicles to their destinations. Components of the cytoskeleton help anchor the cell to neighboring cells, and in some cases, form extensions such as cilia and flagella that aid in cell movement. Cell division would be impossible without the cytoskeleton, as it is used to separate sister chromatids, and also pinches the cell into daughter cells during cytokinesis.

MICROFILAMENTS: COMPOSITION AND ROLE IN CLEAVAGE AND CONTRACTILITY

Microfilaments are the thinnest components of the cytoskeleton, averaging about 6 to 8 nm in diameter. They are composed of protein molecules called actin that join together to form two rod-like polymers which twist around each other to form flexible tension-bearing filaments. These filaments organize into either bundles or networks, and they are involved in maintaining cell shape and events like cytokinesis, muscle contraction, and movement of the cell itself.

During cytokinesis, a cleavage furrow is formed through the contraction of microfilaments. These microfilaments are organized into a ring shape which decreases in size as they contract.

The cytoplasm is constricted until the original cell pinches into two daughter cells. Microfilaments are also involved in muscle contraction. The protein myosin binds to actin filaments forming myofibrils. The two components slide past each other as the cell contracts, and the muscle shortens. Microfilaments also aid in the gross movement of a cell by elongating the plus end (actin polymerization) while shortening the minus end (actin depolymerization).

MICROTUBULES: COMPOSITION AND ROLE IN SUPPORT AND TRANSPORT

Microtubules are the thickest components of the cytoskeleton (around 25 nm in diameter). They are made of a globular protein known as tubulin, which is a dimer made of α-tubulin and β-tubulin. These dimers stack upon each other to form linear rows called protofilaments, and 13 of these protofilaments arrange themselves in a ring to form a hollow tube. Microtubules can lengthen and shorten by polymerization and depolymerization of the tubulin dimers. They extend throughout the cell, helping the cell to resist compressional forces, while also providing a framework for motor proteins to travel on. Kinesins are motor proteins that tend to "walk" toward the plus end of the microtubule and dyneins travel toward the minus end. Many of these motor proteins carry vesicles to their destinations. Microtubules are also the major components of the mitotic spindle which segregates sister chromatids during mitosis. Cilia and flagella are also formed from microtubules which group together in nine pairs that surround a central pair.

INTERMEDIATE FILAMENTS, ROLE IN SUPPORT

Intermediate fibers are components of the cytoskeleton that (at around 10 nm in diameter) are thinner than microtubules but thicker than microfilaments. They are composed of many types of proteins (over fifty), and the types of proteins are specific to certain types of cells. For example, microfilaments made of keratin are found in epithelial cells, and microfilaments made of desmin are found in muscle cells. Lamins are proteins that form the microfilaments that line the inside portion of the nuclear envelope. Unlike their cytoskeletal counterparts, they are not polar, and they are not directly responsible for cell movement. They appear to only play a role in support. They help cells adhere to one another at cell junctions known as desmosomes, and also help to anchor the nucleus and other organelles. Intermediate filaments are specialized to withstand tensile forces, and thereby help to prevent cell distortion under mechanical stress. They do not polymerize and depolymerize the way that microtubules and microfilaments do.

COMPOSITION AND FUNCTION OF CILIA AND FLAGELLA

Both cilia and flagella are structures made of microtubules that extend from some types of cells. In eukaryotic cells, these microtubules are doubled up into pairs, and nine doublets form a ring around a central pair (the "9 + 2" arrangement). Each cilium and flagellum is about 0.25 μm in diameter, but flagella are usually much longer than cilia. Cilia are almost always found in high numbers, while cells rarely have more than a few flagella. Both structures are able to "wave" back and forth through the action of motor proteins called dyneins.

Some cells use cilia for locomotion while cells that are fixed within a tissue may use cilia to sweep materials along the surface. Ciliated cells of the respiratory tract move mucus out of the lungs, and cells of the female reproductive tract use cilia to mobilize the egg. Some cilia can even detect signals and transmit information to the inside of the cell. When cilia move, they do so in back-and-forth strokes, much like oars on a rowboat.

Flagella move differently; they are more whip-like with an undulating, beating pattern. Unlike cilia, they are only used for locomotion. Each human sperm uses a flagellum to move, and (like cilia) they can be found in many types of protists.

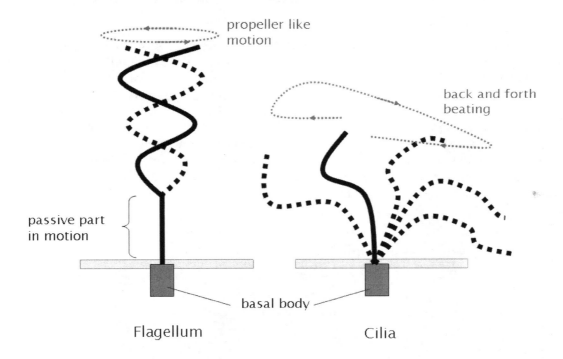

CENTRIOLES, MICROTUBULE ORGANIZING CENTERS

Centrioles are cylindrical structures that are formed from nine triplets of microtubules arranged in a circle around a hollow center. In animal cells, two perpendicular centrioles form an organelle called a **centrosome**. Other types of eukaryotic cells have simple centrosomes, but only animal cells use centrioles to organize their microtubules. Centrosomes are typically found near the nucleus, but they migrate to opposite poles of the cell during cell division. Microtubules extend from the centrioles as the plus ends grow toward the metaphase plate, forming the spindle fibers of the mitotic spindle. Polar fibers extend from one centrosome to the other, while kinetochore fibers attach to the chromosomes, pulling the sister chromatids apart during anaphase.

PLASMA MEMBRANE

GENERAL FUNCTION IN CELL CONTAINMENT

While the plasma membrane is involved in many functions (such as the regulation and transportation of materials, cell to cell recognition, and cell signaling), its most basic function is cell containment. The cell membrane is composed of a double layer of phospholipids that surrounds the cytoplasm of virtually all types of cells. The phospholipids form a fluid-like barrier that is reinforced by cholesterol and protein molecules. This barrier helps to contain the structures and molecules within the cell's interior, and also helps to maintain the desired concentrations of substances on either side of the membrane. Since the phospholipids orient themselves with their fatty acid chains pointed inward, the interior of the membrane is hydrophobic. This property causes the membrane to remain intact in its aqueous environment, while being somewhat impermeable to substances that are soluble in water (with the notable exception of nonpolar gases such as oxygen and carbon dioxide).

> **Review Video: Plasma Membrane**
> Visit mometrix.com/academy and enter code: 943095

PHOSPHOLIPIDS AND PHOSPHATIDS

A phospholipid consists of two nonpolar fatty acid chains bonded to a polar head made of glycerol, a phosphate group, and an organic R-group. (Phosphatids are the simplest phospholipids and lack the functional group on the phosphate.) Phospholipids are amphipathic, meaning that they have both hydrophilic (polar head) and hydrophobic (nonpolar tails) components. Because of this property, they arrange themselves into micelles or bilayers. A micelle is a small spherical structure made of a single layer of phospholipids with the tails pointed inward to form a hydrophobic core. They are used to transport lipid soluble materials. A bilayer is formed when the phospholipids assemble into parallel layers with the tails pointed in toward each other and the heads pointed out. Phospholipid bilayers surround liposomes and other vesicles, and also enclose the organelles in a eukaryotic cell. These bilayers also form cell membranes, which regulate the passage of materials into and out of all types of cells.

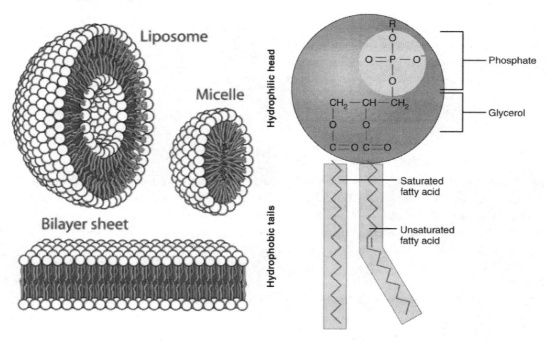

PROTEIN COMPONENTS

The proteins associated with the membrane enable most of the membrane's functions, such as the shuttling of various ions and molecules through the membrane, catalyzing reactions, joining of adjacent cells, cell signaling, cellular support and stability, and cell recognition. Some of these proteins penetrate into the hydrophobic interior of the membrane, and are called **integral** proteins. **Glycoproteins** are integral proteins with an attached sugar chain that aid in cell recognition. When integral proteins extend completely through the membrane, they are called **transmembrane** proteins, and these are often used as receptors for cell signaling. A signal molecule (like a hormone) will bind to the receptor from the extracellular side, and relay a message to the cytoplasmic side. Transmembrane proteins are also required for transport across the membrane. Some transport proteins (called **channel** proteins) have a tunnel-like conformation that allows materials to move passively, while others (**carrier** proteins) change conformation to move materials either by active or passive transport. **Peripheral proteins** are loosely bound to either side of the membrane, and often act as enzymes or receptor proteins. (Note that both of these can also be integral proteins).

OSMOSIS

Osmosis is the diffusion of water across a semipermeable membrane. The net movement of water is down its concentration gradient, meaning it will move from an area of higher water concentration to lower, or lower solute concentration to higher. Osmosis can help to restore balance when the solute cannot cross the membrane (or if it can't cross fast enough to maintain homeostasis). When the extracellular fluid has a higher solute concentration as compared to the cytoplasm, the fluid is described as **hypertonic**. Since there are fewer free water molecules surrounding the cell, the net flow of water will be *out* of the cell. When the extracellular fluid has a lower solute concentration as compared to the cytoplasm, the fluid is described as **hypotonic**. Since there are more free water molecules on the extracellular side of the membrane, the net flow of water will be *into* the cell, causing it to swell and in some cases burst. When the extracellular fluid has the same solute concentration as the cytoplasm, the fluid is described as **isotonic**, and water will move in and out of the cell at equal rates.

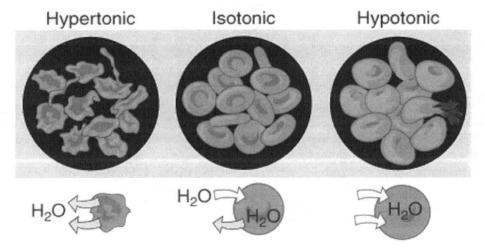

OSMOTIC PRESSURE

A **colligative property** is a property of a solution that depends only on the *amount* of solute, and not the size, mass, or chemical nature of the solute. Osmotic pressure, the minimum amount of pressure required to stop the diffusion of pure water across the membrane, is a colligative property because it is determined by the concentration of solute, as can be seen in the equation:

$$\pi = iMRT$$

- π = osmotic pressure (in atmospheres)
- i = van't Hoff factor (the number of particles formed from one unit of solute)
- M = molar concentration
- R = ideal gas constant
- T = temperature (in Kelvins)

If a vessel is divided into two chambers by a semipermeable membrane, and pure water placed into one chamber while a solution (such as sugar water) is placed in the other chamber, the water level will rise on the side of greater solute concentration. The diffusion of water will continue in this direction until the osmotic pressure becomes too great. The solute concentration will not have changed, but water will have moved from high to low water concentration.

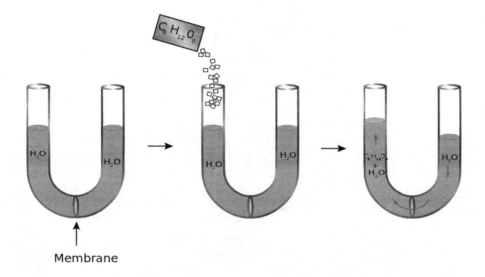

Membrane

PASSIVE TRANSPORT

Passive transport is the movement of substances across a cell membrane without the input of energy. Random motion of particles will lead to the net movement of substances down their concentration gradients in a spontaneous process that leads to an increase in entropy. Simple diffusion, osmosis, and facilitated diffusion are all forms of passive transport. In simple diffusion, substances cross the membrane directly, without the aid of a transport protein. Small, nonpolar molecules such as oxygen gas, carbon dioxide, and uncharged lipids are not repelled by the hydrophobic interior of the membrane.

Osmosis is the passive transport of water across the membrane. Most polar molecules cannot use simple diffusion, but water molecules are small enough to slowly squeeze between the phospholipids. Water can also use channel proteins called aquaporins to increase the rate of osmosis. When proteins are used to transport substances down their concentration gradients, this is called **facilitated diffusion**. Large, polar, and/or charged substances require shielding from the interior of the membrane, and they may use channel or carrier proteins to assist in their transport. None of these processes require ATP, and are driven by the difference in solute concentration.

ACTIVE TRANSPORT

In **active transport**, energy is used to move solutes into or out of the cell. In most forms of active transport, substances are pumped against their concentration gradients from areas of low to high concentration. Active transport is required for processes such as the maintenance of a membrane potential, and the uptake of glucose by intestinal cells even between meals. In **primary active transport**, the pumping of solutes by a carrier protein is directly coupled to the hydrolysis of ATP. In this process, the binding of a phosphate group causes a conformational change in the protein, allowing it to transport solutes across the membrane. **Secondary active transport** relies on ATP to generate an electrochemical gradient, and it is this gradient that directly drives the active transport of a different solute. As one solute moves down its gradient, another is pumped up its gradient. When both solutes move in the same direction, it is called **symport**, and when they move in opposite directions, it is called **antiport**.

Endocytosis and **exocytosis** are types of active transport that employ vesicles to import or export substances. While these processes require ATP, they do not necessarily move solutes up their concentration gradients.

MEMBRANE CHANNELS

Membrane channels belong to a class of transport proteins that form pores to allow the passage of small, charged particles. They are specific to the solutes they transport, and act as a sort of tunnel for particles of a certain size and charge. All channels move substances down their concentration gradient by facilitated diffusion, and therefore do not require energy. Unlike carrier proteins, channels interact very weakly with the solutes they transport, allowing them to move rapidly across the membrane. Channel proteins that allow the passage of water are called aquaporins, and they are always open. Without them, osmosis would occur too slowly to accommodate the needs of the cell. Ion channels, on the other hand, are usually gated; they open and close in response to various stimuli. Voltage-gated channels respond to changes in membrane potential. These types of ion channels are vital to generating electrical impulses in nerve and cardiac cells. Ligand-gated ion channels open in response to the binding of a ligand, such as a hormone or neurotransmitter. Mechanically-gated ion channels respond to a physical stimulus, such as the stretching of the membrane, and are useful in sensory tissues.

EXOCYTOSIS AND ENDOCYTOSIS

Endocytosis and exocytosis are types of vesicular transport that are used for the transport of very large particles, or bulk quantities of smaller particles. Both processes are examples of active transport because the transportation and pinching off of vesicles requires energy. (Note that particles are not necessarily moving up their concentration gradients as in other forms of active transport.) During **exocytosis**, cellular products and wastes are transported via vesicle to the cell membrane where the vesicle fuses, releasing its contents into the extracellular environment. Exocytosis is also the means by which certain membrane components (such as glycoproteins and glycolipids) become incorporated into the cell membrane. **Endocytosis** involves the ingestion of fluid, large particles, or target molecules. During this process the cell membrane folds inward, engulfing the material and pinching off into a vesicle. The ingestion of fluids is called **pinocytosis**, and it is non-specific, meaning it takes in any enzymes and nutrients that happen to be available. **Phagocytosis** is the engulfing of particles, sometimes even entire cells. Immune system cells ingest harmful bacteria by phagocytosis before destroying them. **Receptor-mediated endocytosis** is a form of endocytosis that targets certain molecules (such as LDLs, or low-density lipoproteins) that are in low concentration outside the cell. These molecules bind to receptors on the cell membrane, which then invaginates to form a vesicle.

Endocytosis

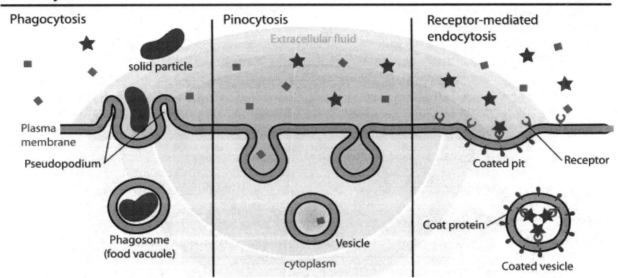

ENDOPLASMIC RETICULUM

ROUGH AND SMOOTH COMPONENTS

Both the rough and smooth endoplasmic reticulum consist of a series of continuous membranes called cisternae, but each type of ER differs in both in structure and function.

The **rough ER** is continuous with the nuclear envelope, and its ribosome-studded cisternae have the appearance of flattened sacs. The ribosomes synthesize polypeptides which are then guided into the lumen of the rough ER before being modified, packaged in a vesicle, and sent to different regions within the cell, often the Golgi apparatus. The Golgi can then further modify the proteins and sort them based on their destinations. Many are shipped out of the cell via exocytosis.

The cisternae of the **smooth ER** are more tubular in shape than the rough ER, and they lack ribosomes. These membranes are continuous with the rough ER and the nucleus. Smooth ER is involved in many tasks, including the synthesis of lipids such as phospholipids and cholesterol. The smooth ER of liver cells detoxifies drugs, and the smooth ER of the muscles regulates and stores calcium ions.

ROUGH ENDOPLASMIC RETICULUM SITE OF RIBOSOMES

Secretory proteins (proteins destined to be exported from the cell) and proteins that are associated with the plasma membrane are synthesized on ribosomes that are bound to the cytoplasmic side of the rough endoplasmic reticulum. These ribosomes are not permanently fixed, and will bind to sites called translocons. Ribosomes that are free in the cytosol are very similar in structure to bound ribosomes, but the proteins they produce remain in the cytosol of the cell. As a polypeptide chain is growing out of a bound ribosome during translation, the chain is fed through a tiny pore into the lumen of the rough ER, where it folds into its proper conformation. Any proteins that do not fold properly into their native shape are recycled. Enzymes in the lumen may modify proteins by covalently bonding a carbohydrate to form a glycoprotein. (The Golgi continues the posttranslational modification of proteins.) Proteins that are shipped to other parts of the cell are first packaged into transport vesicles, and the vesicle will fuse with its target.

MEMBRANE STRUCTURE

The **endoplasmic reticulum** constitutes roughly half of all the plasma membrane in a cell. The membrane system of the rough ER is connected to the outer nuclear membrane, forming flattened sacs (cisternae) that connect to each other in a manner that resembles a multi-story parking garage. These helicoidal sheets are called **Terasaki ramps**. Newly synthesized proteins are packaged in transport vesicles that are coated with protein complexes that help direct each vesicle to its destination. (COPII coating proteins, for example, coat vesicles that fuse with the cis face of the Golgi apparatus.) These vesicles bud from a region of the ER known as transitional ER, where there are few ribosomes. The smooth ER lacks ribosomes altogether, and has a branched tubular structure. Some of these tubules fuse with one another.

MITOCHONDRIA

Mitochondria are described as the "powerhouses" of the cell because they produce most of a cell's ATP. They have two membranes: the outer membrane, which acts a selective barrier, and the inner membrane where most of the ATP is made. The inner membrane is folded into structures called cristae, and it is within these folds that the electron transport chain of aerobic respiration is located. Between the membranes is the intermembrane space where a proton motive force is used to drive **chemiosmosis**: the synthesis of ATP. The protons that are pumped across the intermembrane space during oxidative phosphorylation re-enter the mitochondrial matrix (the interior of the mitochondrion) through the protein ATP synthase, which is located in the inner membrane. The movement of the protons powers ATP synthase, allowing it to phosphorylate ADP. Inside the matrix are ribosomes and mitochondrial DNA. This DNA carries 37 genes (in humans) that are required for normal mitochondrion function. Mitochondria also play a role in apoptosis, or programmed cell death. Proteins associated with the inner mitochondrial membrane move into the cytoplasm in response to oxidative stress and activate other proteins that begin the degradation of the cell.

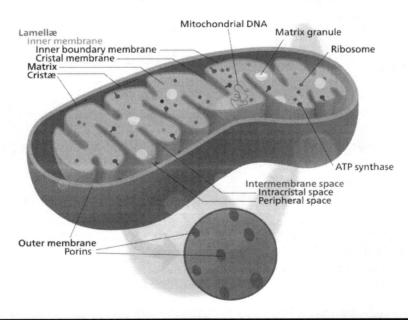

Review Video: Mitochondria
Visit mometrix.com/academy and enter code: 444287

SELF-REPLICATION

Mitochondria are described as semi-autonomous because each one has its own genome and ribosomes, and produces many of its own proteins. They also replicate in a manner similar to that of bacteria; they copy their circular DNA molecules before undergoing fission. However, mitochondria do rely on nuclear genes to produce many of the proteins required for DNA replication and other processes. These proteins are imported from the cytosol.

While the mitochondria are not fully autonomous, it is likely that they evolved from an autonomous heterotrophic prokaryote that established a symbiotic relationship with an ancestral host cell. It was probably engulfed by the host cell (hence the double membrane) and provided that cell with ATP. (This is known as the endosymbiont theory.) Its similarity to bacteria, both in structure and manner of reproduction, suggests that mitochondria were once free-living prokaryotes.

NUCLEAR PARTS OF A CELL

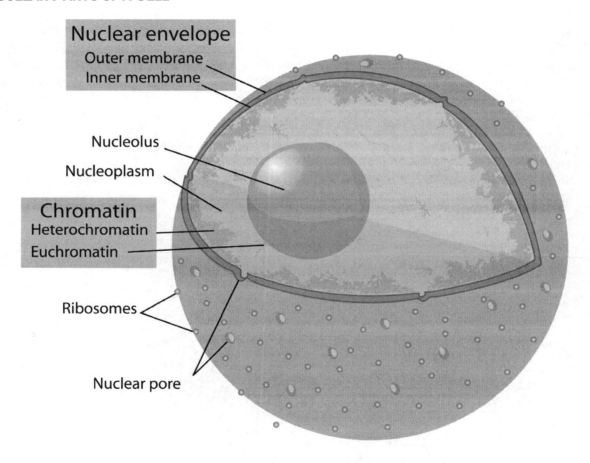

Nucleus (pl. nuclei): This is a small structure that contains the **chromosomes** and regulates the **DNA** of a cell. The nucleus is the defining structure of **eukaryotic cells**, and all eukaryotic cells have a nucleus. The nucleus is responsible for the passing on of genetic traits between generations. The nucleus contains a *nuclear envelope, nucleoplasm, a nucleolus, nuclear pores, chromatin, and ribosomes.*

Chromosomes: These are highly condensed, threadlike rods of **DNA**. Short for **deoxyribonucleic acid**, DNA is the genetic material that *stores information about the plant or animal.*

Chromatin: This consists of the DNA and protein that make up **chromosomes**.

Nucleolus: This structure contained within the nucleus consists of protein. It is small, round, does not have a membrane, is involved in **protein synthesis**, and synthesizes and stores **RNA** (**ribonucleic acid**).

Nuclear envelope: This encloses the structures of the nucleus. It consists of inner and outer membranes made of **lipids**.

Nuclear pores: These are involved in the exchange of material between the nucleus and the **cytoplasm**.

Nucleoplasm: This is the liquid within the nucleus, and is similar to cytoplasm.

COMPARTMENTALIZATION, STORAGE OF GENETIC INFORMATION

The **nucleus** stores most of a cell's genetic information. (DNA is also found in mitochondria and chloroplasts.) Nuclear DNA is enclosed by the nuclear envelope: a double membrane that is perforated with pores. These pores are made of large protein complexes that regulate the passage of materials including RNA, ribosomal subunits, proteins, ions, and signaling molecules. Enclosed in the double membrane is the nucleoplasm (a semifluid), chromatin (DNA and associated histone proteins), and a non-membranous nucleolus which produces the ribosomal subunits. The inner nuclear membrane is covered by a mesh of protein filaments called the nuclear lamina which stabilizes the nucleus while regulating events such as DNA replication and cell division. The outer membrane is continuous with the endoplasmic reticulum.

The nucleus is responsible for the storage of DNA, and is also the site of DNA replication and transcription (the synthesis of RNA). Since gene expression is regulated largely at the level of transcription, the nucleus plays an important role in coordinating the activities of the cell.

NUCLEOLUS: LOCATION AND FUNCTION

The **nucleolus** is the largest structure inside the nucleus, and it is responsible for producing ribosomal subunits. It has no membrane, and is made of three regions: two thread-like fibrillar components and one granular component. The fibrillar center (FC) is where the ribosomal RNA genes are located and transcribed. The dense fibrillar center (DFC) processes the pre-rRNA, and the immature ribosomal subunits are assembled in the granular component (GC). All rRNA is synthesized in the nucleolus except the 5S-rRNA which is made in the nucleoplasm before being incorporated into ribosomal subunits. The subunits are exported from the nucleus through the nuclear pores.

The nucleolus disappears early in mitosis (prophase) and reappears in the final stage (telophase). However, it first appears as ten small units at various chromosome sites called nucleolus organizer regions (NORs) before aggregating into one structure.

NUCLEAR ENVELOPE, NUCLEAR PORES

The **nuclear envelope** is the double membrane that encloses the nucleus, separating the nucleoplasm from the cytoplasm of the cell. There is a 20–40 nm gap between the two phospholipid bilayers called the perinuclear space, and the membranes are joined at the nuclear pores. Each pore is an octagonal aqueous channel made of hundreds of proteins called nucleoporins. These proteins interact with transporter proteins called karyopherins, which shuttle large molecules like RNA and certain proteins back and forth between the nucleus and the cytoplasm. Smaller molecules and ions are able to diffuse through the pore complex without the aid of a transporter. The pores are essential for the import of the enzymes and nucleotides that are required for DNA synthesis and transcription, and the export of mRNA, tRNA, and ribosomal subunits that are required for translation.

The outer membrane of the nuclear envelope is continuous with the endoplasmic reticulum (ER), and the lumen (inner space) of the ER is open to the perinuclear space. This allows for the easy exchange of materials between the two organelles. The nucleoplasmic side of the inner membrane is lined with a network of protein filaments called the nuclear lamina which supports the nucleus, while aiding in the organization of chromatin.

MITOSIS

Mitosis is the stage of the cell cycle in which the nucleus divides. It alternates with a much longer stage called interphase in which the cell performs its normal functions and prepares for division by copying organelles and duplicating chromosomes. If the cell passes the two major regulatory checkpoints of interphase, it proceeds through the four phases of mitosis, as summarized in the table below (though there will be one last checkpoint prior to anaphase). Mitosis is usually followed by cytokinesis, division of the cytoplasm, and results in two genetically identical daughter cells with the same number of chromosomes as the parent cell.

Phase	Description
Prophase	Chromatin condenses into chromosomes The nucleolus and nuclear membrane break down The mitotic spindle begins to form
Metaphase	The spindle aligns the chromosomes along the metaphase plate
Anaphase	Sister chromatids are split at the centromere and pulled toward opposite poles
Telophase	Chromosomes uncoil A nuclear membrane forms around each set of chromosomes A nucleolus forms in each new nucleus The mitotic spindle breaks down Cytokinesis begins (it may also begin during anaphase)

Review Video: Mitosis
Visit mometrix.com/academy and enter code: 849894

At the onset of prophase, chromatin coils tightly into discrete chromosomes that are visible under a light microscope. The chromosomes resemble the shape of an "X", with identical DNA in each sister chromatid. The sister chromatids are bound together along their entire length by protein complexes called cohesins, but by metaphase all cohesins are broken down, except those found at the centromere. As the chromatin condenses, the nuclear envelope begins to disintegrate and the nucleolus disappears. Centrosomes, the microtubule organizing centers of the cell, migrate towards opposite poles of the cell as microtubules polymerize outward. This begins the formation of the mitotic spindle, which continues until metaphase. Protein-based structures called kinetochores form at the centromere to serve as an attachment point for the kinetochore fibers (microtubules) of the spindle. As the kinetochore microtubules attach to each chromosome at the centromere, other microtubules called polar fibers overlap at the center of the cell, never interacting with the chromosomes. By the end of prophase, the nuclear envelope has completely dissolved. This tends to be the longest stage of mitosis.

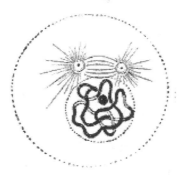

During metaphase, the centrosomes are at opposite poles of the cell, and chromosomes are positioned along an imaginary line between the two centrosomes known as the metaphase plate (sometimes called the spindle equator or equatorial plate). The kinetochore fibers lengthen or shorten as needed to line up the chromosomes, and the movement is assisted by forces exerted by motor proteins. Polar fibers continue to grow until they are sufficiently overlapped in preparation for the next stage of mitosis. Anaphase will only follow metaphase if the chromosomes are properly aligned, and every kinetochore on every sister chromatid is attached to a kinetochore fiber. Metaphase is usually shorter than prophase.

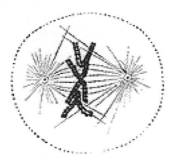

Chromosomes are at their most condensed form during anaphase. The stage begins when an enzyme known as separin cleaves the cohesins that hold sister chromatids together. The kinetochore fibers shorten as a result of depolymerization, splitting the centromeres and pulling the liberated chromosomes toward the centrosomes. As they are dragged through the cytosol, the linear chromosomes bend into a "V" shape as they trail behind the centromere. Meanwhile, the overlapping polar fibers push away from each other, causing the cell to elongate. There is now a complete set of chromosomes at each end of the cell.

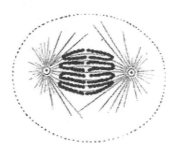

As liberated chromosomes arrive at the poles of the cell, a new nuclear membrane is formed around each group. The polar fibers continue to elongate the cell as the chromosomes uncoil and the nucleoli reform. The microtubules of the spindle are depolymerized and disappear. Cytokinesis begins during either telophase or late anaphase. A cleavage furrow forms near the site of the metaphase plate as a contractile ring of microfilaments beneath the plasma membrane begins to constrict the cell. This will continue after telophase, pinching the parent cell into two identical daughter cells.

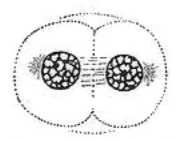

PHASES OF CELL CYCLE: G0, G1, S, G2, M

The **cell cycle** can be described as the life of a cell, beginning with the formation of the cell, and ending with its own division. The phases of the cycle are G_1 (first gap), S (synthesis), G_2 (second gap) and M (the mitotic phase). Many cells, however, enter a non-growing G_0 state in which the cell performs its job but does not divide. This may happen for a number of reasons, and it is not always reversible. Cells that are deficient in nutrients or growth factors may be blocked from proceeding to the S phase, and only called back to the cycle when favorable conditions are restored. Mature liver cells and many adult stem cells exist in a reversible **quiescent** state, and only divide in response to stimuli such as tissue damage. Some cells leave the cell cycle permanently. A cell with damaged DNA, for example, is likely to enter an irreversible state of **senescence**. This allows the cell to avoid apoptosis (programmed cell death), but it will remain in G_0 indefinitely. Other highly differentiated cells such as nerve and cardiac muscle cells permanently leave the cell cycle because they are genetically programmed to do so.

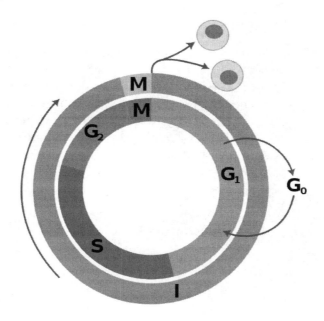

The G_1 (first gap) phase of the cell cycle is the first part of interphase, and it begins immediately after cell division. During this stage, the volume of the cell increases, and the metabolic activities that were inhibited during mitosis are accelerated. The cell begins the task of copying its organelles, synthesizing mRNA, tRNA, and rRNA, and producing the enzymes required for DNA replication, all while continuing to perform its given function. The time duration of this phase varies greatly, but it tends to be the longest phase of the cell cycle, averaging 6-12 hours. Some cells remain in this phase for years. Before the cell is allowed to proceed to the S phase, it is inspected at the G_1 checkpoint. It "passes" if it has grown enough and has sufficient nutrients and growth factors, and the DNA is not damaged. If it "fails" it enters the G_0 phase.

The S (synthesis) phase of the cell cycle falls between G_1 and G_2 of interphase. During this time (which averages 6–8 hours) each molecule of DNA is replicated, doubling the genetic content from 2n to 4n. Note that this does *not* change the ploidy of the cell; the chromosome number remains at 46. Helicases separate the two complementary strands of DNA at multiple sites along each molecule, and DNA polymerases add nucleotides at a rate of about 50 nucleotides per second. By the end of the S phase, there is an identical copy of each DNA molecule, ensuring that each daughter cell that is created during the M phase will have a complete genome. Centrosomes are duplicated during this stage as well, while transcription and protein synthesis are inhibited.

The G_2 (second gap) phase follows DNA replication, and is the final part of interphase. It is characterized by roughly 3–4 hours of cell growth, continued replication of organelles, and protein synthesis. The centrosomes that were duplicated during the S phase begin to mature, as microtubules become more organized and the centrioles elongate. As it prepares for mitosis, the cell performs its usual metabolic functions-but before the cell is allowed to divide, it must pass inspection at the G_2 checkpoint. If any errors are detected in the duplicated chromosomes, the cell cycle is arrested until the DNA can be repaired. Cells that are significantly and irreparably damaged will either enter a state of senescence, or be eliminated through programmed cell death.

Mitosis (nuclear division) and cytokinesis (cytoplasmic division) together make up the M phase of the cell cycle. There is no growth during this phase, and normal metabolic functioning is inhibited to devote the cell's resources to the division process. During mitosis, the chromosomes condense (prophase), align along the metaphase plate (metaphase), split at the centromere and segregate (anaphase), and uncoil as a new nuclear membrane is built around each full set (telophase). Cytokinesis overlaps with the final stages of mitosis.

In animal cells, cytokinesis results from the formation of a contractile ring of actin and non-muscle myosin II filaments. This ring forms around the equator of the cell, directly beneath the plasma membrane, and parallel to the metaphase plate. Myosin is a motor protein that uses ATP to move the actin filaments, causing the ring to contract like a drawstring. As this is happening, vesicles from inside the cell fuse along the cleavage furrow to form a plasma membrane. The two cells become physically separated in a process called abscission. The M phase is the shortest phase of the cell cycle, averaging 1–2 hours.

GROWTH ARREST

Cell growth can be halted in response to signals from both inside and outside the cell. For example, most cells require anchorage to neighboring cells or substrates to proliferate. Cells that exhibit anchorage dependence usually exhibit density-dependent inhibition as well. As they become crowded, the physical constraints may stop the cells from growing. Crowding may also activate signal transduction pathways that arrest cells at certain points in the cell cycle. Growth arrest may also occur in conditions of oxidative stress, infection, or depleted levels of nutrients and/or growth factors. (Growth factors are proteins that stimulate cell growth.) Finally, any cells with damaged or incompletely replicated DNA, or chromosomes that are not properly aligned along the midline of the cell during mitosis, are arrested before they divide by checkpoint proteins. If the problem can be corrected, the cell will be allowed to progress. Cells that are too damaged will either remain in an arrested state permanently, or undergo apoptosis.

REPRODUCTIVE SYSTEM

Gametogenesis is the process by which diploid germ cells give rise to haploid gametes (sex cells). Germ cells are produced in the early stages of embryogenesis, and migrate from the primitive streak to the gonads where they later undergo meiosis. Germ cells are distinguished from somatic cells because they can undergo both mitosis and meiosis. All other cells are restricted to mitosis, and have no potential to produce gametes. Mitosis is a single division that results in two identical cells, each with the same number of chromosomes as the parent cell. In meiosis, a germ cell undergoes two rounds of cell division (meiosis I and meiosis II). During meiosis I, homologous pairs of chromosomes exchange portions of their DNA before they are separated and distributed independently to daughter cells. These events ensure that the daughter cells are genetically unique, and the chromosome number is cut in half. The steps of meiosis II are similar to those of mitosis, and result in four haploid cells. These cells differentiate to give rise to the mature gametes that fuse during fertilization, restoring the diploid number. The production of ova and sperm is more specifically called oogenesis and spermatogenesis, respectively.

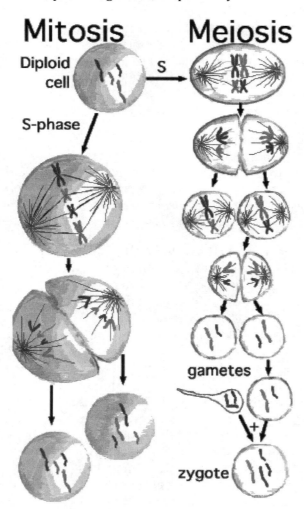

A sperm cell is the smallest of human cells, measuring about 0.05 mm in length. It has three distinct sections: the head, midpiece, and tail; its streamlined form is well suited to its function. The head contains centrioles and a compacted nucleus with tightly coiled DNA. The anterior surface of the head is capped with the **acrosome**, *a* Golgi-derived structure that is packed with enzymes that assist in the penetration of the zona pellucida, and is therefore essential for fertilization. Between 50 and 100 mitochondria spiral around the midpiece, which is the only part of the sperm that contains any mitochondria. The ATP produced by the mitochondria powers the sliding motion of the microtubules within the tail, or **flagellum**, of the sperm, which in turn causes it to undulate. The microtubule-based core of the flagellum is called the **axoneme**, and consists of nine doublets of microtubules arranged around a central pair.

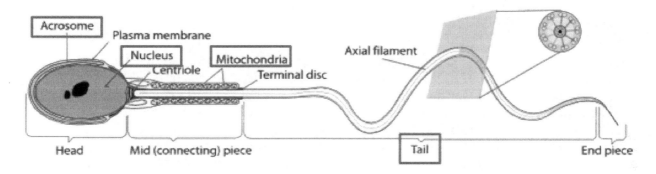

RELATIVE CONTRIBUTION TO NEXT GENERATION

When an oocyte undergoes meiosis and cytokinesis, the cytoplasm divides unequally to produce one large viable ovum. This ensures that nearly all of the resources that are required for the survival of a zygote are present. The ooplasm of the egg contains an abundance of nutrients that will sustain the zygote, and later the daughter cells (blastomeres) that are produced by mitosis. All of the molecules (enzymes, RNA) needed for protein synthesis are present as well. It also contains the organelles, with the exception of the centrioles, which are degraded during oogenesis. These structures are instead donated by the sperm cell. Sperm cells do contain mitochondria, but they are left behind when the midpiece and tail are released from the head during fertilization. Any paternal mitochondria that manage to enter the egg are quickly destroyed, leaving only maternal mitochondria. Each gamete contributes 22 autosomes (non-sex chromosomes) and one sex chromosome to the zygote. The egg always contributes an X chromosome, and the sperm contributes either an X or a Y chromosome.

REPRODUCTIVE SEQUENCE: FERTILIZATION; IMPLANTATION; DEVELOPMENT; BIRTH

Fertilization usually occurs in the fallopian tube within 24 hours of ovulation. Of the hundreds of millions of sperm that are ejaculated, an average of 200 reach the secondary oocyte. When a sperm makes contact with the oocyte, it burrows through the corona radiata and binds to receptor proteins in the zona pellucida. The acrosome releases enzymes that allow the sperm to pass through the zona pellucida to the membrane of the oocyte. Here, actin filaments extend from the sperm to form a tubular structure called the acrosomal apparatus through which its pronucleus is passed. (The midpiece and tail are left behind.) Entry of the pronucleus stimulates the cortical reaction; enzymes from cortical granules beneath the membrane of the oocyte diffuse into the zona pellucida, causing it to harden, and preventing fertilization by more than one sperm. Another block to polyspermy is the depolarization of the oocyte membrane that occurs in response to calcium ions that are released when the sperm meets the membrane. The oocyte then divides unequally by meiosis II to produce an ovum and a nonviable polar body. The pronucleus of the sperm fuses with the pronucleus of the ovum, and a zygote (fertilized egg) is formed.

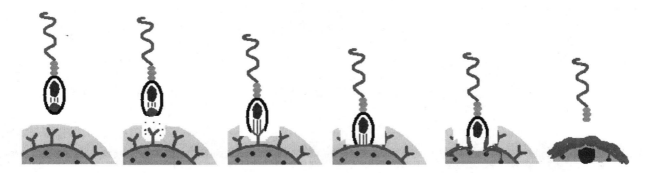

After fertilization, the zygote develops into a cluster of cells called a **morula**. The morula is pushed from the fallopian tube to the uterine cavity by peristalsis (muscle contractions) and the wave-like motions of cilia. It floats freely in the uterus for around 3 days, using uterine secretions as nourishment. The cells of the morula begin to differentiate and give rise to a blastocyst with a fluid-filled cavity and two types of cells. The inner cell mass will give rise to the embryo, and the outer trophoblasts develop into the placenta. Degeneration of the zona pellucida, followed by "zona hatching", occurs around six days after fertilization in preparation for implantation. As this transformation happens, the blastocyst secretes human chorionic gonadotropin (hCG) which stimulates the production of other hormones. These hormones help to maintain the corpus luteum (preventing menses) and prepare the endometrium for implantation. About one week after ovulation, the blastocyst (now over 200 cells) attaches to the endometrium, and outer cells of the trophoblast fuse to form large multinucleated syncytiotrophoblasts that extend like fingers (called chorionic villi) into the endometrium. Fetal blood vessels form inside these villi. About two weeks after fertilization, the blastocyst is fully implanted, and the endometrium is now called the decidua (the maternal contribution to the placenta).

During the pre-embryonic stage of development, the zygote undergoes **cleavage**, dividing mitotically to form a morula. The morula continues to divide and differentiate into a fluid-filled blastocyst. The blastocyst implants in the uterine wall, and the embryonic stage of development commences. During **gastrulation**, the cells of the embryo are reorganized to form the embryonic germ layers (ectoderm, mesoderm, and endoderm) that will produce the tissues and organs of the embryo. A neural plate derived from the ectoderm invades the mesoderm to form the neural tube in a process called **neurulation**. **Organogenesis** continues with the development of a rudimentary heart that beats at around the third week. The digestive system and other internal organs form, as well as the placenta and umbilical cord. By the end of eight weeks, the organ systems have formed and the embryo is now a fetus. During the fetal stage, development continues with the differentiation of the reproductive organs, coordinated movements of limbs, ossification of bones, and an increase of subcutaneous fat. Birth normally occurs around 40 weeks post fertilization.

The fetus must adapt quickly as it transitions from an intrauterine environment to an extrauterine environment. This transition is facilitated by hormones, notably cortisol and catecholamines. Before birth, the neonate relies on oxygen from the mother's blood, and its lungs are collapsed and fluid-filled. As labor approaches, the secretion of fluid from the fetal lungs decreases, while reabsorption increases. At birth, the lungs fill with air and the rest of the fluid leaves the lungs. This first breath triggers critical circulatory changes. Pulmonary resistance decreases, pulmonary blood flow increases, and the shunts that cause the blood to bypass the lungs and liver close or constrict. (The

foramen ovale that bypasses the lungs closes at first breath. The **ductus arteriosus**, which also bypasses the lungs, and the **ductus venosus** that bypasses the liver, both constrict at birth and close soon after.) The neonate will no longer receive nourishment from the placenta, and will rely on mother's milk and stores of glycogen in the liver. The neonate must also expend energy to keep warm, and so increases its metabolic rate through muscle movements and the burning of brown fat.

TISSUES FORMED FROM EUKARYOTIC CELLS

EPITHELIAL CELLS

Epithelial cells come in a variety of shapes and functions, but they share the characteristic of being avascular. They are nourished by the diffusion of oxygen and nutrients from capillaries in the underlying layer of connective tissue called the basement membrane. Epithelial tissues are the lining and covering tissues of the body, and depending on their location may be involved in protection, absorption, secretion, and/or filtration. These tissues are classified according to the shape and arrangement of their cells:

	Description	Name
Cell Shape	flattened, scale-like	Squamous
	cube-shaped	Cuboidal
	long, thin	Columnar
Arrangement	single layer of cells	Simple epithelia
	appearance of multiple layers as a result of differences in cell shape and location	Pseudostratified
	multiple layers of cells	Stratified epithelia

There are **many** types of epithelial tissues in the body. Stratified squamous epithelial tissues are found in locations that experience friction, such as the mouth, esophagus, and exterior skin. Simple columnar epithelia line the digestive tract, and harbor mucus-producing goblet cells. Simple squamous epithelia form membranes where filtration or diffusion occurs, such as the alveoli of the lungs. These are merely a few examples.

CONNECTIVE TISSUE CELLS

Connective tissues are the most abundant tissues in the body. Most connective tissues are highly vascular, the exceptions being ligaments, tendons, and cartilage. In general, they support and protect the body, and are characterized by the presence of a nonliving matrix. This matrix is secreted by the cells of the connective tissue and it consists of ground substance (water, proteins, and carbohydrates) and protein fibers such as collagen, elastin, or reticular fibers. The consistency of these connective tissues varies greatly from one tissue type to another. Blood is a connective tissue made of blood cells and plasma, and it transports oxygen, carbon dioxide, nutrients, and wastes. Adipose tissue is made of fat cells that cushion and insulate the body. Osseous tissue, or bone, consists of osteocytes surrounded by a hard matrix of calcium salts and collagen. Cartilage, like bone, is a connective tissue that provides support, but it is made of cells called chondrocytes, and is more flexible. Ligaments and tendons are made of dense fibrous connective tissue, which is made mostly of collagen fibers.

MECHANISMS OF DEVELOPMENT

CELL–CELL COMMUNICATION IN DEVELOPMENT

Cell-cell communication is crucial for the proper development of an embryo. When cells are "competent" they are able to receive signals from adjacent or nearby cells, inducing them to become a certain type of cell. (Competence is not a permanent state, and may change during the course of development.) A developing cell may also secrete inducing factors of its own. Cells that secrete signal molecules are called **inducers**, and cells that differentiate in response to those signals are called **responders**. Most of these signals are growth factors that only act on cells of a specific tissue. **Autocrine** signals are self-generated; they act on the same cell that secreted them. **Paracrine** signals diffuse to cells in close proximity. **Endocrine** signals enter the blood and travel to distant tissues. **Juxtacrine** signals require direct contact between cells. When the contact is made, signals from one cell bind to the receptors of another. Sometimes, two different tissues respond to each other's signals, promoting differentiation in each other. This is called reciprocal induction.

CELL MIGRATION

Cell migration is required for normal embryonic development; it begins during gastrulation and continues throughout life. Any errors in the migration pathway can lead to malformations, diseases, or even demise of the embryo. Migration is initiated by signaling molecules that trigger the detachment of cells from their substrate. The cell polarizes to define a leading edge, while actin filaments of the cytoskeleton polymerize to push the cell forward in a crawling motion. Rearrangement of the cytoskeleton forms flat, sheet-like projections called **lamellipodia** at the leading edge. Sometimes, finger-like projections called **filopodia** extend beyond the lamellipodia in the direction of motion. Contraction of the cell occurs when actin interacts with myosin. Chemical messengers continually influence the direction and rate of motion, ensuring that cells reach the intended site in the body at the right time. Some cells migrate individually, while others (such as epithelial and mesenchymal cells) migrate collectively.

PLURIPOTENCY: STEM CELLS

Potency describes the ability of a cell to differentiate. Only totipotent cells (the zygote and cells that arise after the first few divisions) have complete potency, but pluripotent stem cells still have great differentiation potential. They can develop into any cell type, with the exception of placental cells. As the zygote and subsequent blastomeres undergo cleavage, the once totipotent cells give rise to two lineages: the cells of the trophoblast, and the embryonic stem cells that give rise to the primary germ layers (the ectoderm, mesoderm, and endoderm). All of the hundreds of types of human cells stem from these germ layers - however, pluripotent cells cannot form an entire organism because they can't produce the needed placental tissues.

Because of the malleability of pluripotent cells, they can used therapeutically in the treatment of various diseases. Researchers have identified ways to reprogram somatic cells in a way that reverses the differentiation process. These induced pluripotent stem cells, or iPS cells, provide an alternative to the harvesting of stem cells from an embryo.

GENE REGULATION IN DEVELOPMENT

Differential gene expression is the mechanism for cell specialization and ultimately the development of an organism. Many factors collectively determine which genes are expressed and *when* they are expressed. In cell-cell communication, target cells detect and respond to signals (such as growth factors) released by other cells. When a signaling molecule binds to a membrane receptor, it causes a conformational change in the receptor. The signal transduction pathway continues with the phosphorylation of cytoplasmic proteins, which leads to the activation of transcription factors. Transcription factors bind to DNA and either promote or suppress gene expression.

Other strategies exist to regulate gene expression as well. **Epigenetic regulation** involves the methylation of DNA and modification of the histone proteins that it wraps around. These heritable modifications alter the structure of the chromosome. (Regions of DNA that are more condensed are less accessible to RNA polymerase.)

Regulation continues beyond the level of transcription. For example, coding regions (exons) of messenger RNA can be spliced together in different orders to produce different proteins from the same transcript. The proteins that are produced during translation may also require activation at a later time.

PROGRAMMED CELL DEATH

Programmed cell death, or apoptosis, is an important part of embryonic development. It is induced by signals that activate proteases called caspases. Caspases cleave certain cytoplasmic proteins, setting a series of events in motion. The cell shrinks and loses its anchorage to adjacent cells. Chromatin condenses as the cell membrane bulges out into protrusions called blebs. The DNA and organelles are broken down into fragments, and the blebs break free of the cell, taking a portion of the cytoplasm with them. The blebs, now called apoptotic bodies, are engulfed and digested by phagocytic cells. No intracellular components leak out during this process (unlike necrosis, in which an injured cell releases its contents into the surroundings).

This regulated process is used to eliminate abnormal, mispositioned, or misplaced cells. It also helps to sculpt certain structures. For example, many of the precursors to neural cells are eliminated in order to create a more direct pathway for electrical impulses. Apoptosis also helps to shape the hands and feet. If the process is incomplete, toes or fingers may be fused in a condition known as syndactyly. Sometimes, apoptosis occurs as a result of teratogenic agents, leading to malformations or fetal death.

SENESCENCE AND AGING

Senescence is a progressive decline in function as a result of biological aging. The term can be used to describe an organism as a whole, or the irreversible state of a cell that can no longer divide but remains physiologically active. Senescence can be brought on by the activation of an oncogene or the deactivation of a tumor suppressor gene, as a way to reduce the threat of cancer. This non-proliferative state can also be induced by oxidative stress, DNA damage, and telomere shortening. **Telomeres** are repetitive non-coding sequences of DNA found at the ends of chromosomes that protect the coding sequences. Every time a cell divides, the chromosomes shorten because DNA polymerase cannot replicate the end portion. Eventually the telomeres are lost and the cell must enter a state of senescence to prevent damage to important genes. An enzyme called telomerase *can* add nucleotides to these problematic end portions, but it is only found in certain types of cells, such as embryonic stem cells, germ cells, cancerous cells, and even adult stem cells (in low amounts). The proportion of senescent cells tends to increase with age, but evidence shows that senescence is also a strategy used during embryonic development to halt the growth of certain tissues, thereby helping to shape the embryo.

TERMS OF DIRECTION

- **Medial** means *nearer to the midline* of the body. In anatomical position, the little finger is medial to the thumb.
- **Lateral** is the opposite of medial. It refers to structures *further away from the body's midline*, at the sides. In anatomical position, the thumb is lateral to the little finger.
- **Proximal** refers to structures *closer to the center* of the body. The hip is proximal to the knee.
- **Distal** refers to structures *further away from the center* of the body. The knee is distal to the hip.

- **Anterior** refers to structures in *front*.
- **Posterior** refers to structures *behind*.
- **Cephalad** and **cephalic** are adverbs meaning towards the *head*. **Cranial** is the adjective, meaning of the *skull*.
- **Caudad** is an adverb meaning towards the *tail* or posterior. **Caudal** is the adjective, meaning of the *hindquarters*.
- **Superior** means *above*, or closer to the head.
- **Inferior** means *below*, or closer to the feet.

THE THREE PRIMARY BODY PLANES

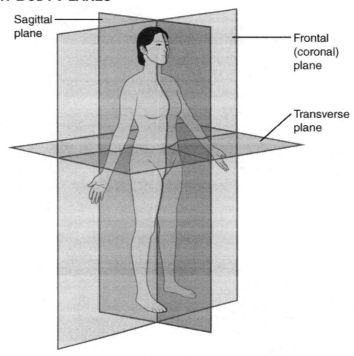

The **transverse (or horizontal) plane** divides the patient's body into imaginary upper (*superior*) and lower (*inferior or caudal*) halves.

The **sagittal plane** divides the body, or any body part, vertically into right and left sections. The sagittal plane runs parallel to the midline of the body.

The **coronal (or frontal) plane** divides the body, or any body structure, vertically into front and back (*anterior* and *posterior*) sections. The coronal plane runs vertically through the body at right angles to the midline.

Respiratory System

GENERAL FUNCTION

The respiratory system includes the nose, mouth, nasal cavity, sinuses, pharynx, larynx, trachea, bronchial tree, and lungs. These organs facilitate the delivery of oxygen to the cells of the body for use in cellular respiration. The **conductive zone** brings inhaled air to the **respiratory zone** where gas exchange occurs. As oxygen is loaded into the blood, carbon dioxide is removed. Essential to this process are the diaphragm and intercostal muscles which are used to enlarge the chest cavity during pulmonary respiration (breathing). External respiration is the exchange of gas between the lungs and the blood. Internal respiration is the exchange of gas between the blood and tissues. Secondary functions of the respiratory system include pH regulation of the blood, thermoregulation, odor detection, and the production of speech.

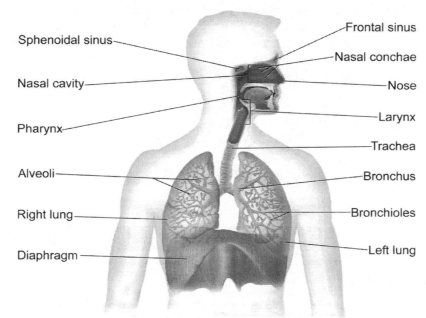

The Respiratory System

GAS EXCHANGE, THERMOREGULATION

Gas exchange is the loading of oxygen into pulmonary blood, and the removal of carbon dioxide. Inhaled air moves from through the mouth or nose to the pharynx, larynx, trachea, right / left main bronchi, and bronchioles, and then the alveoli. It is here that gases diffuse down their partial pressure gradients across a shared membrane between the capillaries and alveoli called the respiratory membrane. Oxygen diffuses into the blood where it is delivered to tissues throughout the body, and carbon dioxide diffuses out of the blood as a waste product of cellular respiration.

The respiratory system is also involved in **thermoregulation**: the regulation of body temperature. Capillaries within the respiratory tract, particularly the nasal passages and trachea, can constrict to conserve heat and dilate to release heat. The exhalation of warm, moistened air also helps to cool the body.

PROTECTION AGAINST DISEASE: PARTICULATE MATTER

A secondary role of the respiratory system is protection against disease and filtration of particulate matter. Some particles are filtered by nostril hairs and others get caught in mucus. Lysozymes within the mucus help to break down the trapped debris, and the cilia that line the respiratory tract then sweep it away. Immunoglobulin A (IgA) is also produced in the mucosal lining, and these antibodies aid in immune defenses by neutralizing pathogens. Mast cells within the respiratory tract release inflammatory chemicals that increase blood flow to the region, and alert the immune system to a threat. Large phagocytic cells called macrophages can also help to protect the lungs by engulfing small cells and particulates.

STRUCTURE OF LUNGS AND ALVEOLI

The lungs are spongy, porous organs that occupy most of the thoracic cavity. A serous membrane called the pleura lines the thoracic cavity (**parietal pleura**) as well as the surface of the lungs (**visceral pleura**). The three-lobed right lung is separated from the two-lobed left lung by the **mediastinum**. The trachea forks into primary bronchi which enter the left and right lung (along with blood and lymphatic vessels) at a region called the **hilum**. Each primary bronchus splits repeatedly into secondary bronchi, tertiary bronchi, and bronchioles to form the bronchial tree. The terminal bronchioles further divide into respiratory bronchioles, which are characterized by the presence of some alveoli. The respiratory bronchioles lead into alveolar ducts, which terminate in alveolar sacs.

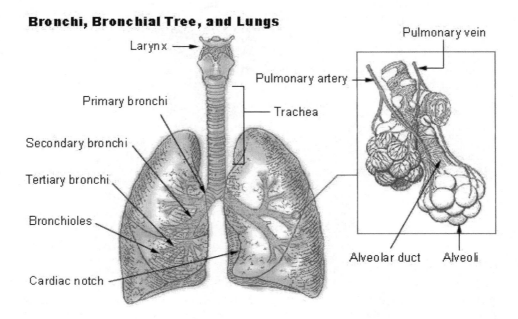

Bronchi, Bronchial Tree, and Lungs

Larynx

Primary bronchi

Secondary bronchi

Tertiary bronchi

Bronchioles

Cardiac notch

Pulmonary vein

Pulmonary artery

Trachea

Alveolar duct

Alveoli

Within the alveolar sacs of the bronchi are clusters of **alveoli**: microscopic pouches where gas exchange occurs. The lungs contain hundreds of millions of these sacs, with a combined surface area that averages 70 m². The wall of each alveolus consists of a single layer of epithelial cells, most of which are type I cells. These squamous cells are involved in gas exchange. Type II cells are cuboidal cells that secrete surfactant to prevent the alveoli from collapsing. The alveolar walls are perforated by pores that connect adjacent alveoli, providing an alternate route for the passage of air in case of blocked ducts. The outer surfaces are covered with a network of capillaries. The basement membrane of a capillary fuses with the alveolar basement membrane to form the **respiratory membrane** (which also includes the capillary and alveolar epithelial cells).

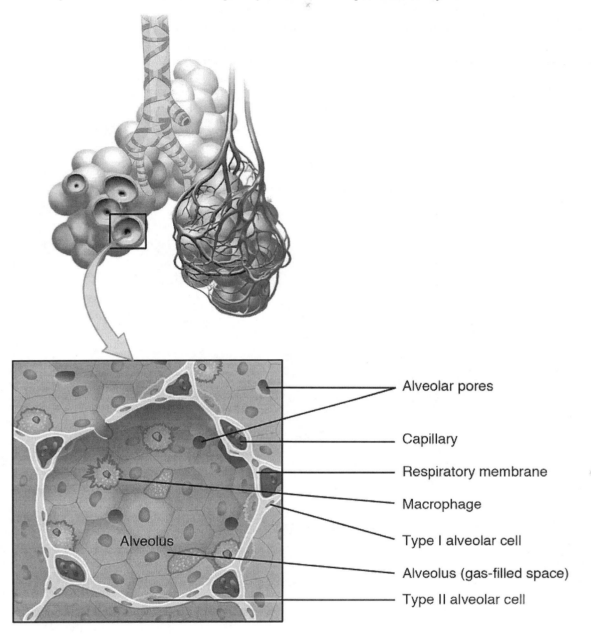

BREATHING MECHANISMS

The diaphragm is a thin, dome-shaped muscle that separates the abdominal cavity from the thoracic cavity. This muscle, along with the external and internal intercostal muscles of the rib cage, are responsible for changing the volume, and therefore the pressure, of air in the lungs. This mechanism of breathing follows **Boyle's law**: the pressure and volume of a gas have an inverse relationship, assuming the temperature is constant.

When the diaphragm and external intercostals contract, the volume of the thoracic cavity increases, and the rib cage and sternum elevate and expand outward. The increase in volume results in a decrease in intrapleural pressure, and air enters the lungs in a process called **inspiration**. This is called **negative-pressure breathing** because the pressure in the lungs is lower than atmospheric pressure (and gases move down the pressure gradient). **Expiration** is usually a more passive process, and it is achieved by simply relaxing the same muscles that facilitated inhalation. As the volume of the thoracic cavity decreases, intrapleural pressure increases, and air leaves the lungs. Air can be forcibly pushed out through the contraction of the internal intercostals and abdominal muscles.

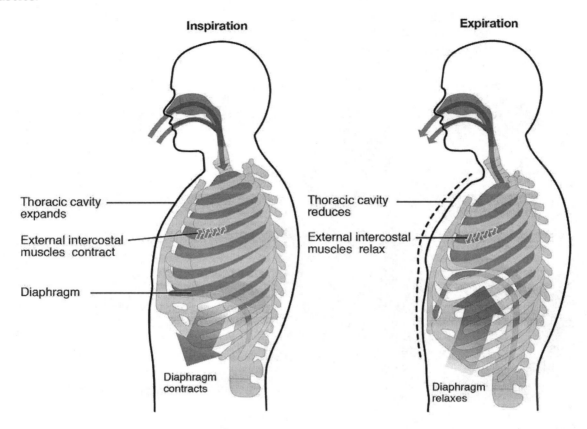

Cardiovascular System

FUNCTIONS

The circulatory system is primarily associated with the transport of oxygen, nutrients, hormones, ions, and fluids throughout the body, as well as the removal of metabolic wastes.

Oxygen moves down its partial pressure gradient from the air into the blood of the alveolar capillaries, where most of it binds to hemoglobin molecules in the red blood cells. A small amount dissolves in the blood. Without oxygen, cells would be unable to transfer the energy in glucose to ATP during cellular respiration.

The carbon dioxide that is produced during cellular respiration is transported away from tissues and diffuses out of the alveolar capillaries. Like oxygen, carbon dioxide can dissolve in blood or bind to hemoglobin, but most travels in the form of bicarbonate ions. Other metabolic waste products such as urea are brought to the kidneys to be filtered. The kidneys also help to regulate the levels of fluids and ions in the blood.

Digested nutrients such as glucose, amino acids, and fats are circulated to target cells where they are absorbed. Hormones released by endocrine glands also reach their target cells in this way. Lipid-soluble molecules require the use of a carrier protein to be transported in blood.

ROLE IN THERMOREGULATION

The circulatory system plays an important role in thermoregulation. The human body maintains an average temperature of around 98.6 °F (37 °C), which is optimal for metabolic processes and defense against pathogens. Heat exchange occurs at the surface of the skin, where blood vessels can dilate or constrict in response to signals from the brain.

Sensory neurons called thermoreceptors detect changes in temperature and send impulses to the hypothalamus, which then sends signals to the effectors - the smooth muscles that surround cutaneous arterioles. If the body temperature is too warm, the smooth muscle relaxes, and the arterioles dilate. Vasodilation allows more blood to flow through the capillary beds near the surface of the skin, and more heat is lost to the surroundings. If the temperature is too cool, the smooth muscle contracts, and the arterioles constrict. Vasoconstriction reduces the volume of blood that flows near the body's surface, which minimizes heat loss to the surroundings. Sweating and shivering also help to control body temperature.

THE HEART

The wall of the heart is a composed of three layers of tissue. The outer layer is the **epicardium**, which protects the heart and secretes lubricating serous fluid. The middle layer is the muscular **myocardium**, which contracts to pump blood. The innermost layer is the **endocardium**, which lines the chambers and valves.

The heart is a four-chambered organ. The superior "receiving" chambers are the atria. The **right atrium** receives blood from the vena cava, and the **left atrium** receives blood from the pulmonary veins. The muscular "discharging" chambers are the ventricles. The **right ventricle** pumps blood into the pulmonary trunk, and the **left ventricle** pumps blood into the aorta.

The **tricuspid valve** (also called the right atrioventricular valve, or right AV valve) prevents backflow into the atrium when the ventricle contracts. The **pulmonary semilunar valve** prevents the return of blood into the right ventricle. The **bicuspid valve** (also called the left AV valve, or mitral valve) prevents blood from entering the left atrium when the ventricle contracts. The **aortic semilunar valve** stops the backflow of blood into the right ventricle as it leaves through the aorta.

The path of blood through the heart is traced in the diagram below:

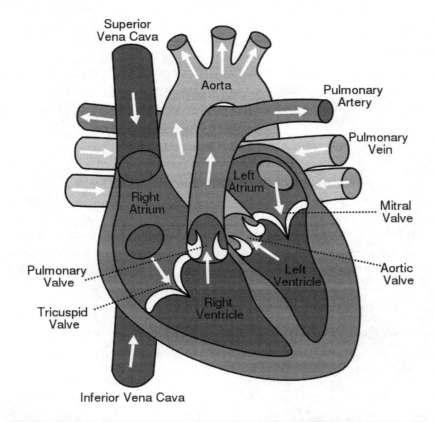

Review Video: The Heart
Visit mometrix.com/academy and enter code: 451399

ENDOTHELIAL CELLS

The thin inner lining of blood vessels (and the lymphatic vessels) is called the **endothelium**. This tissue lines the entire circulatory system, including the interior of the heart. It is composed of a single layer of squamous endothelial cells that are connected by tight junctions and adherens junctions. This allows the endothelium to act as a selectively permeable barrier between the blood and the surrounding tissue, though some vessels have pores and gaps that allow the passage of larger molecules. The smoothness of the endothelium reduces friction between the blood and the vessel wall. Endothelial cells also play a role in vasoconstriction by releasing peptides called endothelins that cause the smooth muscle within the vessel walls to contract. They also secrete chemicals that inhibit the coagulation of blood, but if the endothelium is damaged they release different chemicals required for clot formation.

SYSTOLIC AND DIASTOLIC PRESSURE

Blood pressure is the force per unit area that is exerted by the blood on the walls of the vessels. Unless otherwise indicated, blood pressure refers specifically to the pressure within the major arteries, since arterioles, capillaries, venules, and veins have progressively less pressure. Blood pressure is often expressed as two numbers, and in units of millimeters of mercury (mmHg). The first number refers to the **systolic pressure**, or the maximum pressure that is exerted during **systole**. During this time, the ventricles contract, forcing blood into the aorta and pulmonary trunk.

As the blood enters the arteries, the elastic walls stretch to accommodate the increased volume, and then return to their normal diameter during **diastole**. Diastole is the period in which the ventricles relax and blood pressure is at its lowest point. The normal average blood pressure for an adult at rest is 120/80 mmHg, where 120 is the systolic bp, and 80 is the diastolic bp. High blood pressure can damage the walls of the blood vessels and increase the risk of heart disease, heart failure, and stroke. Low blood pressure is only concerning if it occurs suddenly, or if it causes noticeable symptoms such as lightheadedness or fainting.

SYSTEMIC AND PULMONARY CIRCULATION

The **systemic circuit** carries blood from the muscular left ventricle of the heart to the aorta, which gives rise to the arteries that eventually branch into arterioles and then the capillary beds within the tissues of the body. Oxygen and nutrients enter the tissues, and carbon dioxide and other wastes enter the blood. Deoxygenated blood leaves the capillary beds through venules, which merge into larger veins. The blood then enters the right atrium through the superior and inferior vena cava. Because this circuit is much longer than the pulmonary circuit, blood pressure is *higher*. Unlike the pulmonary circuit, blood in the arteries carries *more* oxygen than blood in the veins. When oxygen levels are low, vessels dilate to promote blood flow to tissues that need it.

Systemic Circuit

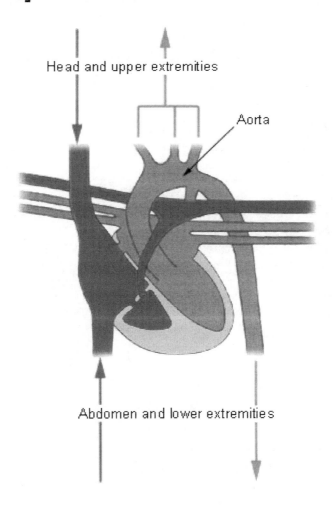

Head and upper extremities

Aorta

Abdomen and lower extremities

The **pulmonary circuit** is the part of the circulatory system that carries blood from the heart to the lungs and back to the heart. When deoxygenated blood is expelled from the right ventricle, it moves through the pulmonary trunk, which bifurcates into the right and left pulmonary arteries. Each branch extends into the lungs, eventually giving rise to arterioles and then the capillaries where gas exchange occurs by diffusion. Oxygenated blood leaves the capillaries through venules which fuse into veins, finally merging into four pulmonary veins that return blood to the left atrium. Note that in the pulmonary circuit, the arteries have *less* oxygen than the veins. Low blood oxygen in the pulmonary circuit triggers vasoconstriction, which redirects blood to better ventilated parts of the lung.

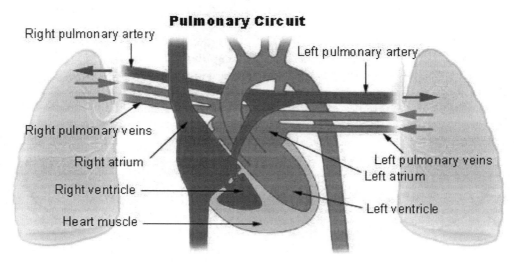

ELECTRICAL CONDUCTION SYSTEM

The electrical conduction system of the heart generates and propagates the electrical impulses that sustain the rhythmic electrical contractions of the heart. The entire system is composed of the sinoatrial (SA) and atrioventricular (AV) nodes and the internodal pathways, the Bundle of His, as well as the right and left bundle branches and the anterior and posterior fascicles. First, the SA node generates a spontaneous electrical impulse that stimulates atrial contraction, corresponding to the P wave on the ECG. Next, the electrical impulse reaches the AV node and slows in velocity. This corresponds to the PR segment on the ECG. The electrical impulse travels through the Bundle of His and the bundle branches, then to the Purkinje fibers. The Purkinje fibers carry the electrical impulse that stimulate the ventricles to depolarize and contract, corresponding to the QRS complex.

ELECTROCARDIOGRAMS

CARDIAC CYCLE AND THE ECG RELATIONSHIP

Each heart beat is seen as three major waves or complexes on an ECG. The heart rhythm begins in the sinoatrial node and lead to atrial depolarization. The P wave represents depolarization of the atria on an ECG. This is followed by the QRS interval, which represents depolarization of the ventricle. Next follows the ST segment and T wave, corresponding to repolarization of the ventricle. A small U wave may follow the T wave and represents further repolarization of the ventricle.

The first phase of the cardiac cycle is seen as the **P wave** on the ECG and corresponds to the wave of depolarization that spreads from the sinoatrial node to the atria, representing activation of the atria. The normal length of the P wave is 0.08 to 0.1 seconds in duration. The appearance of the P wave is smooth and round. The first segment of the P wave represents activation, or contraction, of the right atrium, followed by activation of the left atrium. The activation of the atrioventricular node is represented by the middle of the P wave. Absent P waves may suggest certain arrhythmias.

The **Q wave** is seen as a negative wave on an ECG, marking the beginning of the QRS complex. A normal duration of the Q wave is small, but the actual value will depend on which lead is used to measure the wave in an ECG. However, this value may often be less than 0.03 seconds. An enlarged Q wave suggests abnormal conduction in the ventricles or a myocardial infarction.

The **R wave** is a positive wave on an ECG and is the predominant portion of the QRS complex. It may or may not be preceded by a Q wave. If a second positive wave is seen following the R wave, it is termed the R' wave. The **S wave** is a negative wave that follows the R wave in the QRS complex seen on an ECG. Together with the Q wave, the R and S waves represent ventricular depolarization.

The **T wave** is a positive wave following the S wave on the ECG that represents ventricular repolarization, or recovery of the ventricle. It is the final major wave of the cardiac cycle seen on an ECG. It is longer than the QRS complex, indicating that repolarization takes longer than depolarization during the cardiac cycle. The T wave is smooth and round, similar in shape to the P wave. Abnormal T waves may indicate heart disease or electrolyte imbalances. The T wave may be followed by a small **U wave** that still represents the final repolarization of the ventricles.

PR INTERVAL

The PR interval on an ECG represents the period from the beginning of atrial depolarization to the beginning of ventricular depolarization. The PR interval also includes activation of the bundle of His and bundle branches. The PR interval is measured from the beginning of the P wave to the beginning of the QRS complex. A normal PR interval ranges from 0.12 to 0.20 seconds. If the PR interval is shorter than 0.12 seconds, the heart is said to have "accelerated conduction." If a first degree AV block or heart block is present, the interval is longer than 0.20 seconds. The PR interval may also vary with heart rate, decreasing in length as heart rate increases. Further, the PR interval increases with age, being short in childhood and lengthening into adulthood.

QRS COMPLEX

Together, the Q, R, and S waves comprise the QRS complex that indicates depolarization, or activation, of both the right and left ventricles. A normal QRS complex is 0.06 to 0.1 seconds in duration. This indicates that ventricular depolarization occurs very rapidly. A long QRS interval suggests impaired conduction in the ventricles. The Q wave precedes the R wave on an ECG and is a negative wave. The R wave is a positive wave.

The S wave is a negative wave, seen after the R wave in an ECG. On an ECG, the shape of the QRS complex will change depending on which recording electrodes are used. In some instances, all three waves (Q, R, and S) are not visible.

ST SEGMENT

The ST segment follows the QRS interval and corresponds to the period in which the ventricle is completely depolarized. It is measured from the end of the QRS complex to the beginning of the T wave. This approximately corresponds to the plateau phase of the action potential. The J point is the junction of the QRS complex and the ST segment. This point is usually a 90° angle with the S wave. The ST segment may be depressed or elevated and can be used to diagnose ventricular ischemia or hypoxia.

QT INTERVAL

The QT interval represents the entire action potential, the time for both ventricular depolarization and repolarization. The normal QT interval lasts 0.2 to 0.4 seconds. At increased heart rates, this interval shortens. Long QT intervals may be indicative of arrhythmias.

MEASURING HEART RATE

Heart rate can easily be calculated on ECG graph paper is the heartbeat occurs at regular intervals. Usually, there are the same number of P waves and QRS complexes and they occur at regular intervals. To calculate the heart rate, simply count the number of horizontal squares on the graph paper between recurring waves or cycles. Counting the number of cardiac cycles in six seconds and multiplying this number by 10 may also determine heart rate.

If the heart rate is less than 100 beats per minute, only the large squares on the ECG graph paper need to be counted to determine time. If, however, the heart rate is greater than 100 beats per minute, it is best to consider the smaller squares when measuring the time interval.

CARDIAC ARRHYTHMIAS

Cardiac arrhythmias, abnormal heart beats, in adults are frequently the result of damage to the conduction system during major cardiac surgery or as the result of a myocardial infarction.

Bradyarrhythmias are pulse rates that are abnormally slow:

- **Complete atrioventricular block** (A-V block) may be congenital or a response to surgical trauma.
- **Sinus bradycardia** may be caused by the autonomic nervous system or a response to hypotension and decrease in oxygenation.
- **Junctional/nodal rhythms** often occur in post-surgical patients when absence of P wave is noted but heart rate and output usually remain stable, and unless there is compromise, usually no treatment is necessary.

Tachyarrhythmias are pulse rates that are abnormally fast:

- **Sinus tachycardia** is often caused by fever and infection.
- **Supraventricular tachycardia** (200-300 BPM) may have a sudden onset and result in congestive heart failure.

Conduction irregularities are irregular pulses that often occur post-operatively and are usually not significant.

Premature contractions may arise from the atria or ventricles.

> **Review Video: Pulse**
> Visit mometrix.com/academy and enter code: 342004

ARTERIAL AND VENOUS SYSTEMS (ARTERIES, ARTERIOLES, VENULES, VEINS)

The walls of all blood vessels (except the capillaries) consist of three layers: the innermost **tunica intima**, the **tunica media** consisting of smooth muscle cells and elastic fibers, and the outer **tunica adventitia**.

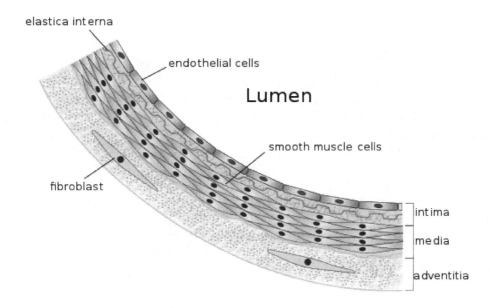

Vessel	Structure	Function
Elastic arteries	Includes the aorta and major branches Tunica media has more elastin than any other vessels Largest vessels in the arterial system	Stretch when blood is forced out of the heart, and recoil under low pressure
Muscular arteries	Includes the arteries that branch off of the elastic arteries Tunica media has a higher proportion of smooth muscle cells, and fewer elastic fibers as compared to elastic arteries	Regulate blood flow by vasoconstriction / vasodilation
Arterioles	Tiny vessels that lead to the capillary beds Tunica media is thin, but composed almost entirely smooth muscle cells	Primary vessels involved in vasoconstriction / vasodilation Control blood flow to capillaries
Venules	Tiny vessels that exit the capillary beds Thin, porous walls; few muscle cells and elastic fibers	Empty blood into larger veins
Veins	Thin tunica media and tunica intima Wide lumen Valves prevent backflow of blood	Carry blood back to the heart

PRESSURE AND FLOW CHARACTERISTICS

Blood pressure is highest in the main arteries of the systemic circuit, particularly the aorta. The pressure decreases progressively as blood flows through the arterioles, capillaries, venules, and veins. The blood pressure is lowest in the vena cava. The steepest *drop* in blood pressure (as opposed to absolute pressure) occurs at the arterioles. The large reduction in diameter from artery to arteriole results in an increase in resistance as blood moves against the vessel wall. This slows down the flow of blood, and decreases the pressure.

Blood flow can be described as turbulent or laminar. Turbulence is an unsteady, swirling flow of blood that can occur during periods of high velocity, when the blood encounters an obstruction, or when the vessels take a sharp turn or narrow suddenly. Turbulent flow usually produces sounds, while laminar flow is silent. Laminar flow is the steady, streamlined flow of blood that occurs throughout most of the circulatory system.

CAPILLARY BEDS

MECHANISMS OF GAS AND SOLUTE EXCHANGE

Capillaries have only a single layer of endothelial cells that rest on a basement membrane. Capillary beds are groups of interconnected capillaries that facilitate the exchange of gas and solutes between the blood and interstitial fluid. Nutrients and oxygen enter the interstitial fluid, and carbon dioxide and other wastes enter the capillary blood. Gases and lipid-soluble substances can cross the endothelial cell membranes by simple diffusion, but ions and large particles often require the help of transport proteins or vesicular transport. Sometimes materials move through **intercellular clefts**: channels between adjacent endothelial cells. Capillaries with a nonporous continuous endothelium are called **continuous capillaries**. These are the most common types of capillaries in the body, and also the most impermeable. **Fenestrated capillaries** have pores that increase their permeability and are found in the kidneys and small intestine. **Sinusoidal capillaries** have a discontinuous endothelium that permits the passage of large particles and even blood cells. They are the most permeable of the capillaries.

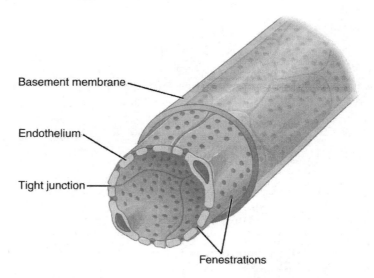

SOURCE OF PERIPHERAL RESISTANCE

Peripheral resistance is the resistance of the vessels to the flow of blood as a result of friction. As resistance increases, the rate of blood flow decreases. The main factors that affect peripheral resistance are diameter and length of the vessel, and volume and viscosity of the blood.

Resistance is most affected by changes in the *diameter* of the vessel. The relationship is inverse; as radius decreases, the resistance increases proportionally to the fourth power of the radius. For example, if the radius of a blood vessel is cut in half due to the buildup of plaque, resistance increases by a factor of 16. As such, vasoconstriction and vasodilation are critical to maintaining the appropriate level of resistance and flow. As *length* of the vessel increases, the resistance increases proportionally due to the increased surface area. As a person gains weight, the new blood vessels that nourish the new adipose tissue cause the total resistance of the system to increase. Blood volume and blood viscosity are usually not subject to sudden changes, but the effects of such changes are fairly intuitive. A decrease in either of these factors results in a decrease in resistance and an increase in flow rate.

COMPOSITION OF BLOOD

PLASMA, CHEMICALS, BLOOD CELLS

Blood is a mixture of plasma, chemicals, and blood cells. The clear, straw-colored liquid portion that makes up 55% of the blood is called **plasma**, and the remaining 45% consists of **formed elements**: the red and white blood cells and platelets.

Plasma is a solution of water, plasma proteins (albumin, antibodies, clotting proteins), carbohydrates, amino acids, lipids, vitamins, salts, gases, hormones, and waste products. About 92% of plasma is water.

Most of the cells in the blood are **red blood cells** (RBCs, or erythrocytes). These biconcave cells lack organelles, leaving room for hemoglobin - a protein to which oxygen and carbon dioxide can bind. The percentage of red blood cells by volume is called **hematocrit**, and averages about 42% for women and 46% for men. Less than 1% of blood consists of white blood cells and platelets. White blood cells (WBCs, or leukocytes) are the only blood cells with nuclei. Unlike RBCs, they are not confined to the blood and can move in and out of vessels. There are many types of WBCs, and all are specialized to fight pathogens in different ways. **Platelets** (thrombocytes) are cell fragments that initiate clotting, and they outnumber WBCs about 40:1.

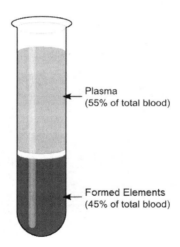

Plasma
(55% of total blood)

Formed Elements
(45% of total blood)

ERYTHROCYTE PRODUCTION AND DESTRUCTION; SPLEEN, BONE MARROW

Erythropoiesis (the production of red blood cells) occurs in the red bone marrow. When oxygen levels are low, the hormone **erythropoietin** (produced by the kidneys and liver) targets the marrow, stimulating **myeloid stem cells** to differentiate into **erythroblasts**. These immature RBCs divide many times, filling up with newly synthesized hemoglobin. The nuclei condense, and are ejected along with other organelles until only some endoplasmic reticulum remains. These cells are called **reticulocytes**, and they are released into the blood. After 1-2 days, the rest of the endoplasmic reticulum is lost, and mature **erythrocytes** are formed. Note that these cells are incapable of division.

After about 120 days, old and damaged RBCs are recognized and engulfed by phagocytes that are concentrated in the liver, spleen, and bone marrow. Hemoglobin is broken down into its four globin polypeptide chains and heme groups. Amino acids are released from the chains and enter the blood. The iron within the heme groups is either stored as ferritin in the liver or returned to the marrow to make more hemoglobin. The rest of the heme group is degraded to bilirubin and excreted in the bile.

Leukocytes (White Blood Cells)

Lymphocytes are a special type of white blood cell that play an important role in the immune system. B cells and T cells are the two types of lymphocytes.

A monocyte is another type of white blood cell. These cells are characterized by a well-defined nucleus. They play an important role in the body's immune response to pathogens. These cells are also produced in the bone marrow.

A granulocyte is a type of white blood cell that has granules in its cytoplasm. There are three types of granulocytes: basophils, eosinophils, and neutrophils. Approximately 75% of all white blood cells are granulocytes. The types of granulocytes are distinguished by their ability to be stained with various types of stains in the laboratory. Basophils are stained black by basic stains, eosinophils are stained red by acid stains, and neutrophils are stained pale lilac by neutral pH stains. Basophils play an important role in allergies and allergic reactions, as well as in inflammation. Eosinophils play an important part in the defense against infection by parasites, and neutrophils take part in the defense against infection from microorganisms.

Leukocyte	Maturation Series
Granulocytes	Myeloid progenitor
	Myeloblast (10-20 mm): oval nucleus with no granules evident in cytoplasm.
	Promyelocyte (10-20 mm): Granules in cytoplasm.
	Myelocyte (10-18 mm): Large oval nucleus. Primary granules evident but secondary more prevalent.
	Metamyelocyte (10-18 mm): Kidney-shaped nucleus with primary and secondary (most prevalent) granules.
	Band: U-shaped nucleus, secondary or neutrophilic or basophils granules most common.
	Segmented cells (14 mm): 2-5 joined lobes.
Monocyte:	Myeloid progenitor
	Monoblast (12-20 mm) with large oval nucleus and lymphoid dendritic cells
	Promonocyte (from monoblast)
	Monocyte
	Macrophage and myeloid dendritic cell.
Lymphocyte:	Common lymphoid progenitor
	Lymphoblast (10-20 mm) with large round nucleus.
	Prolymphocyte
	Small lymphocyte and natural killer cell
	B and T lymphoctyes (from small lymphocyte)

BLOOD TYPES

In the ABO blood group, there are 4 main blood types as follows: A, B, O and AB. These blood types are categorized based on whether or not A and B red cell antigens are present. Individuals with blood type A have A antigens. Individuals with blood type B have B antigens. Individuals with blood type AB have A and B antigens. Individuals with blood type O have neither A nor B antigens. Blood also contains antibodies to the antigens. Individuals with type A blood produce anti-B antibodies. The opposite is true of individuals with type B blood. Individuals with type AB blood produce no antibodies. Those with type O blood produce anti-A and anti-B antibodies. In the Rhesus group of blood types an individual is either positive or negative for the Rh factor. The Rh factor is an antigenic substance.

COAGULATION AND CLOTTING MECHANISMS

When a blood vessel is damaged, the smooth muscle constricts at the site of injury and platelets adhere to the exposed collagen of the vessel wall. The platelets develop spine-like projections, and release chemicals to attract other platelets and promote further vasoconstriction. A plug is formed as platelets aggregate, but this is rarely a sufficient fix without the coagulation of the blood.

There are two clotting mechanisms: extrinsic and intrinsic. In the extrinsic clotting mechanism, damaged tissue releases thromboplastin, which triggers a cascade of reactions that results in the production of an enzyme called prothrombin activator. Prothrombin activator is also produced by the slower-acting *intrinsic* clotting mechanism. When blood encounters a foreign substance or tissue, the Hageman factor (also called coagulation factor XII) is activated, leading to the production of prothrombin activator. From here, the clotting pathways are the same. Prothrombin activator converts prothrombin to thrombin using calcium as a cofactor. Thrombin splits fibrinogen to form fibrin, but also stimulates its own production (a positive feedback loop). Fibrin is a fibrous protein that forms a mesh-like network that traps more platelets and red blood cells. This forms a clot that seals the injured region of the blood vessel.

OXYGEN TRANSPORT BY BLOOD

Almost all oxygen is transported by molecules of **hemoglobin** (Hb) that are found within erythrocytes, though 1.5% of blood oxygen is dissolved in the plasma. Hemoglobin has a protein component and a heme component. The protein component consists of four polypeptide chains known as globin (two alpha chains and two beta chains). Associated with each chain is a heme group that gives blood its red color. The heme group consists of a single iron atom surrounded by a complex organic ring called **protoporphyrin**. When blood passes through the capillaries of the lungs, it picks up oxygen. Each iron atom binds a molecule of oxygen - so one hemoglobin can bind up to four molecules of oxygen, and each erythrocyte carries around 250 million molecules of hemoglobin. The oxygenated form of hemoglobin is called **oxyhemoglobin**.

Hemoglobin can also transport up to four carbon dioxide molecules, though CO_2 binds to amino acids within the globin, not iron. Only about 23% of carbon dioxide is transported in this form, known as **carbaminohemoglobin**. Roughly 70% travels in the form of bicarbonate ions (as seen in the bicarbonate buffer system), and the rest is dissolved in the plasma.

NERVOUS AND ENDOCRINE CONTROL

Heart rate and blood pressure are greatly influenced by the nervous and endocrine systems. The sympathetic division of the autonomic nervous system increases the heart rate by releasing norepinephrine (NE), which acts on the SA node of the heart. The parasympathetic division has the opposite effect. The vagus nerves that innervate the heart release acetylcholine (ACh), which slows the heart rate. Central and peripheral chemoreceptors also help to regulate heart rate by monitoring levels of pH, carbon dioxide, and oxygen.

Blood pressure is regulated by baroreceptors in the aortic arch and carotid arteries (both of which detect high blood pressure) and also the venae cavae, pulmonary veins, and atrial walls (all of which detect low blood pressure). When high blood pressure is detected, the blood vessels dilate and heart rate decreases to restore homeostasis. Blood pressure is also regulated by hormones of the endocrine system. When blood pressure drops, the kidneys secrete a hormone called renin which initiates a series of reactions that ultimately cause the release of aldosterone from the adrenal glands. Aldosterone promotes the reabsorption of water, increasing the plasma volume.

Gastrointestinal System

Mechanical digestion begins in the mouth with the voluntary act of chewing (mastication). Skeletal muscles of the mouth and pharynx aid in swallowing (deglutition), which consists of three phases: the voluntary buccal phase and the involuntary pharyngeal and esophageal phases. The muscularis externa of the digestive tract consists of two layers of muscle tissue (three in the stomach) that contract radially and then relax to squeeze food in one direction. This involuntary propulsive process is called **peristalsis**. Peristalsis moves food from the pharynx to the esophagus to the stomach where an extra muscle layer helps to churn and mix the food. Another involuntary process called **segmentation** occurs in the intestines (in addition to peristalsis). In segmentation, non-adjacent portions of the digestive tract contract and relax to move the chyme back and forth. Haustral contractions in the large intestine are a form of segmentation that moves chyme from one haustrum to the next. Mass peristalsis describes the movements that occur two to four times a day to push large amounts of chyme toward the rectum. Movement along the digestive tract is also controlled by the gastroesophageal sphincter, pyloric sphincter, and anal sphincters.

INGESTION

When food is ingested, it is immediately moistened by saliva. This lubricating fluid is secreted by hundreds of minor salivary glands that are scattered throughout the oral cavity, and three pairs of major salivary glands: the parotid, submandibular, and sublingual glands.

Saliva contains a variety of solutes, many of which are enzymes. **Salivary amylase** begins the chemical breakdown of polysaccharides into simpler sugars, and **lingual lipase** begins the breakdown of fats. The effects of salivary enzymes are minimal, however, compared to the digestion that occurs later in the stomach and small intestine. Saliva contains antimicrobial agents as well. **Lysozyme** is an enzyme that works together with immunoglobulin A to break down the cell walls of many bacteria. Other components of saliva include bicarbonate ions that help the saliva to maintain a pH that is optimal for salivary enzymes, as well as other ions. **Mucin** is a protein that helps to form a gel-like coating that lubricates the bolus of food.

ESOPHAGUS AND TRANSPORT FUNCTION

The esophagus is a 25-cm tube extending from the pharynx to the stomach that functions as a passageway for food. It is not involved in digestion or absorption of nutrients, but it does secrete mucus to lubricate the esophagus and aid in the transport of food. The esophagus (and the alimentary canal that follows) has a wall that consists of four layers: the mucosa, submucosa, muscularis externa, and adventitia. Most of the digestive tract has a muscularis externa made of smooth muscle tissue, but the upper third of the esophagus is composed of skeletal muscle, and is under voluntary control. The middle portion is a mixture of both skeletal and smooth muscle, and the lower third is entirely smooth muscle. Food does not simply "fall" into the stomach; it is pushed along by **peristalsis**: an involuntary process in which the muscles in the wall of the digestive organ rhythmically contract and relax. The upper esophageal sphincter at the superior end of the esophagus and the lower esophageal sphincter at the inferior end control the passage of food by contracting and relaxing.

STOMACH

STORAGE AND CHURNING OF FOOD

The stomach is a muscular organ that can stretch to accommodate a high volume of food. While some chemical digestion does occur, the primary role of the stomach is the storage and mechanical breakdown of food. The inner surface (mucosa) is folded into a series of ridges called rugae that allow the stomach to expand as it fills with food. The stomach holds about 1 liter after a typical meal, but can stretch to accommodate nearly four times that amount. It churns and pummels food for an average of three to four hours with the help of a third muscle layer in the muscularis externa that is unique to the stomach. As the food is mixed with gastric juices, it turns into a creamy paste called chyme. A valve called the pyloric sphincter regulates the passage of chyme into the small intestine.

PRODUCTION OF DIGESTIVE ENZYMES, SITE OF DIGESTION

The mucosa of the stomach contains gastric glands which open into numerous gastric pits. There are four types of cells in these glands: mucous cells, parietal cells, chief cells, and endocrine cells. **Endocrine cells** (G cells) release hormones such as gastrin into the blood, and do not contribute to gastric juices. The rest of the glands are exocrine, and secrete their products into the stomach.

Parietal cells secrete intrinsic factor, which is required for the absorption of vitamin B_{12} in the small intestine. They also release hydrochloric acid (HCl), which lowers the pH of gastric juice to an average range of 1 to 3. This acidic environment is required for the activation of pepsinogen, which is secreted by the **chief cells**. The active form of pepsinogen is called pepsin - a digestive enzyme that breaks down proteins into smaller peptide chains. Chief cells also secrete gastric lipase, which continues the digestion of fats (though most fat and protein digestion occurs in the small intestine).

The **mucous cells** secrete bicarbonate-containing mucus to protect the stomach from the acidity and digestive enzymes.

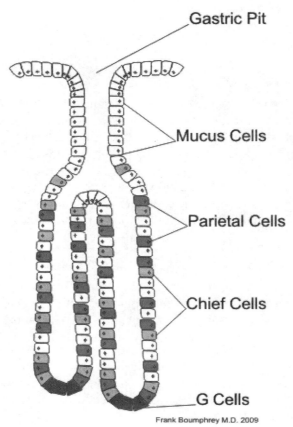

Frank Boumphrey M.D. 2009

STRUCTURE (GROSS)

The stomach is a muscular organ located in the left superior region of the abdomen. The gastroesophageal sphincter (also called the lower esophageal or cardioesophageal sphincter) found at the junction between the esophagus and stomach helps to prevent the reflux of acidic contents. The stomach itself can be divided into four main parts: the cardiac region, the fundus, the body, and the pylorus. The **cardiac region** is the area where food is emptied into the stomach. The **fundus** is the most superior region of the stomach, and the **body** is the largest, most central region. The body curves toward the right to form a "J" shape, with a lesser curvature and a greater curvature. It then narrows into a funnel-shaped region called the **pylorus**. The wider end of the pylorus is called the pyloric antrum and the narrow portion is the pyloric canal. The pyloric sphincter is the valve that regulates the release of small amounts of chyme into the small intestine. Other features of the stomach include the gastric folds (rugae) of the mucosa that allow the stomach to stretch and expand. The stomach is also characterized by an inner oblique layer of smooth muscle that is not seen in the rest of the alimentary canal.

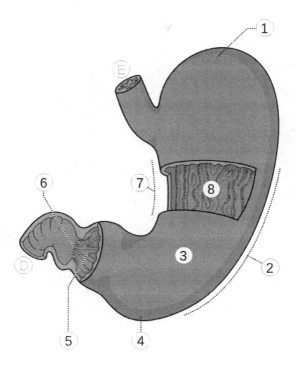

- 1. Fundus
- 2. Greater curvature
- 3. Body
- 4. Pyloric region
- 5. Pyloric antrum
- 6. Pyloric canal
- 7. Lesser curvature
- 8. Rugae
- E. Esophagus
- D. Duodenum of small intestine

LIVER

STRUCTURAL RELATIONSHIP OF LIVER WITHIN GASTROINTESTINAL SYSTEM AND THE PRODUCTION OF BILE

The liver is an essential component of the gastrointestinal system, but is not a part of the alimentary canal. This large, four-lobed organ acts as an accessory organ by performing many functions such as the production of bile, nutrient metabolism, and detoxification.

The primary digestive function of the liver is the synthesis of bile. Bile is a yellow-green solution of bile salts, pigments (mainly bilirubin from the breakdown of hemoglobin), cholesterol, and electrolytes. Only the bile salts play a role in digestion, and they do so mechanically (not enzymatically) by emulsifying fats into smaller globules called micelles that can be acted on by lipases in the small intestine. Bile also enhances the absorption of the fat-soluble vitamins A, D, E, and K. Liver cells synthesize bile salts from cholesterol.

Bile is stored and concentrated in the gallbladder. When food enters the small intestine, a hormone called cholecystokinin (CCK) signals the gallbladder to contact, and the bile is squeezed into the common bile duct. This duct joins with the pancreatic duct at the hepatopancreatic ampulla (ampulla of Vater) and bile spills into the duodenum via the duodenal papilla. Bile can also flow directly from the liver to the duodenum.

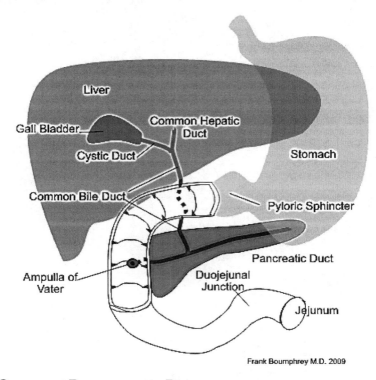

Frank Boumphrey M.D. 2009

ROLE IN BLOOD GLUCOSE REGULATION, DETOXIFICATION

The liver performs many metabolic functions, including the regulation of blood glucose concentration (which averages 100 mg/dl). Blood from the digestive tract enters the liver through the hepatic portal vein. If the blood sugar is too high, the liver polymerizes glucose to form glycogen in a process called **glycogenesis**. If blood sugar is too low, liver cells break down stored glycogen and release glucose monomers in a process called **glycogenolysis**. In cases of prolonged fasting, the liver can produce glucose from non-carbohydrate sources such as proteins and fats. This is called **gluconeogenesis**.

The liver also has a vital role in detoxification. Ammonia (a toxic waste product of the metabolism of amino acids) is converted to urea in the liver and excreted by the kidneys. Hormones that are circulating in the blood are inactivated by the liver and eliminated by the kidneys as well. The liver also breaks down exogenous compounds, such as drugs and alcohol.

PANCREAS

PRODUCTION OF ENZYMES AND TRANSPORT OF ENZYMES TO SMALL INTESTINE

The **pancreas** is a triangular-shaped organ with both endocrine and exocrine functions. (As an endocrine gland, it releases insulin, glucagon, and somatostatin into the blood.) It is located below the stomach, and extends from the duodenum to the spleen. Its role in digestion is the production and secretion of digestive juices. When chyme reaches the duodenum, enteroendocrine cells secrete cholecystokinin (CCK), which stimulates the acinar cells of the pancreas to release enzyme-rich juices. Secretin is secreted as well, which stimulates the duct cells to release a bicarbonate-rich solution that raises the pH. This provides the optimal environment for enzymes released by the pancreas. Pancreatic amylase digests starch, and pancreatic lipase digests fats. Proteases are released in their inactive form, but are activated in the small intestine. These activated protein-digesting enzymes include trypsin, carboxypeptidases A and B, and chymotrypsin. Nucleases digest nucleic acids. Pancreatic juice is emptied into the main pancreatic duct, which merges with the common bile duct at the hepatopancreatic ampulla. Juices enter the duodenum at the duodenal papilla. There is also an accessory pancreatic duct that empties directly into the duodenum at the minor papilla.

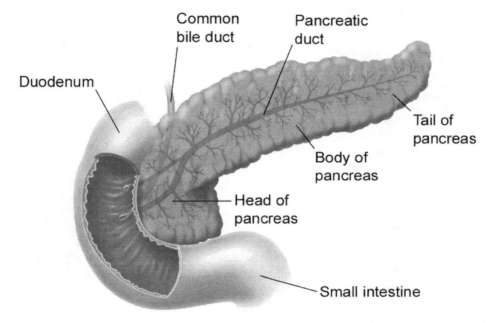

National Cancer Institute

SMALL INTESTINE

The small intestine is a long tube that extends from the pyloric sphincter to the ileocecal valve. Pancreatic enzymes and enzymes of the small intestine continue the digestion of food so the nutrients are small enough to be absorbed. These enzymes (called brush border enzymes) are embedded in the **microvilli**: tiny folds of the apical cell membrane that increase surface area. The core of each microvillus consists of actin filaments that extend out from the cytoplasm. Finger-like projections of the mucosa (villi) and deep circular folds of the mucosa and submucosa (plicae circulares) also increase the surface area available for absorption.

Absorption of water and food molecules occurs mostly in the jejunum and ileum of the small intestine. Amino acids and most sugars are taken into the intestinal cells using cotransport with sodium ions (secondary active transport). Lipid components and water are absorbed into the cells by simple diffusion. Short-chain fatty acids, sugars, amino acids, water, and electrolytes enter the bloodstream by diffusing into capillaries within the villi and traveling to the liver.

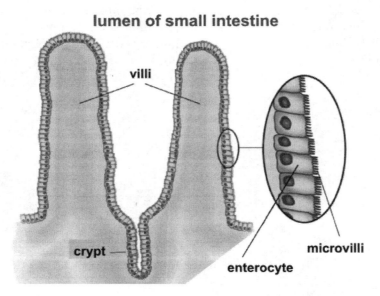

PRODUCTION OF ENZYMES, SITE OF DIGESTION AND NEUTRALIZATION OF STOMACH ACID

Most of the chemical digestion of food occurs in the small intestine. Brush border enzymes of the microvilli (as well as pancreatic enzymes) break down carbohydrates, fats, proteins, and nucleic acids into smaller components which are then absorbed. Some mechanical digestion occurs in the small intestine as well. Peristalsis moves chyme toward the small intestine, while segmentation pushes it back and forth to help mix enzymes into the chyme. Brunner's glands in the duodenum secrete bicarbonate-containing fluid that (with the help of alkaline pancreatic juice) neutralizes the acidic chyme, providing the optimal pH for enzyme activity.

Brush border enzymes and the substrates that they break down are summarized in the table below.

Brush border enzyme	Substrate
Dextrinase	Oligosaccharides
Glucoamylase	Oligosaccharides
Maltase	Maltose (disaccharide)
Lactase	Lactose (disaccharide)
Sucrase	Sucrose (disaccharide)
Aminopeptidase	Peptides
Dipeptidase	Dipeptides
Nucleosidase	Nucleotides
Phosphatase	Nucleotides

STRUCTURE (ANATOMIC SUBDIVISIONS)

The small intestine is subdivided into three regions: the duodenum, jejunum, and ileum. At about 25 cm, the C-shaped **duodenum** is the shortest segment, but it has the widest diameter. It receives chyme from the stomach and neutralizing digestive juices from the pancreas. Most of the chemical digestion of food occurs here. It does not play a large role in absorption, with the exception of iron. The **jejunum** is the main site of absorption. It averages 2.5 meters in length, and is characterized by prominent plicae circulares, long villi, and dense microvilli. The longest segment of the small intestine is the **ileum**. It averages 3.5 meters in length, but is the most narrow in diameter. Small aggregates of lymphatic cells called Peyer's patches are common in this segment, but they can be found throughout the small intestine. The primary role of the ileum is to absorb vitamin B_{12}, bile salts, and any nutrients that were not absorbed by the jejunum. It has few circular folds, and they disappear altogether in the distal region. It terminates at the ileocecal valve, which controls the movement of chyme into the large intestine.

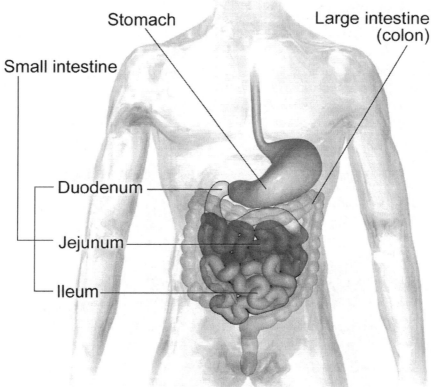

Anatomy of Small Intestine

LARGE INTESTINE

ABSORPTION OF WATER

The large intestine specializes in the absorption of vitamin K, biotin, sodium ions, chloride ions, and water. By the time chyme reaches the large intestine, most of the water (approximately 80%) has already been absorbed by the small intestine. As the chyme is pushed through the colon 90% of the remaining liquid is absorbed, leaving a mass of indigestible food, water, and bacteria. If the feces are excreted before enough water is absorbed, they leave as diarrhea. Constipation results when too much water is absorbed.

BACTERIAL FLORA

The large intestine does not secrete digestive enzymes, but there are hundreds of species of resident bacteria that can digest certain materials left in chyme. These beneficial microbes are nourished by small amounts of cellulose and other carbohydrates, and they release gases such as carbon dioxide and methane as waste products of fermentation. The bacteria also release vitamin K, biotin, thiamin, riboflavin, and vitamin B_{12}. Vitamin K (required for the synthesis of clotting proteins) and biotin (a cofactor for many enzymes) are absorbed for use in the body. Resident gut flora also help to keep populations of pathogenic bacteria in check. The appendix *may* serve as a reservoir for beneficial species of bacteria, though it is often infected with harmful microbes.

STRUCTURE (GROSS)

The large intestine is the portion of the alimentary canal that begins at the **ileocecal valve** and terminates at the anus. It is larger in diameter than the small intestine, but much shorter in length - averaging 1.5 meters. The first portion of the large intestine is a pouch called the **cecum**, and it receives chyme from the small intestine. It is also the site of a blind-ended tube called the **appendix**. The middle portion of the large intestine is the **colon**, which can be further subdivided into the ascending colon (right side of the body), transverse colon (extends across the abdominal cavity), descending colon (left side of the body), and sigmoid colon. The sigmoid colon lies in the pelvic cavity and becomes the **rectum**, which opens to the anus. There are no villi in the large intestine, but there are pouch-like sacculations called **haustra** that are separated by folds called plicae semilunares. These pouches are formed by the contraction of smooth muscle within the muscularis layer. The walls of the large intestine are lubricated by mucus, which is secreted by goblet cells.

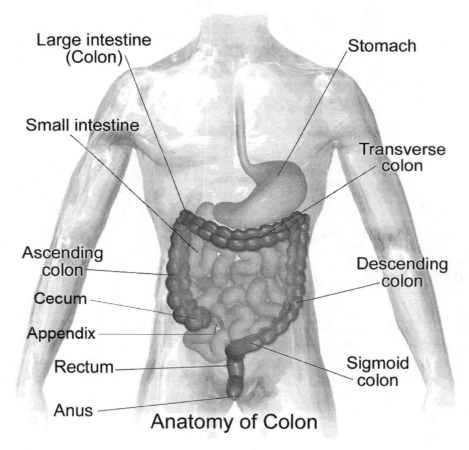

Anatomy of Colon

RECTUM: STORAGE AND ELIMINATION OF WASTE, FECES

The final 12 to 15 cm of the large intestine is called the rectum. In humans, it curves to conform to the shape of the sacrum and coccyx bone. The **anal canal** is the last portion of the rectum, and it ends with an involuntary internal sphincter and a voluntary external sphincter. A dilated region (superior to the anal canal) called the **rectal ampulla** functions as a storage area for feces before they are eliminated in the process of defecation. Feces consist of bacteria, water, undigested material, epithelial cells, and bile (which accounts for the brown coloration). As this material accumulates, the walls of the rectum expand and stretch receptors send signals that cause the rectal muscles to contract, the internal sphincter to relax, and the external sphincter to contract. At this point, the decision can be made to eliminate or delay elimination.

THE ENTERIC NERVOUS SYSTEM

The network of neurons buried in the lining of the gastrointestinal tract that controls the function of the digestive system is called the **enteric nervous system** (ENS). The ENS can operate independently of the brain and spinal cord, and communicates with the CNS through the parasympathetic and sympathetic nervous systems. The parasympathetic nervous system stimulates digestive activities, while the sympathetic nervous system inhibits them.

The ENS is divided into two main parts: the submucosal and myenteric plexuses. The **submucosal plexus** is embedded in the connective tissue of the submucosa. It functions in regulating local secretions, absorption, contraction of submucosal muscle, and blood flow. The **myenteric plexus** is located between the circular and longitudinal layers of the muscularis externa. This network exerts control over the motility of the GI tract. It increases the tone, as well as the rate, intensity, and velocity of contractions.

Nervous System

MAJOR FUNCTIONS

The nervous system is responsible for coordinating and controlling all of the activities of the body. It is composed of a complex network of neurons and the neuroglial cells that support them. Neurons are responsible for carrying out the **sensory**, **integrative**, and **motor** functions of the nervous system. Sensory receptors detect changes in the internal and external environment, such as pain, pressure, light, or temperature. During integration, the information is brought to the central nervous system where it is processed and interpreted. The motor function refers to the voluntary or involuntary response that is carried out by effectors, such as the contraction of a muscle, or the secretion of products by gland cells. These rapid responses are essential for the maintenance of homeostasis, heart rate, breathing, regulation of temperature, movement, sensations, memory, emotion, language, and more.

> **Review Video: The Nervous System**
> Visit mometrix.com/academy and enter code: 708428

HIGH LEVEL CONTROL AND INTEGRATION OF BODY SYSTEMS

The nervous system is responsible for the integration of body systems. The central nervous system (CNS) consists of the brain and spinal cord. It is considered the control/integration center because it combines sensory information from various sources. It communicates with the rest of the body via the peripheral nervous system (PNS). The **afferent** division of the PNS brings information *to* the CNS, and the **efferent** division delivers messages *from* the CNS to muscles or glands.

The nervous system works particularly closely with the endocrine system. Nerve impulses send information about the condition of the body to the hypothalamus, which regulates the release of hormones from the pituitary. The pituitary, or "master gland," controls other glands of the endocrine system. All body systems ultimately require direction from the nervous system to function properly and maintain homeostasis. Heart rate, digestion, body temperature, movement, and higher functions such as cognitive ability, memory, emotion, and fine motor skills are under the control of the nervous system.

ADAPTIVE CAPABILITY TO EXTERNAL INFLUENCES

The nervous system is the first body system to respond to changes in the environment. The receptors of afferent neurons (sensory neurons) are specialized to detect certain types of stimuli, and these neurons transmit action potentials to the CNS where a motor response may be called for. Sensory receptors are found nearly everywhere in the body. They can be classified by location, morphology (free vs. encapsulated nerve endings), the nature of the stimuli they detect (pressure, chemicals, light, temperature), and rate of adaptation.

Sensory adaptation refers to the change in sensitivity that occurs when receptors are exposed to a prolonged stimulus. Adaptation rates vary greatly across the different types of receptors, but they can be classified into two main groups. **Phasic** receptors quickly adapt to a constant stimulus, meaning that action potentials decrease over time and eventually stop. This explains the loss of sensation of clothes against the skin, or how an odor seems to disappear when the source is still present. Most tactile and chemoreceptors are phasic. **Tonic** receptors adapt slowly, constantly alerting the CNS of the stimulus with action potentials. Proprioceptors (receptors that provide feedback about position and movement of the body) are tonic receptors, as are photoreceptors (light-detecting receptors) and nociceptors (pain receptors).

ORGANIZATION OF VERTEBRATE NERVOUS SYSTEM

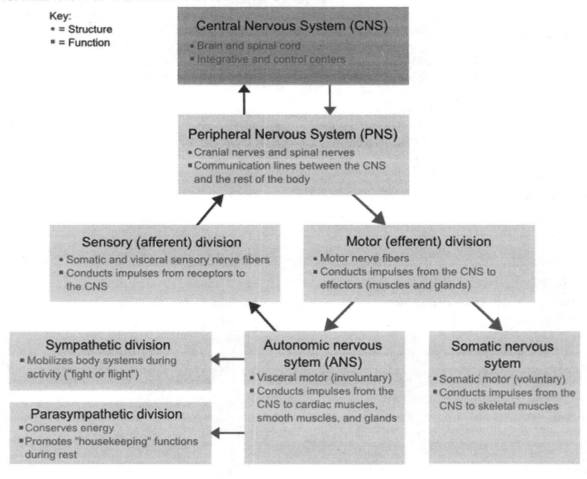

The nervous system is divided into two main parts: the central nervous system (CNS), which consists of the brain and spinal cord, and the peripheral nervous system (PNS), which consists of nervous tissues (nerves, ganglia) that are outside the CNS. The CNS integrates sensory information, and the PNS sends information to and from the CNS, allowing it to communicate with the rest of the body. Afferent neurons of the PNS transmit impulses to the CNS, and efferent neurons transmit impulses to effectors.

The PNS is further divided into the autonomic system (ANS) and somatic nervous system (SNS). The SNS controls voluntary movements, such as the contraction of skeletal muscles. The ANS controls involuntary movements, such as the contraction of smooth and cardiac muscles, and glandular secretions. The ANS has two subdivisions that tend to work antagonistically (though there are exceptions). The sympathetic division activates the "fight or flight" response, preparing the body for action by increasing heart rate, dilating pupils and bronchial tubes, and suppressing functions that are not required for immediate survival. The parasympathetic division activates the "rest and digest" functions by decreasing heart rate, constricting pupils and bronchial tubes, and promoting digestion.

SYMPATHETIC AND PARASYMPATHETIC NERVOUS SYSTEMS: ANTAGONISTIC CONTROL

The autonomic nervous system has two divisions, sympathetic and parasympathetic, and they tend to have antagonistic effects when they both innervate the same organ. Both divisions use a two-neuron pathway, consisting of a preganglionic neuron which runs from the CNS to a ganglion, and a postganglionic neuron which innervates the effector.

The sympathetic nervous division is responsible for triggering the "fight or flight" response. Preganglionic neurons of the sympathetic nervous system release acetylcholine (ACh), which is the stimulus for the release of norepinephrine from postganglionic neurons. Norepinephrine acts on target tissues, prompting a rapid and unified response. The heart rate increases, respiration rate increases, blood flow to the heart and skeletal muscle increases, pupils dilate, and glycogen is broken down.

The parasympathetic nervous division is responsible for the "rest and digest" response. *Both* pre- and postganglionic neurons of the parasympathetic nervous system release acetylcholine. The parasympathetic nervous system stimulates events that are slower-paced, and less essential for immediate survival. The heart rate and respiration rate decrease, blood flow is directed to digestive organs, peristalsis is promoted, pupils constrict, and glycogen is synthesized.

SENSOR AND EFFECTOR NEURONS

Sensory neurons are the afferent neurons that deliver impulses to the CNS. They are sometimes classified by the type of stimulus that they respond to. **Mechanoreceptors** respond to changes in pressure or tension. Cutaneous touch receptors such as Meissner's corpuscles, Merkel's disks, Pacinian corpuscles, and Ruffini endings are all mechanoreceptors, as are the muscle spindles that detect stretching of skeletal muscle and the receptors of the inner ear that detect vibrations. **Chemoreceptors** such as olfactory and taste receptors detect the presence of chemicals. **Photoreceptors** such as the rod and cone cells of the eye respond to light. **Thermoreceptors** sense both absolute temperature, and changes in temperature. **Nociceptors** detect pain.

Sensory neurons can also be categorized by location. **Exteroceptors** near the body surface transmit information about the external environment. **Proprioceptors** within the inner ear, skeletal muscles, and joints provide information about movement, position, and equilibrium. **Interoceptors** of visceral organs and blood vessels provide information about internal stimuli.

Once the sensory information has been processed, **effector neurons** (motor neurons) transmit the impulse away from the CNS to activate muscles and glands. All motor neurons of the somatic division run directly from the CNS to the effector without synapsing with another neuron. The autonomic division uses two-neuron pathways.

CENTRAL NERVOUS SYSTEM

BRAIN

The brain consists of the hindbrain, midbrain, and forebrain. The hindbrain includes the medulla oblongata, cerebellum, and pons. The midbrain integrates sensory signals and orchestrates responses to these signals. The forebrain includes the cerebrum, thalamus, and hypothalamus. The cerebral cortex is a thin layer of grey matter covering the cerebrum. The brain is divided into two hemispheres, with each responsible for multiple functions. The brain is divided into four main lobes, the frontal lobe, the parietal lobe, the occipital lobe, and the temporal lobes. The frontal lobe located in the front of the brain is responsible for a short term and working memory and information processing as well as decision-making, planning, and judgment. The parietal lobe is located slightly toward the back of the brain and the top of the head and is responsible for sensory input as well as spatial positioning of the body. The occipital lobe is located at the back of the head just above the brain stem. This lobe is responsible for visual input, processing, and output; specifically nerves from the eyes enter directly into this lobe. Finally, the temporal lobes are located at the left and right sides of the brain. These lobes are responsible for all auditory input, processing, and output.

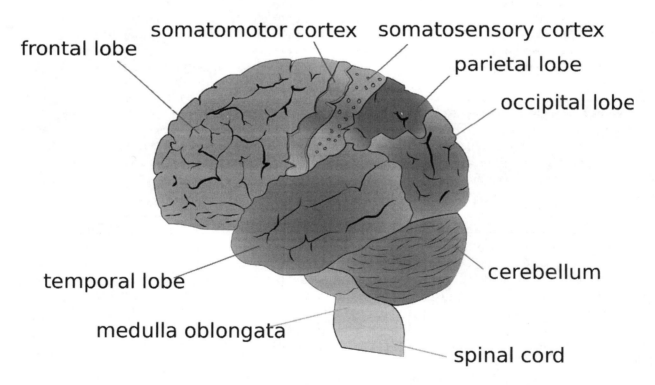

The cerebellum plays a role in the processing and storing of implicit memories. Specifically, for those memories developed during classical conditioning learning techniques. The role of the cerebellum was discovered by exploring the memory of individuals with damaged cerebellums. These individuals were unable to develop stimulus responses when presented via a classical conditioning technique. Researchers found that this was also the case for automatic responses. For example, when these individuals were presented with a puff of air into their eyes, they did not blink, which would have been the naturally occurring and automatic response in an individual with no brain damage.

The posterior area of the brain that is connected to the spinal cord is known as the brain stem. The midbrain, the pons, and the medulla oblongata are the three parts of the brain stem. Information from the body is sent to the brain through the brain stem, and information from the brain is sent to the body through the brain stem. The brain stem is an important part of respiratory, digestive, and circulatory functions.

The midbrain lies above the pons and the medulla oblongata. The parts of the midbrain include the tectum, the tegmentum, and the ventral tegmentum. The midbrain is an important part of vision and hearing. The pons comes between the midbrain and the medulla oblongata. Information is sent across the pons from the cerebrum to the medulla and the cerebellum. The medulla oblongata (or medulla) is beneath the midbrain and the pons. The medulla oblongata is the piece of the brain stem that connects the spinal cord to the brain. So, it has an important role with the autonomous nervous system in the circulatory and respiratory system.

Encased in cranial bones that form of base of the cavity and the skull cap the top, the **cranial cavity** contains the brain, the 12 cranial nerves, and the pituitary gland. The meninges (comprised of the dura mater, arachnoid mater, and pia mater) line the cavity and surround the brain and the spinal cord and contain cerebrospinal fluid between the arachnoid mater and pia mater in the subarachnoid space. The meninges and cerebrospinal fluid protect and cushion the dorsal cavity. The vascularized pia mater is adhered to the surface of the brain and the spinal cord. The middle layer, the arachnoid mater, contains connective tissue but not nerves or blood vessels. The enervated, vascularized dura mater is the outer layer that lies next to the bones and folds inward in places in the cavity and separates the brain into different compartments. The dura mater has two layers: The endosteal lines the cranial bones; the meningeal layer, which lines the endosteal layer within the cranium, lines the vertebral cavity.

CRANIAL NERVES

The cranial nerves are 12 pairs of nerves that come from the brain and brainstem and control the senses, muscles, and internal organs. Cranial nerve names, functions and types are as follows:

Nerve	What It Controls	Sensory/ Motor/Both
I Olfactory	Smell	S
II Optic	Sight	S
III Oculomotor	Moves the eye up, down, left, right and diagonally; adjusts the pupil and lens of the eye	M
IV Trochlear	Moves the eye up, down, left, right, and diagonally	M
V Trigeminal	Largest of the cranial nerves; chewing, face sensation.	B
VI Abducens	Moves the eye up, down, left, right, and diagonally	M
VII Facial	Facial expression and anterior two-thirds of the tongue	B
VIII Vestibulocochlear	Sound	S
IX Glossopharyngeal	Swallowing, saliva, and taste	B
X Vagus	Control of the peripheral nervous system	B
XI Accessory	Swallowing and movement of the head and neck	M
XII Hypoglossal	Speech and swallowing; tongue muscles	M

Mnemonic for nerve names: Oh, once one takes the anatomy final, very good vacations are heavenly.

Mnemonic for whether nerves are sensory/motor/both: Some say my mother bought my brother some bad beer, my, my.

SPINAL CORD

The spinal cord is a column of nerve fibers that connects the brain to the rest of the body. It is encased in the bony structure of the vertebrae, which protects and supports it. Its nervous tissue functions mainly with respect to limb movement and internal organ activity. Major nerve tracts ascend and descend from the spinal cord to the brain. The vertebrae and spinal cord are contained within the vertebral cavity. The meninges extend from the cranial cavity to enclose the vertebral cavity. The spinal cord is divided into 5 regions: cervical, thoracic, lumbar, sacral, and coccyx.

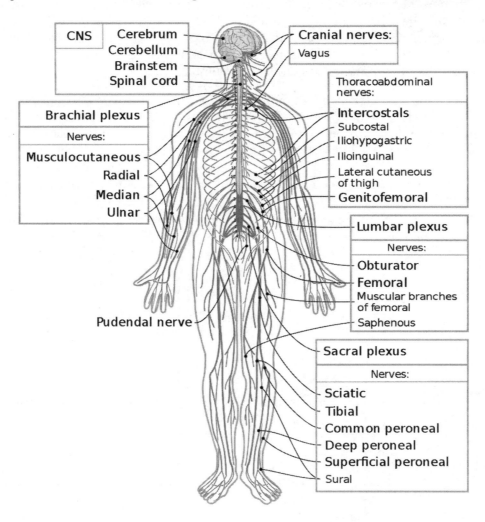

ROLE OF SPINAL CORD AND SUPRASPINAL CIRCUITS

The spinal cord is a major reflex center that connects the afferent and efferent pathways. It is made of an exterior layer of white matter that surrounds an interior core of grey matter. The white matter consists of glial cells and myelinated bundles of axons that form tracts to and from the brain. There are no cell bodies or dendrites in white matter. Grey matter consists mostly of interneurons, but also contains motor neurons and glial cells. (The axons are mostly unmyelinated, giving the tissue its grey appearance.) The cell bodies of afferent neurons reside in dorsal root ganglia, just outside the spinal cord. Afferent fibers enter into the posterior/dorsal aspect of the spinal cord (a region called the posterior grey horn) through the anterior root, while efferent fibers exit on the anterior/ventral aspect (the anterior grey horn) through the posterior root. Spinal neurons usually innervate structures that are inferior to the neck.

Not all reflexes are mediated by spinal neurons. Supraspinal circuits require input from the brain or brainstem, and are involved in actions such as the blinking and gagging reflexes.

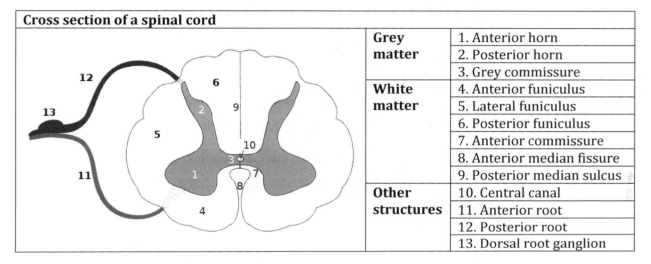

Cross section of a spinal cord		
Grey matter	1. Anterior horn	
	2. Posterior horn	
	3. Grey commissure	
White matter	4. Anterior funiculus	
	5. Lateral funiculus	
	6. Posterior funiculus	
	7. Anterior commissure	
	8. Anterior median fissure	
	9. Posterior median sulcus	
Other structures	10. Central canal	
	11. Anterior root	
	12. Posterior root	
	13. Dorsal root ganglion	

REFLEXES

A **reflex** is a nearly instantaneous, unconscious, and involuntary response to a stimulus. The stimulus (for example, the sensation of heat when one touches a hot stove) is detected by the receptors of afferent neurons, and sensory information is sent to interneurons in the spinal cord. (Interneurons are entirely restricted to the central nervous system, and act as bridges between sensory and motor neurons.) From here, the signal travels along motor neurons to the effectors (the muscles of the arm and hand). Before the signal for pain has reached the brain, the hand has already been withdrawn. While reflexes do not require conscious thought, some have pathways that involve the brain. The brain can sometimes override reflex actions - for example, trying not to blink during an eye exam. Sometimes, a reflex involves a direct link between the sensory and motor neuron - for example, the patellar reflex, or knee-jerk reaction. This is referred to as a monosynaptic reflex. Polysynaptic reflexes are more complex because they involve interneurons.

FEEDBACK LOOP, REFLEX ARC

A reflex arc describes a neural pathway that triggers a reflex action. It begins with a **receptor** - the site or organ that receives the stimulus. A **sensory neuron** carries the impulse along the afferent pathway to the **integration center** within the central nervous system. Interneurons process the information and pass the impulse to a **motor neuron**. The impulse travels along the efferent pathway to the **effector** - the responding muscle or gland.

Most reflexes attempt to maintain homeostasis by inhibiting a change in condition; this is called negative feedback. The maintenance of body temperature is one of many examples. As body temperature changes, thermoreceptors send information to the hypothalamus. If body temperature is too high, a command is sent to dilate blood vessels and release sweat. If the temperature is too low, the body shivers and blood vessels constrict. Positive feedback loops are less common, and sometimes harmful because they enhance the stimuli rather than inhibit them. A beneficial form of positive feedback occurs during childbirth. When the cervix is stretched by the descending fetus, impulses are sent to the pituitary, which sends a command to increase uterine contractions. The more the fetus is pushed, the more the cervix stretches. This positive feedback loop continues until birth.

PRIMITIVE REFLEXES

A **primitive reflex** is an involuntary reaction to a stimulus. Reflexes develop in utero and become integrated as we age. If a primitive reflex has not integrated and disappeared by a certain age, that is often seen as a sign of a neurological issue or brain damage. There are seven primitive reflexes seen in a newborn.

Reflex	Characteristics	Integrated
Moro	Early fight-or-flight reflex. It is stimulated by a sudden lack of support when the baby feels as though it is falling. This is tested by holding the torso and head of the baby off the exam table and then letting the head and shoulders drop quickly several inches. The baby will look startled, extend its arms and legs out, bring them back in, and cry.	3 months
Rooting	Present even before birth. When the baby is stimulated by a touch to the cheek on either side, the baby will turn his head to that direction in preparation to suck.	4 months
Palmar	This is caused when the baby's palm is stimulated. The baby will make a fist and grasp the object, and the fist will tighten as you try to remove the object.	6 months
Plantar/Babinski Reflex	The bottom of the foot is stroked firmly moving from the heel to the toes. The big toe bends back toward the foot, and the toes splay out.	2 years
Asymmetrical Tonic Neck Reflex	This is known as the fencing reflex. When the baby is on his back and his head is turned to one side, the arm and leg extend in the direction that the baby is facing and the other arm and leg flex.	3 months
Spinal Galant Reflex	The baby is on her stomach and is stimulated firmly on one side of her spine in a downward motion. The hips will laterally flex toward the stimulus. This is thought to assist in rolling and crawling.	9 months
Symmetrical Tonic Neck Reflex	The chin of the baby is tipped to his chest. The arms flex, and the legs will extend. Present at birth then disappears and returns at 6 months.	11 months to 1 year.

INTEGRATION WITH ENDOCRINE SYSTEM: FEEDBACK CONTROL

The nervous system is closely integrated with the endocrine system. Both systems control the body - the nervous system through electrical impulses, and the endocrine system though slower-acting, but longer-lasting hormones. The two systems are linked via the hypothalamus, a region in the brain that controls the autonomic nervous system as well as the pituitary gland. In fact, neurons within the hypothalamus have axons that extend through the infundibulum and terminate in the posterior pituitary. The hypothalamus produces oxytocin and antidiuretic hormone (ADH), but these hormones are stored in and secreted by the posterior pituitary. The release of other important hormones from the anterior pituitary is also regulated by the hypothalamus. Pituitary hormones go on to control other endocrine glands and body functions. Hormones travel through the bloodstream to target tissues, eliciting responses that are important for growth, development, metabolism, and the maintenance of homeostasis. An example of the interaction between the two systems can be seen in the letdown of milk during nursing. As a baby begins to nurse, the stimulus sends an impulse to the hypothalamus, causing the pituitary to release oxytocin into the blood. The hormone targets the mammary gland, inducing it to release milk.

NERVE CELL

CELL BODY: SITE OF NUCLEUS, ORGANELLES

The cell body, or soma, of a neuron contains the organelles that are responsible for the metabolic activities of the neuron. The interior of the cell body contains a nucleus with a prominent nucleolus. The DNA within the nucleus encodes the information for the many proteins that are needed for the neuron to function. The neuronal cytoplasm contains most of the organelles that are characteristic of animal cells (cytoskeleton, rough and smooth endoplasmic reticulum, Golgi bodies, lysosomes, peroxisomes, and mitochondria). There are relatively high numbers of mitochondria to support the high metabolic needs of the neuron. Granular Nissl bodies (made of rough ER and clusters of free ribosomes) synthesize proteins for use within the cell. Notably absent in mature neurons are centrioles, as differentiated neurons have lost their ability to divide.

Various projections (dendrites and/or an axon) extend from the cell body, and neurons can be classified according to these structural differences.

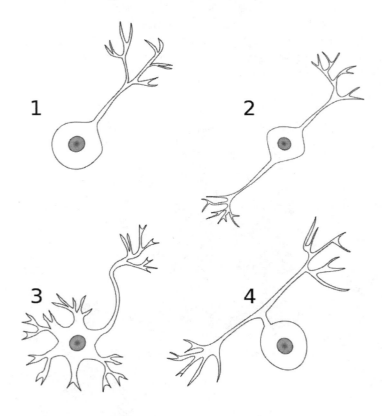

1: unipolar (many sensory neurons are unipolar)

2: bipolar (rare - associated with retina and inner ear)

3: multipolar (most common - interneurons and motor neurons)

4: pseudounipolar (sensory neurons)

DENDRITES: BRANCHED EXTENSIONS OF CELL BODY

Dendrites are relatively short, branched extensions of the cell body that receive incoming chemical signals (neurotransmitters) from the other neurons. These tree-like projections taper with every branch, maximizing the surface area for synaptic inputs. Many dendrites have tiny protrusions called dendritic spines that synapse with a single axon. The cytoplasm within the dendrites contains the same organelles as the cell body, with the exception of the nucleus.

The neurotransmitters that are released from axon terminals of the presynaptic cell cross the synaptic cleft, where they bind to receptor sites on the dendrites of the postsynaptic cells. These signals may be excitatory or inhibitory, and the net effect of these signals determines whether the neuron is inhibited or triggered to fire (in which case the chemical message will be converted to an electrical impulse that travels down the axon).

AXON: STRUCTURE AND FUNCTION

An axon is a smooth, cable-like nerve fiber that is specialized to conduct electrical impulses away from the soma. Most neurons have one long axon, but the axon's length can vary, and some neurons have no axon at all. The axon emerges from a slightly elevated structure called the **axon hillock** that connects the soma to the axon. The cytoplasm of the axon is called **axoplasm**, and it lacks the Golgi bodies, Nissl bodies, and ribosomes found in dendritic cytoplasm. Since there is little to no translation, proteins must be imported from the soma. The axon often splits into **collaterals** that allow one neuron to interact with more than one cell. At the end of each axon are highly branched structures called **axon terminals**. These club-shaped endings contain synaptic vesicles filled with neurotransmitters. When an action potential is generated at the axon hillock, it propagates along the axon. When it reaches the axon terminals, the neurotransmitters are released to a target cell.

MYELIN SHEATH, SCHWANN CELLS, INSULATION OF AXON

The axons of many neurons are sheathed in a lipid-based coating called **myelin**. Myelin insulates the axon much like the coating on electrical wire. It also increases the rate at which an impulse can travel. There are intermittent gaps in the sheath called nodes of Ranvier that allow the impulse to jump quickly from one node to the next.

Neurons of the peripheral nervous system are myelinated by **Schwann cells**. These glial cells curve around the axon, wrapping their plasma membranes around it like a bandage to form multiple lipid-rich layers. The nucleus and cytoplasm remain outside the myelin sheath, but are encased in the outer **neurilemmal** sheath of the Schwann cell. Axons of very small diameter may be supported by Schwann cells, but are not myelinated by them. These are called non-myelinating Schwann cells. **Oligodendrocytes** are responsible for sheathing the neurons of the central nervous system. Unlike Schwann cells, a single oligodendrocyte can myelinate dozens of axons by extending its membrane in multiple directions and wrapping around the axons. White matter of the CNS is made mostly of myelinated axons, while the axons associated with grey matter are unmyelinated.

Multiple sclerosis, the leukodystrophies, and many other diseases result from damaged myelin. Without the proper insulation, the neurons of affected individuals cannot effectively conduct an impulse.

NODES OF RANVIER: PROPAGATION OF NERVE IMPULSE ALONG AXON

Nodes of Ranvier are uninsulated gaps between myelinated portions of the axon that increase the rate of conduction. These exposed portions are about 1 μm in length, and they contain a high density of voltage gated sodium and potassium channels. The channels open to allow the passage of these ions, depolarizing the membrane. Since ions are unable to diffuse through the myelin, the action potential must jump to the next node. This is called **saltatory propagation**. This type of conduction is faster and more efficient than the continuous conduction that is seen along the entire length of an unsheathed axon. Large-diameter myelinated axons conduct impulses much faster (80–120 m/s) than thin unmyelinated axons (0.5–10 m/s). While rapid conduction has its benefits, myelinated axons have less neuroplasticity than unmyelinated axons; that is, they are more limited in their ability to form new connections with other neurons.

GLIAL CELLS, NEUROGLIA

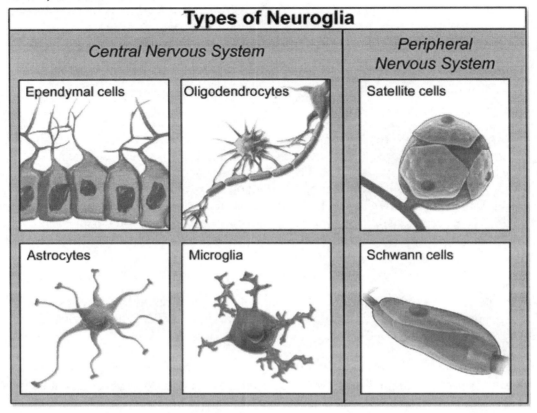

Types of Neuroglia

Central Nervous System

Ependymal cells

Oligodendrocytes

Astrocytes

Microglia

Peripheral Nervous System

Satellite cells

Schwann cells

Glial cells, also called neuroglia, support and protect neurons within the central and peripheral nervous system. Despite their inability to conduct impulses, there are many more glial cells than neurons within nervous tissue. Glia also have the ability to divide, and so nearly all brain tumors arise from them.

	Glial Cell	Characteristics	Function
CNS	Astrocytes	The most abundant cells found in neural tissue	Anchor neurons and facilitate exchange of materials between capillaries and neurons Uptake excess ions and neurotransmitters
	Microglia	Relatively few extensions	Phagocytic - immune defense, digest dead neurons and debris
	Oligodendrocytes	Extensions wrap around axons of CNS neurons	Produce myelin sheaths that insulate CNS neurons and speed up neurotransmission
	Ependyma	Form the epithelial lining of the ventricles and central canal of the spinal cord	Circulate cerebrospinal fluid (CSF) and facilitate exchange of materials between the CSF and interstitial fluid of brain and spinal cord
PNS	Schwann cells	Extensive lipid membranes wrap around PNS axons to form layers	Produce the myelin sheaths that insulate PNS neurons Speed up neurotransmission
	Satellite cells	Surround the soma of neurons within PNS ganglia	Protect and cushion PNS neurons

Synapse: Site of Impulse Propagation Between Cells

A **synapse** is a communicating junction between two neurons, or between a neuron and an effector (muscle or gland). The synapse consists of a presynaptic element, a tiny gap called the synaptic cleft, and a postsynaptic element. Impulses are transmitted across the synaptic cleft through the action of neurotransmitters. Synapses can be classified according to the nature of the postsynaptic element. **Axodendritic** synapses terminate on the dendrites of a postsynaptic neuron. **Axosomatic** synapses terminate on a postsynaptic soma. **Axoaxonic** synapses are rare, terminating on a postsynaptic axon.

They can also be classified by the mode in which the impulse is transmitted. Most synapses are unidirectional **chemical** junctions, using neurotransmitters to send messages to the postsynaptic cell. When the impulse reaches the axon terminals, the vesicles that store the neurotransmitters fuse with the plasma membrane, releasing the signals into the synaptic cleft before they bind to receptors on the postsynaptic target. At this point, the postsynaptic membrane will either be excited (depolarized) or inhibited (hyperpolarized). Bidirectional **electrical** synaptic junctions do not use neurotransmitters. They are linked by gap junctions that allow the flow of ions between cells. Electrical synapses are faster, always excitatory, and more rare.

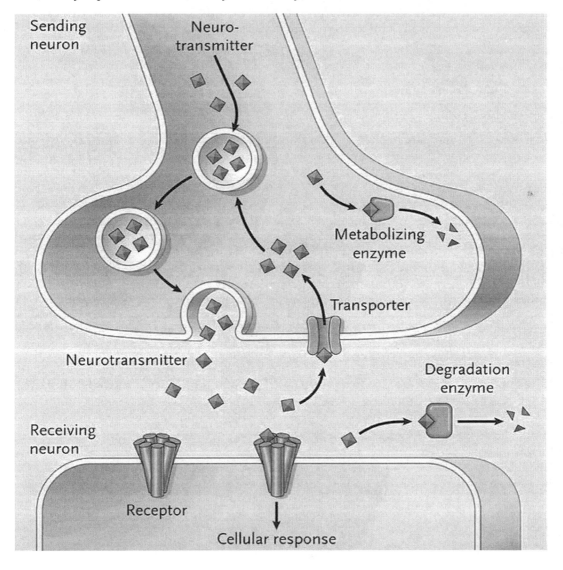

When an action potential reaches the axon terminal, voltage-gated calcium channels open in response to the depolarization of the membrane. Calcium ions enter, triggering the release of neurotransmitters by exocytosis. The neurotransmitters diffuse across the synaptic cleft, binding to receptors in the target cell and eliciting either an excitatory or an inhibitory response. The neurotransmitters are then recycled back to the presynaptic cell, are degraded by enzymes, or diffuse away from the synaptic cleft to prevent overstimulation.

Common neurotransmitters and their actions are summarized below:

Neurotransmitter	Action
Acetylcholine (ACh)	Stimulates skeletal muscle
Norepinephrine (NE)	Influences mood and sleep patterns
Dopamine	Associated with mood, attention, reward system, and movement
Histamine	Works with the hypothalamus, promotes wakefulness
Serotonin	Many roles–mostly inhibitory. Influences sleep, mood, hunger, arousal
GABA	The major inhibitory neurotransmitter
Glutamate	The major excitatory neurotransmitter

Muscular System

IMPORTANT FUNCTIONS

SUPPORT: MOBILITY

The muscle system is made up of skeletal, smooth, and cardiac muscles that contract to produce nearly all body movements. Skeletal muscles are used for voluntary actions. Walking, jumping, smiling, eye movements, and the maintenance of posture are all under the control of the somatic nervous system. The muscles that coordinate voluntary movements are attached to bone by tendons, and the bone is moved when the muscle shortens. Skeletal muscles also work with the tendons, ligaments, and bone to support and stabilize the joints.

Contraction of smooth muscle is involuntary, and therefore under autonomic control. Smooth muscle in the gastrointestinal tract contracts rhythmically to propel food along the gastrointestinal tract. This is called peristalsis. Blood pressure is regulated by contraction and relaxation of the smooth muscle within the vessel wall. Vasoconstriction increases blood pressure and decreases blood flow, while vasodilation decreases blood pressure and increases blood flow. Cardiac muscle of the heart contracts to pump blood throughout the body.

PERIPHERAL CIRCULATORY ASSISTANCE

The return of blood to the heart is assisted by a system called the **skeletal muscle pump**. Large peripheral veins in the legs and arms have valves that prevent the backflow of blood. When the skeletal muscles around these deep veins contract, the vessel is compressed, and blood is forced through the valves in the direction of the heart. Exercising these muscle groups increases the rate of blood flow.

The **thoracic pump** also facilitates venous return. During inspiration, contraction of the diaphragm and intercostal muscles expands the thoracic cavity. The increased volume results in a decrease in pressure, which is transmitted to the right atrium. This drop in pressure helps the blood to return to the heart. Also, when the pressure in the thoracic cavity decreases, the pressure in the abdominal cavity increases, squeezing the blood in the inferior vena cava toward the heart.

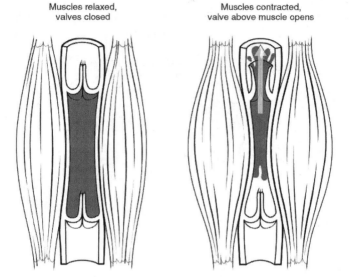

Muscles relaxed,
valves closed

Muscles contracted,
valve above muscle opens

THERMOREGULATION (SHIVERING REFLEX)

When thermoreceptors detect a drop in temperature, impulses are sent to the posterior hypothalamus, which then sends signals to the effectors. Smooth muscles in the walls of the cutaneous arterioles contract involuntarily to reduce the blood flow near the surface of the skin. This minimizes heat loss to the environment. Arrector pili muscles also contract, causing hairs to stand on end in an attempt to trap warm air. If the core body temperature drops, the shivering reflex is triggered by the posterior hypothalamus. Shivering is involuntary shuddering, caused by the rapid contracting and relaxing of skeletal muscles. Contraction of these muscles requires the hydrolysis of ATP, and this exothermic reaction releases energy in the form of heat. Some heat is also generated as a result of friction between the sliding filaments of the muscle.

When thermoreceptors detect a rise in temperature, the anterior hypothalamus tells the smooth muscles that surround cutaneous arterioles to relax. Vasodilation allows more blood to flow near the surface of the skin, and heat is lost to the environment.

MOVEMENT

SAGITTAL PLANE OF MOTION

The sagittal plane passes through the body from front to back, dividing the body into left and right sides.

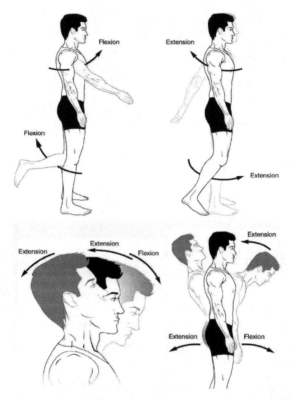

Flexion	Decrease the angle between two body parts (bending the elbow)
Extension	Increasing the angle between two body parts (straightening the elbow)
Dorsiflexion	Ankle flexion (moving the toes toward the shin)
Plantar flexion	Ankle extension (moving the toes toward the ground/pointing the toes)

FRONTAL PLANE OF MOTION

The frontal plane passes through the body from left to right, dividing the body into anterior and posterior.

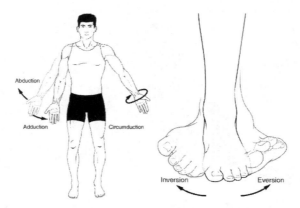

Adduction	Movement toward the midline/to the body (bringing the arm to the body).
Abduction	Moving away from the midline Think of someone being abducted or taken away (moving the arm away from the body).
Elevation	Scapula movement, superior movement (shoulder shrug).
Depression	Scapula movement, inferior movement (shoulder shrug).
Inversion	Lifting the medial border of the foot. Bring the sole of the foot to face inward.
Eversion	Lifting the lateral border of the foot. Bring the sole of the foot to face outward.

TRANSVERSE PLANE OF MOTION

The transverse plane passes through the body in a line parallel to the floor, dividing the body into top and bottom.

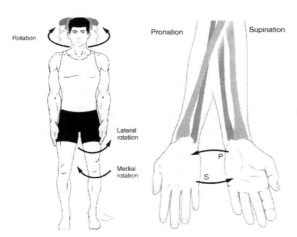

Pronation	Rotating the hand and wrist medially from the bone. If laying on the back, the hand would have the palm to the floor.
Supination	Rotating the hand and wrist laterally from the bone. If laying on the back, the palm and wrist would be facing toward the ceiling.
Horizontal adduction	The angle between two joints decreases on the horizontal plane.
Horizontal abduction	The angle between two joints increases on the horizontal plane.
Rotation	Pivoting or twisting on the axis (turning the head left or right).

MAJOR MUSCLES OF THE BODY

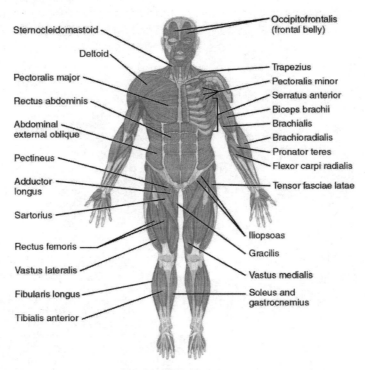

Major muscles of the body.
Right side: superficial; left side:
deep (anterior view)

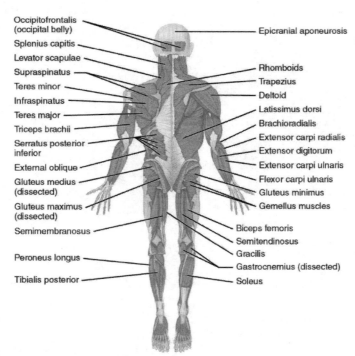

Major muscles of the body.
Right side: superficial; left side:
deep (posterior view)

STRUCTURE OF THREE BASIC MUSCLE TYPES: STRIATED, SMOOTH, CARDIAC

Skeletal muscle is under somatic (voluntary) control and does not display myogenic activity. (Skeletal muscles require external stimulation to contract.) They are involved in the movement of bone, support, thermoregulation, and venous return to the heart. These muscles are **striated**; the muscle fibers have alternating regions of light and dark bands. A single skeletal myocyte is cylinder-shaped and has many nuclei.

Smooth muscle is under autonomic (involuntary) control and is capable of using myogenic mechanisms to contract (independent of nervous stimulation). Smooth muscle tissue is found in the walls of hollow organs and vessels, and aids in the movement of substances such as food and blood. The cells are spindle-shaped, non-striated, and uninucleated.

Like smooth muscle, cardiac muscle is under autonomic control and exhibits myogenic activity. Cardiac muscle tissue is found in the walls of the heart, and is required for the pumping of blood. The cells are branched, striated, and usually uninucleate (but may have two nuclei). They are connected to each other by intercalated discs with gap junctions that allow the cells to communicate.

MUSCLE STRUCTURE AND CONTROL OF CONTRACTION

T-TUBULE SYSTEM

Transverse tubules, or **T-tubules**, are tunnel-like invaginations of the **sarcolemma** - the plasma membrane of striated muscle cells. The membranes of this system contain a high concentration of ion channels, allowing them to play an important role in muscle contraction. When an action potential propagates along the sarcolemma, the T-tubules help to depolarize the cell by carrying the impulse to the **sarcoplasmic reticulum** (SR) that surrounds the **myofibrils** in a muscle cell. The SR is a form of smooth endoplasmic reticulum that is specialized to store and release calcium ions. The t-tubules are sandwiched between two enlarged chambers of the SR called **terminal cisternae**. This "sandwich" makes up a structure called the **triad**. When the impulse reaches the SR, the calcium channels in the SR membrane open, releasing calcium ions that ultimately cause contraction of the muscle. ATP-powered calcium pumps within the SR membrane pump Ca^{2+} back into the SR to relax the muscle.

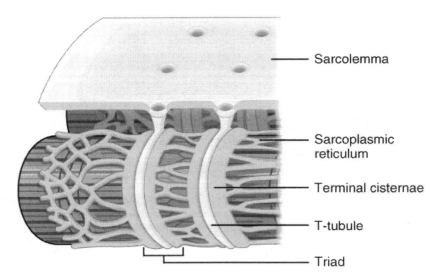

CONTRACTILE APPARATUS

The **contractile apparatus** describes a unit within muscle tissue that is specialized for contraction. The structure of the contractile apparatus is similar among striated muscle tissues, and consists of a repeating unit called a **sarcomere**. Tens of thousands of these sarcomeres lie end to end to form a **myofibril**. One sarcomere is separated from another by a boundary called the **Z line**, where a network of proteins serves as a point of anchorage for **actin** (thin filaments). Six thin filaments surround a single thick myosin filament. The filaments themselves do not change length during contraction; their arrangement allows them to slide over each other when myosin heads pull on the thin filaments, causing the sarcomeres to shorten, and the muscle to contract. Note that while smooth muscle cells do contain actin and myosin, the filaments are disorganized, and no sarcomeres are present.

CONTRACTILE VELOCITY OF DIFFERENT MUSCLE TYPES

There are three main types of skeletal muscle fibers: slow-twitch oxidative (SO - type I), fast-twitch oxidative-glycolytic (FOG - type IIa), and fast-twitch glycolytic (FG - type IIb). Most muscles consist of an even blend of these fibers, but the proportions vary in certain muscles, depending on function. For example, muscles associated with maintaining posture will have a high percentage of slow-twitch fibers, while muscles in the lower legs of a sprinter will have a high percentage of fast-twitch fibers.

The characteristics of each type of fiber are summarized in the following table:

	Slow Twitch, Type I	**Fast Twitch, Type IIa**	**Fast Twitch, Type IIb**
Fiber Diameter	Smaller	Intermediate	Larger
Capillary density	High	Moderate	Low
Myoglobin Concentration / Color	High / Red	Moderate / Red-Pink	Low / White
Metabolism	High aerobic capacity, low anaerobic capacity	Both aerobic and anaerobic capabilities	Low aerobic capacity, high anaerobic capacity
Concentration of Mitochondria	High	Moderate	Low
Resistance to Fatigue	High	Moderate	Low
Contractile Velocity	Slow	Rapid	Rapid
Force Production	Low	Moderate	High
General Use	Prolonged, low-intensity aerobic activities / maintenance of posture	Moderate intensity activities, such as running	Short bursts of activity, such as sprinting or heavy lifting

REGULATION OF CARDIAC MUSCLE CONTRACTION

Cardiac muscle demonstrates myogenic activity. The pacemaker cells of the sinoatrial (SA) node of the heart generate their own action potential, which then travels to the atrioventricular (AV) node (the secondary pacemaker), the bundle of His, the bundle branches, and finally the Purkinje fibers. Gap junctions between adjacent cardiac cells facilitate the transmission of the action potential from one cell to the next. As the impulse travels through the sarcolemma of a cardiac muscle cell, voltage-gated calcium ion channels open, allowing the entry of extracellular Ca^{2+}. The inflow of Ca^{2+} triggers the release of even more Ca^{2+} from the sarcoplasmic reticulum. Calcium ions cause the cardiac muscle to contract in a similar manner to skeletal muscle cells (the sliding filament mechanism). Note that skeletal muscle cells do not generate their own action potential, and the action potential is more prolonged in cardiac cells.

While the heart is autorhythmic, the muscle contraction is further regulated by the autonomic nervous system. Sympathetic stimulation increases heart rate, while parasympathetic stimulation (the vagus nerve) decreases heart rate. The endocrine system influences heart rate as well. Epinephrine secreted from the adrenal medulla and thyroxine from the thyroid gland both increase heart rate.

OXYGEN DEBT: FATIGUE

Oxygen debt is the amount of oxygen required to restore metabolic conditions to resting levels. Muscle activity is powered by the hydrolysis of ATP. In a resting state, aerobic respiration provides enough ATP for muscles to function. Stored ATP is quickly used up during intense exercise, and a molecule called **creatine phosphate** phosphorylates ADP to produce ATP. Anaerobic respiration also supplies ATP relatively quickly, but only for a short amount of time. If oxygen is available, aerobic respiration synthesizes ATP. When oxygen levels become depleted, **lactic acid** (a byproduct of anaerobic respiration) begins to accumulate. The buildup of lactic acid, along with the depletion of ATP and oxygen, causes muscle fatigue. Lactic acid that does not remain in the muscles is brought to the liver, where it is converted into glucose. The amount of oxygen required to accomplish this task, and to replenish the levels of ATP and creatine phosphate, is called oxygen debt.

NERVOUS CONTROL

SYMPATHETIC AND PARASYMPATHETIC INNERVATION

Involuntary muscle tissues (smooth, cardiac) are innervated by motor neurons of the sympathetic and parasympathetic divisions of the autonomic nervous system. Motor pathways of the ANS consist of *two* neurons: a preganglionic and a postganglionic neuron. The cell body of a preganglionic neuron resides in the central nervous system and synapses with the cell body of one or more postganglionic neurons within an autonomic ganglion. Postganglionic nerve fibers are shorter than presynaptic fibers, and they extend to the effectors. *Pre*ganglionic neurons of both the sympathetic and parasympathetic systems release acetylcholine (ACh). *Post*ganglionic neurons of the parasympathetic division release ACh, but those of the sympathetic division release norepinephrine (NE).

In general, the sympathetic and parasympathetic systems tend to have antagonistic effects on the muscles (and glands) they innervate. The sympathetic division induces a fight or flight response, which causes the heart rate and blood pressure to increase, and blood to be diverted away from the digestive system. The parasympathetic division induces a rest and digest response, which causes the heart rate and blood pressure to decrease, and promotes digestion.

VOLUNTARY AND INVOLUNTARY MUSCLES

The peripheral nervous system is divided into the somatic and autonomic nervous systems. Voluntary muscles are composed of skeletal muscle tissue and are under the control of the somatic nervous system. Most voluntary muscles are connected to bone. These muscles usually contract in response to a conscious thought process, but they are also involved in certain involuntary reflexes, such as the knee jerk reflex. The motor cortex of the brain is responsible for generating most of the nerve impulses that initiate voluntary movements.

Involuntary muscles are innervated by motor neurons of the autonomic nervous system. These muscles include the smooth muscles found in the walls of hollow organs such as the intestines and blood vessels, as well as the cardiac muscle of the heart. The lower part of the brainstem called the medulla oblongata sends signals to involuntary muscles that play a role in digestion, vasodilation/vasoconstriction, heart rate, respiratory rate, and other visceral functions.

MOTOR NEURONS, NEUROMUSCULAR JUNCTION, MOTOR END PLATES

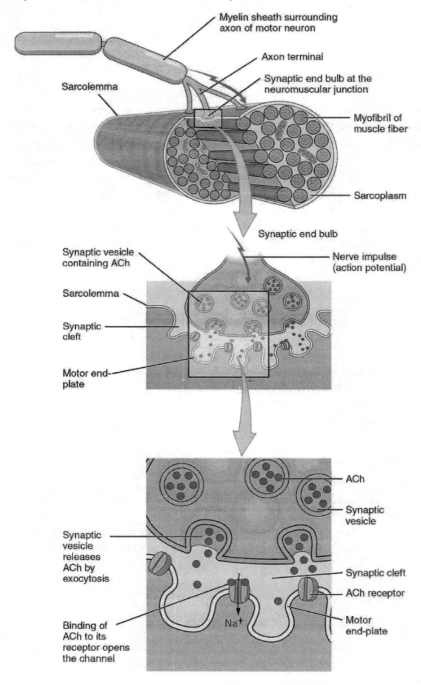

The stimulus for skeletal muscle cell contraction comes from motor neurons, and the synapse between the neuron and muscle cell is called the **neuromuscular junction**. A single motor neuron can form synapses with multiple muscle cells. The neuron and the muscle cells that it innervates are collectively called a **motor unit**. This arrangement allows a large group of cells to contract together. All the motor neurons that innervate the same muscle make up a **motor pool**.

When an action potential reaches an axon terminal, voltage-gated calcium ions in the membrane are opened, and Ca^{2+} enters. These ions bind to synaptic vesicles that store acetylcholine (ACh), causing them to fuse with the membrane and release ACh into the synaptic cleft. ACh binds to nicotinic receptors on a folded portion of the sarcolemma known as the motor end plate. The permeability of the muscle cell changes, and the cell depolarizes. The action potential is taken into the muscle cell via T-tubules, causing calcium channels in the sarcoplasmic reticulum to open. The release of calcium into the sarcoplasm causes the muscle to contract.

Reproductive System

MALE AND FEMALE REPRODUCTIVE STRUCTURES AND THEIR FUNCTIONS

MALE GENITALIA

The internal male genitalia include the epididymides, vasa deferentia, and accessory glands including the seminal vesicles, prostate gland, and Cowper's glands (the bulbourethral glands). The **epididymis** is a convoluted tube attached to the outside of a testicle that nourishes sperm as they finish maturing, and stores them until ejaculation. From here the sperm pass through the **vas deferens** (sperm duct), **ejaculatory duct**, and **urethra**, and exit through the penis. The **seminal vesicles** secrete fluid into the ejaculatory duct that makes up roughly 60% of the volume of semen. The contents of this mildly alkaline fluid include fructose, prostaglandins, and proteins. Secretions of the **prostate gland** (about 30% of semen volume) nourish the sperm and increase their motility. **Cowper's glands** secrete a lubricating fluid that makes up 2–5% of semen volume.

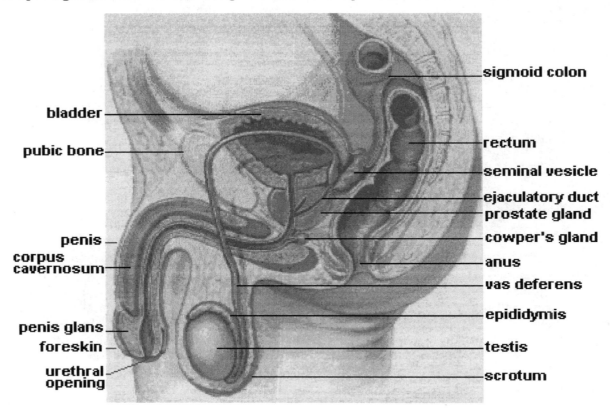

The external male genitalia include the penis and scrotum. The **penis** is the erectile organ responsible for delivering sperm to the female. It consists of three cylinders of spongy tissue: a pair of **corpora cavernosa** and the **corpus spongiosum** that surrounds the urethra. The **scrotum** is the sac that protects the sperm-producing testes and keeps them at the proper temperature.

FEMALE GENITALIA

The internal female genitalia include the ovaries, the fallopian tubes, the uterus, and the vagina. The **ovaries** produce oocytes, and also secrete sex hormones. When an oocyte is released during ovulation, it is "captured" by the **fallopian tube**, also known as the uterine tube or oviduct, which is not directly connected to the ovaries. Fertilization typically occurs in the fallopian tube, and implantation of the fertilized egg usually occurs in the endometrium of the uterus. The **uterus** is a muscular, pear-shaped organ that nourishes and protects the developing embryo. The neck of the uterus that opens to the vagina is called the **cervix**. The **vagina** is a muscular canal that receives the penis during intercourse. During childbirth, the baby passes through the vagina - also called the birth canal.

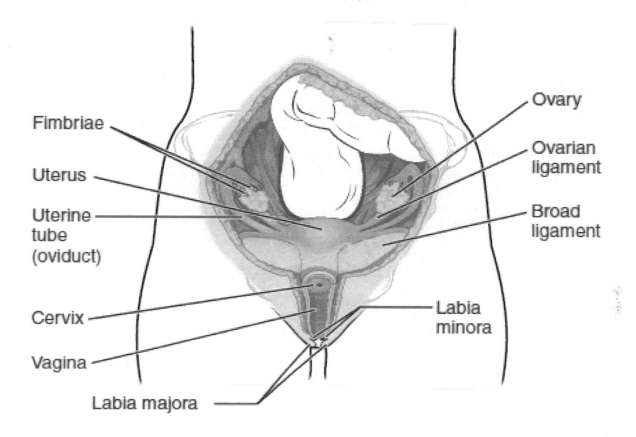

The external female genitalia include the structures of the **vulva**. These include the mons pubis, the labia majora and labia minora, Bartholin's glands, and the clitoris. The **mons pubis** is a mound of fatty tissue that lies over the pubic bone. The skin folds that form the **labia** help to protect the more delicate tissues beneath. **Bartholin's glands** produce a fluid that lubricates the vagina. The **clitoris** consists of erectile tissue full of nerve endings that contribute to sexual arousal.

GONADS

The gonads are the components of the reproductive system that produce gametes (sex cells) and secrete hormones. The male gonads are the **testes**. These structures are housed in the scrotum and encapsulated by a fibrous layer of connective tissue called the **tunica albuginea**. Thin layers of tissue extend from the tunica albuginea and divide the testes into 250 to 300 compartments called **lobules**. Each lobule contains –one to four **seminiferous tubules** - the sites of spermatogenesis. The epithelial lining of these tubules consists of the **spermatogenic cells** that give rise to sperm, as well the cells that nourish them (**sustentacular cells**, also called **Sertoli cells**). **Interstitial cells** (**Leydig cells**) around the seminiferous tubules produce testosterone, which stimulates the production of sperm. The seminiferous tubules join together to form a network of channels called the **rete testis** that bring maturing sperm cells to the **efferent ducts** where they exit the testes and enter the **epididymis**.

The female gonads are the **ovaries**. Ovaries are oval-shaped structures that rest in slight depressions on either side of the uterus known as the **ovarian fossae**, and they are held in position by several peritoneal ligaments. Each ovary is covered by two types of tissue: a layer of simple cuboidal epithelium known as the **germinal epithelium**, and the underlying **tunica albuginea**. The ovary is subdivided into the outer cortex and the inner medulla. The **cortex** has a granular appearance due to the presence of thousands of nourishing **follicles** in various stages of development. Each of these saclike follicles contains an oocyte. Initially, the oocyte is surrounded by a single layer of **follicular cells**, but as the follicle matures, the cells give rise to a multi-layer of estrogen-producing **granulosa cells**. After ovulation, a gland called the **corpus luteum** forms, and it secretes progesterone and small amounts of estrogen. This gland disappears unless pregnancy occurs. The interior of the ovary, or **medulla**, is made of loose areolar connective tissue, and contains many blood vessels, lymphatic vessels, and nerves that enter and leave through the **hilum**.

DIFFERENCES BETWEEN MALE AND FEMALE STRUCTURES

Many of the structures within the male and female reproductive are "homologous" to each other because they share a common developmental pathway. But these structures become specialized for different roles in reproduction.

The male reproductive system is designed to produce sperm and deliver it to the female for fertilization. Most of the male reproductive structures are external, which helps to keep the sperm at the optimal temperature. The testes produce much higher levels of testosterone than female gonads, and they produce millions of gametes per day after puberty. The male urethra is a common passageway for both urine and semen.

In contrast, the female reproductive system is designed to nurture a developing embryo. The reproductive structures are housed internally. The ovaries produce much higher levels of estrogen than male gonads. They contain all of the oocytes that they will ever have before birth, and only one is released per month during ovulation. The female urethra is not connected to the reproductive system.

SEXUAL DEVELOPMENT

Sex determination occurs at birth; two X chromosomes will give rise to a female, and XY gives rise to a male. The SRY gene on the Y chromosomes is responsible for the development of the male reproductive organs and the repression of female reproductive organs. In the absence of the Y chromosome, the embryo will be female. **Wolffian ducts** give rise to male internal reproductive structures, and **Mullerian ducts** give rise to female internal reproductive structures. As one system develops, the other is broken down. Seven weeks after conception, the differences in external genitalia become evident. At puberty, there is a surge in development as the hypothalamus releases gonadotropin releasing hormone (GnRH). This triggers the secretion of luteinizing hormone (LH) and follicle stimulating hormone (FSH) from the anterior pituitary gland. These gonadotropins increase the production of sex hormones, which allow the male and female reproductive organs to mature. Spermatogenesis begins in males, and ovulation and menstruation begin in females. Secondary sex characteristics emerge as well. Males develop facial, axillary, and pubic hair, and the voice deepens as the larynx grows. Females develop pubic hair and begin to ovulate and menstruate, and the hips become wider.

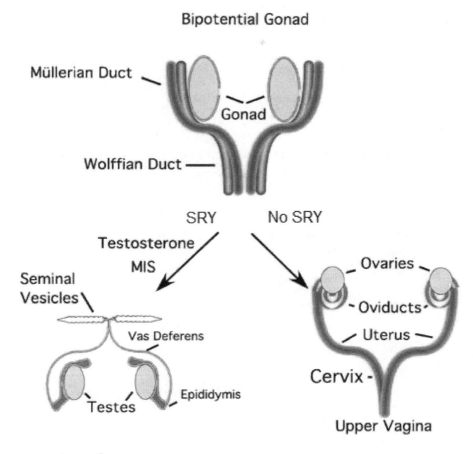

FEMALE REPRODUCTIVE CYCLE

The female reproductive cycle is characterized by changes in both the ovaries and the uterine lining (endometrium).

The ovarian cycle has three phases: the follicular phase, ovulation, and the luteal phase. During the **follicular phase**, FSH stimulates the maturation of the follicle, which then secretes estrogen. Estrogen helps to regenerate the uterine lining that was shed during menstruation. **Ovulation**, the release of a secondary oocyte from the ovary, is induced by a surge in LH. The **luteal phase** begins with the formation of the corpus luteum from the remnants of the follicle. The corpus luteum secretes progesterone and estrogen, which inhibit FSH and LH. Progesterone also maintains the thickness of the endometrium. Without the implantation of a fertilized egg, the corpus luteum begins to regress, and the levels of estrogen and progesterone drop. FSH and LH are no longer inhibited, and the cycle renews.

The uterine cycle also consists of three phases: the proliferative phase, secretory phase, and menstrual phase. The **proliferative phase** is characterized by the regeneration of the uterine lining. During the **secretory phase**, the endometrium becomes increasingly vascular, and nutrients are secreted to prepare for implantation. Without implantation, the endometrium is shed during **menstruation**.

PREGNANCY, PARTURITION, LACTATION

Pregnancy: When a blastocyst implants in the uterine lining, it releases hCG. This hormone prevents the corpus luteum from degrading, and it continues to produce estrogen and progesterone. These hormones are necessary to maintain the uterine lining. By the second trimester, the placenta secretes enough of its own estrogen and progesterone to sustain pregnancy and the levels continue to increase throughout pregnancy, while progesterone decreases.

Parturition: The precise mechanism for the initiation of parturition (birth) is unclear. Birth is preceded by increased levels of fetal glucocorticoids, which act on the placenta to increase estrogen and decrease progesterone. Stretching of the cervix stimulates the release of oxytocin from the posterior pituitary gland. Oxytocin and estrogen stimulate the release of prostaglandins, and prostaglandins and oxytocin increase uterine contractions. This positive feedback mechanism results in the birth of the fetus.

Lactation: During pregnancy, levels of the hormone prolactin increase, but its effect on the mammary glands is inhibited by estrogen and progesterone. After parturition, the levels of these hormones decrease, and prolactin is able to stimulate the production of milk. Suckling stimulates the release of oxytocin, which results in the ejection of milk.

Integumentary System

STRUCTURE

The **epidermis** is the outermost layer of skin. The keratinocytes of the stratum basale are the stem cells of the epidermis. The give rise to cells that differentiate as they move toward the surface.

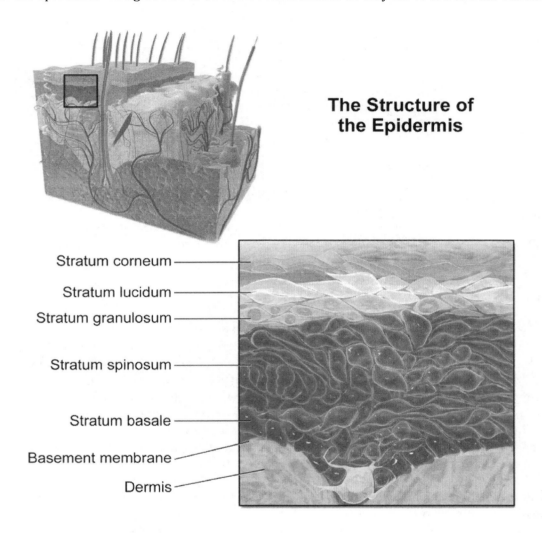

The Structure of the Epidermis

Stratum corneum
Stratum lucidum
Stratum granulosum
Stratum spinosum
Stratum basale
Basement membrane
Dermis

The **stratum basale** is the deepest layer of the epidermis. It usually contains just a single layer of cuboidal or columnar cells that adhere to the basement membrane. These are the most nourished cells because they are closest to the capillaries of the dermis. The **stratum spinosum** consists of eight to ten layers of spiny cells that are connected by structures called **desmosomes**. There is limited mitotic activity in the deeper portion of this layer. The **stratum granulosum** consists of two to five layers of slightly flattened cells containing granules of keratohyalin. The cells in the superficial portion of this layer lose their nuclei. The **stratum lucidum** consists of two to five layers of dead, flattened keratinocytes, and is only present in the palms and the soles of feet. These cells contain **eleiden** - a translucent, water-resistant protein derived from keratohyalin. The **stratum corneum** is the most superficial layer, and it consists of 15 to 30 layers of dead, keratin-containing squamous cells. This layer helps to prevent water loss from the body.

The types of cells found in the epidermis and dermis:

Cell Type	Location	Description
Keratinocytes	Epidermis	The most common type of cell in the epidermis. Arise from stem cells in the stratum basale They flatten and die as they move toward the surface of the skin Produce keratin - a fibrous protein that hardens the cell and helps make the skin water resistant
Melanocytes	Epidermis	Produces melanin - a pigment that gives skin its color and protects against UV radiation
Langerhans cells	Epidermis	Antigen-presenting cells of the immune system (phagocytes) More common in the stratum spinosum than in any other layer of the epidermis
Merkel cells	Epidermis	Cutaneous receptors, detect light touch Located in the stratum basale
Fibroblasts	Dermis	Secrete collagen, elastin, glycosaminoglycans, and other components of the extracellular matrix
Adipocytes	Dermis	Fat cells
Macrophages	Dermis	Phagocytic cells that engulf potential pathogens
Mast cells	Dermis	Antigen-presenting cells that play a role in the inflammatory response (release histamine)

FUNCTIONS OF THE INTEGUMENTARY SYSTEM

HOMEOSTASIS, OSMOREGULATION, AND THERMOREGULATION

The skin functions in homeostasis in a variety of ways. Different types of *sensory receptors* in the skin can detect touch, pressure, temperature, and pain. This system allows the body to sense changes in the environment and to respond appropriately. As a *physical barrier*, the skin can prevent infectious microbes or harmful substances from entering the body. (Pathogens that do manage to enter are subject to a second line of defense: macrophages and other cells of the immune system.) The skin also helps to shield the body from ultraviolet radiation. When the body is exposed to the sun, melanocytes respond by increasing the production of melanin. The integumentary system has many mechanisms for *thermoregulation*, including vasoconstriction and vasodilation of superficial capillaries, and sweating and evaporation. While the skin is not the primary organ involved in *osmoregulation*, it does play an important role. The skin helps prevent water loss from the underlying tissues, as well as the excessive uptake of water from outside the body. It also excretes salts and metabolic wastes such as urea and ammonia through sweat. The ducts of eccrine sweat glands reabsorb many of the sodium ions before they are lost during perspiration.

When the body is cold, it responds by contracting a small smooth muscle in the dermis called the **arrector pili**. This muscle pulls on the hair follicle, causing the hair to stand erect. When many hairs stand up simultaneously, it helps to trap a warm layer of air which has an insulating effect. However, this effect may be minimal in humans.

A better insulator comes in the form of adipose tissue. Beneath the dermis is a layer of subcutaneous tissue known as the **hypodermis** (which is considered separate from the skin). It helps to anchor the skin to the underlying organs, and consists mainly of loose connective tissue, specifically adipose tissue. This layer of fat cells provides insulation from heat and cold.

SWEAT GLANDS, LOCATION IN DERMIS

There are two types of sweat glands (also called sudoriferous glands) in the body: eccrine glands and apocrine glands. The secretory portion of these glands lies in the dermis. Apocrine sweat glands tend to lie deeper in the dermis than eccrine sweat glands because eccrine sweat glands secrete sweat directly onto the skin, while the ducts of apocrine glands empty into hair follicles. Apocrine sweat glands are found only in certain regions of the body, and their function is not clear; they play no role in thermoregulation. They only activate at the onset of puberty in response to sex hormones. Eccrine glands, however, are found nearly everywhere, and the secretion and evaporation of sweat helps to cool the body. The release of sweat is regulated by the hypothalamus. When body temperature rises above normal, the hypothalamus sends signals telling the eccrine sweat glands to secrete until enough heat has been removed. Hormones play a role in the degree to which the body sweats, which may explain why men sweat more than women.

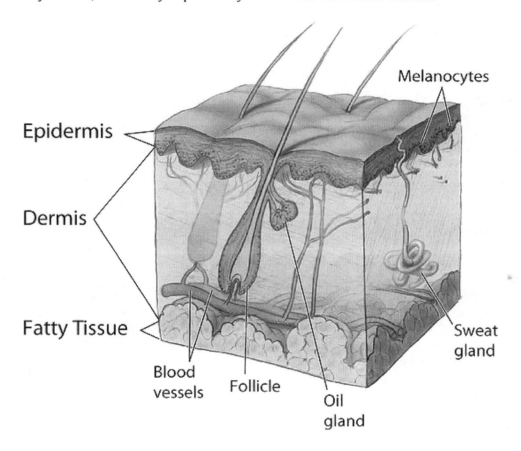

VASOCONSTRICTION AND VASODILATION IN SURFACE CAPILLARIES

When body temperature rises, arterioles in the dermis can promote heat loss by dilating in response to signals from the hypothalamus. This allows more blood to enter capillary beds near the surface of the skin, and heat is lost to the surroundings, primarily through radiation. Conduction and convection can also cool the body, assuming the surrounding temperature is cooler than the body. If the body temperature is too low, the adrenal medulla secretes the hormones epinephrine and norepinephrine, which act on the arterioles, causing them to constrict. This reduces the volume of warm blood that flows near the body's surface, minimizing heat loss at the skin surface.

PHYSICAL PROTECTION

NAILS, CALLUSES, HAIR

Nails are dense plates of hardened keratinocytes that protect the distal ends of fingers and toes. Each nail is composed of modified epidermal tissue that grows from the nail matrix. The nail itself does not have sensory receptors, but pressure can still be detected. Nails also aid in the grasping and manipulation of objects, while protecting delicate tissues beneath.

When a region of the skin experiences repeated mechanical abrasion, the stratum basale responds by increasing the rate of mitosis, which soon leads to an overdevelopment of the stratum corneum (hyperkeratosis). The buildup of dead cells forms a protective pad called a callus.

Hair provides a variety of protective functions as well. It shields the scalp from ultraviolet light, and offers some cushioning in case of injury. It also helps to insulate the skull. Hairs of the nostrils, ears, eyebrows, and eyelashes help to trap foreign particles. Hairs can also act as sensory receptors, allowing a quick response to possible injury.

PROTECTION AGAINST ABRASION, DISEASE ORGANISMS

The skin is continually subject to minor abrasions, but it is protected by the keratin-filled cells of the epidermis. The outer cells of the stratum corneum lose their connection to neighboring cells and slough off when exposed to mechanical stress. Keratinocytes, along with glycolipids produced by the stratum granulosum, form a seal that keeps harmful chemicals and pathogenic organisms from entering the body. The secretions of sweat and sebaceous glands mix together on the surface of the skin to form the **acid mantle**. The low pH of these secretions, along with antimicrobial agents and enzymes, helps to prevent infection. There are also beneficial microorganisms that populate the surface of the skin that outcompete harmful microbes. Within the layers of skin are dendritic cells and other white blood cells that are ready to engulf disease-causing organisms.

Endocrine System

The endocrine system consists of all the glands and tissues that secrete chemical messengers called hormones. The endocrine system works closely with the faster-acting nervous system to coordinate and regulate important processes including growth, development, metabolism, immune function, reproduction, response to stress, and water and electrolyte balance. In short, the endocrine system is essential for the maintenance of homeostasis in the body. When hormones are secreted into the extracellular fluid, they diffuse into the bloodstream and are carried throughout the body. Only cells with receptors that are specific to the secreted hormones are affected. This specificity allows hormones to control targeted tissues and organs - often other endocrine glands (these are called tropic hormones). Major glands of the endocrine system include the hypothalamus, pineal gland, pituitary gland, thyroid, parathyroid glands, thymus, adrenal glands, gonads, and pancreas. Certain cells within the heart, kidneys, gastrointestinal tract, and placenta also have endocrine functions.

An **endocrine gland** produces hormones and secretes them directly into the blood without the use of a duct. (*Endo* = within, *crine* = separate or secretion.) When the hormones are first released by the gland, they enter the interstitial fluid before diffusing into nearby capillaries. The circulatory system then delivers the hormones to target organs. By contrast, **exocrine glands** release non-hormone products such as sweat, oil, tears, and bile through ducts to their target locations - usually a cavity or epithelial surface inside or outside the body. Unlike hormones, exocrine products do not bind to receptors.

Hormones are molecules that bind to receptors and deliver regulatory messages. Many of these signaling molecules are steroids derived from cholesterol. These include the sex hormones and corticosteroids. The rest are non-steroids, and include amines, peptides, and proteins.

HORMONE SOURCES OF THE HEAD AND NECK

The **hypothalamus** is the link between the nervous system and the endocrine system. It is located in the brain, superior to the pituitary and inferior to the thalamus. The hypothalamus communicates with the pituitary by secreting "releasing hormones" (RH) and "inhibiting hormones" (IH). Hormones of the hypothalamus include:

Hormone	Action
GnRH - gonadotropin RH	Stimulates anterior pituitary to release LH and FSH
GHRH - growth hormone RH	Stimulates anterior pituitary to release GH
GHIH - growth hormone IH (somatostatin)	Inhibits the release of GH from the anterior pituitary
TRH - thyrotropin RH	Stimulates anterior pituitary to release thyrotropin (TSH)
PRH - prolactin RH	Stimulates anterior pituitary to release prolactin
PIH - prolactin IH (dopamine)	Inhibits the release of prolactin from the anterior pituitary
CRH - corticotropin RH	Stimulates anterior pituitary to release ACTH
Oxytocin	Targets the uterus - stimulates contractions. Targets the mammary glands - milk secretion
ADH - antidiuretic hormone (vasopressin)	Targets the kidneys and blood vessels - increases water retention

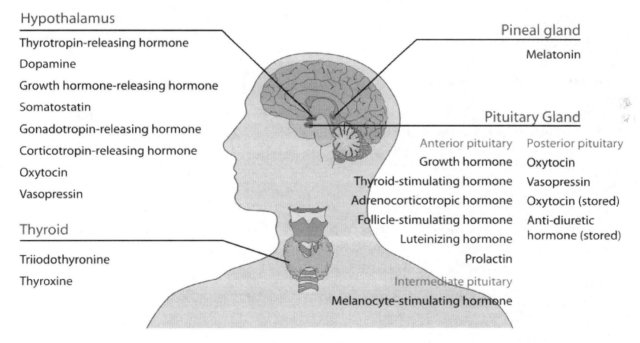

The **pituitary** is nicknamed the "master gland" because many of the hormones it secretes act on other endocrine glands. It is located within the sella turcica of the sphenoid bone, beneath the hypothalamus. This pea-sized gland hangs from a thin stalk called the infundibulum, and it consists of an anterior and posterior lobe - each with a different function.

Source	Hormone	Action
Pituitary gland (anterior)	TSH - thyroid stimulating hormone (thyrotropin)	Targets the thyroid - stimulates the secretion of thyroid hormones
	ACTH - adrenocorticotropic hormone	Targets the adrenal cortex - stimulates the release of glucocorticoids and mineralocorticoids
	GH - growth hormone	Targets muscle and bone - stimulates growth
	FSH - follicle stimulating hormone	Targets the gonads - stimulates the maturation of sperm cells and ovarian follicles
	LH - luteinizing hormone	Targets the gonads - stimulates the production of sex hormones; surge stimulates ovulation in females
	PRL - prolactin	Targets the mammary glands - stimulates production of milk
Pituitary gland (posterior)	Oxytocin (produced in hypothalamus; stored and released by posterior pituitary)	Targets the uterus - stimulates contractions Targets the mammary glands - stimulates milk secretion
	ADH - antidiuretic hormone (vasopressin) (produced in hypothalamus; stored and released by posterior pituitary)	Targets the kidneys and blood vessels - increases water retention

Source/Description	Hormone	Action
Pineal gland Situated between the two hemispheres of the brain where the two halves of the thalamus join.	Melatonin	Targets the brain - regulates daily rhythm (wake and sleep)
Thyroid gland Butterfly-shaped gland; the point of attachment between the two lobes is called the isthmus. The isthmus is on the anterior portion of the trachea, with the lobes wrapping partially around the trachea.	T_3 - triiodothyronine	Targets most cells - stimulates cellular metabolism
	T_4 - thyroxine	Targets most cells - stimulates cellular metabolism
	Calcitonin	Targets bone and kidneys - lowers blood calcium
Parathyroid gland Four small glands that are embedded in the posterior aspect of the thyroid.	PTH - Parathyroid hormone	Targets bone and kidneys - raises blood calcium

HORMONE SOURCES OF THE ABDOMEN

Source/Description	Hormone	Action
Thymus gland Located between the sternum and the heart, embedded in the mediastinum. It slowly decreases in size after puberty.	Thymosin	Targets lymphatic tissues - stimulates the production of T-cells
Pancreas The head of the pancreas is situated in the curve of the duodenum and the tail points toward the left side of the body. The pancreas is mostly posterior to the stomach.	Insulin	Targets the liver, muscle, and adipose tissue - decreases blood glucose
	Glucagon	Targets the liver - increases blood glucose
	GHIH - growth hormone IH (somatostatin)	Inhibits the secretion of insulin and glucagon
Adrenal medulla Located on top of the kidneys. The adrenal medulla is the inner part of the gland.	Epinephrine and norepinephrine	Target heart, blood vessels, liver, and lungs - increase heart rate, increase blood sugar (fight or flight response)
Adrenal cortex The adrenal cortex is the outer portion of the adrenal gland.	Mineralocorticoids (aldosterone)	Target the kidneys - increase the retention of Na^+ and excretion of K^+
	Glucocorticoids	Target most tissues - released in response to long-term stressors, increase blood glucose (but not as quickly as glucagon)
	Androgens	Target most tissues - stimulate development of secondary sex characteristics

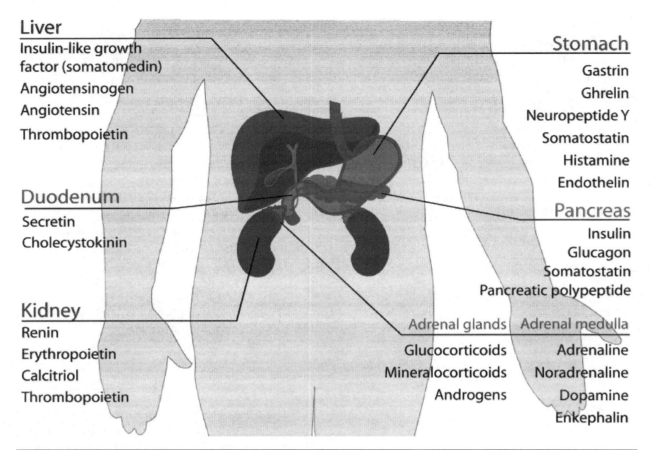

Liver
Insulin-like growth factor (somatomedin)
Angiotensinogen
Angiotensin
Thrombopoietin

Duodenum
Secretin
Cholecystokinin

Kidney
Renin
Erythropoietin
Calcitriol
Thrombopoietin

Stomach
Gastrin
Ghrelin
Neuropeptide Y
Somatostatin
Histamine
Endothelin

Pancreas
Insulin
Glucagon
Somatostatin
Pancreatic polypeptide

Adrenal glands
Glucocorticoids
Mineralocorticoids
Androgens

Adrenal medulla
Adrenaline
Noradrenaline
Dopamine
Enkephalin

Source/Description	Hormone	Action
GI tract Cells within the mucosa of the small intestine and stomach release hormones to control much of the digestion process.	Gastrin	Targets the stomach - stimulates the release of HCl
	Secretin	Targets the pancreas and liver - stimulates the release of digestive enzymes and bile
	CCK - cholecystokinin	Targets the pancreas and liver - stimulates the release of digestive enzymes and bile
Kidneys Bean-shaped organs located in the lumbar region, one on each side of the sagittal plane.	Erythropoietin	Targets the bone marrow - stimulates the production of red blood cells
	Calcitriol	Targets the intestines - increases the reabsorption of Ca^{2+}
Heart Situated just left of the midline of the body, between the lungs	ANP - atrial natriuretic peptide	Targets the kidneys and adrenal cortex - reduces reabsorption of Na^+, lowers blood pressure
Adipose Tissue Located under the layers of skin and throughout the body.	Leptin	Targets the brain - suppresses appetite

HORMONE SOURCES OF THE REPRODUCTIVE SYSTEM

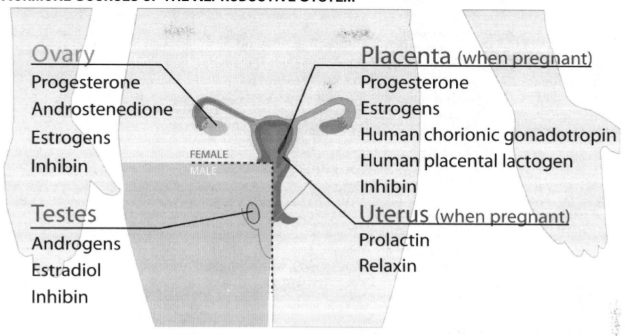

Ovary
Progesterone
Androstenedione
Estrogens
Inhibin

FEMALE
MALE

Testes
Androgens
Estradiol
Inhibin

Placenta (when pregnant)
Progesterone
Estrogens
Human chorionic gonadotropin
Human placental lactogen
Inhibin

Uterus (when pregnant)
Prolactin
Relaxin

Source/Description	Hormone	Action
Ovaries The ovaries rest in depressions in the pelvic cavity on each side of the uterus. (Note that ovaries produce testosterone in small amounts.)	Estrogen	Target the uterus, ovaries, mammary glands, brain, and other tissues - stimulate uterine lining growth, regulate menstrual cycle, facilitate the development of secondary sex characteristics
	Progesterone	Targets mainly the uterus and mammary glands - stimulates uterine lining growth, regulates menstrual cycle, required for maintenance of pregnancy
	Inhibin	Targets the anterior pituitary - inhibits the release of FSH
Placenta Attached to the wall of the uterus during pregnancy	Estrogen, progesterone, and inhibin	(See above)
	Human chorionic gonadotropin (hCG)	Targets the ovaries - stimulates the production of estrogen and progesterone
Testes Located within the scrotum, behind the penis.	Testosterone	Targets the testes and many other tissues - promotes spermatogenesis, secondary sex characteristics
	Inhibin	(See above)

MAJOR TYPES OF HORMONES

Hormones can be broadly classified into lipid-soluble hormones (steroids) and water-soluble hormones (non-steroids). Steroid hormones are derived from cholesterol, and their base structure consists of four fused carbon rings. They are released by the adrenal cortex, testes, ovaries, and the placenta. Major types of steroid hormones include the **sex hormones** (estrogens, androgens, progesterone) and the **corticosteroids** (glucocorticoids and mineralocorticoids). Since these hormones are lipid-soluble, they can diffuse through the cell membrane and bind to the nuclear receptors that regulate transcription.

Non-steroid hormones tend to elicit faster responses than steroid hormones. They cannot diffuse into the cell, and instead bind to receptors on the cell membrane, activating second-messenger systems. These hormones are classified into amines, peptides, and proteins. **Amines** are derivatives of the amino acids tyrosine or tryptophan, and include epinephrine, norepinephrine, thyroxine, and melatonin. **Peptide hormones** are short chains of amino acids. Common examples include oxytocin, somatostatin, and antidiuretic hormone. **Protein hormones** such as insulin, growth hormone, and parathyroid hormone consist of longer chains - generally over 100 amino acids. Hormones can also be **glycoproteins**. Follicle-stimulating hormone, thyroid-stimulating hormone, and luteinizing hormone all have carbohydrate attachments.

Genitourinary System

ROLES IN HOMEOSTASIS

BLOOD PRESSURE

When osmoreceptors detect an increase in blood osmolality, or when baroreceptors detect a decrease in blood pressure, the pituitary gland secretes **antidiuretic hormone** (ADH). ADH stimulates the reabsorption of water in the kidney so that less water is excreted in the urine. This increases the volume and pressure of the blood.

The **renin-angiotensin-aldosterone system** (RAAS) is another mechanism by which blood pressure is regulated. When granular juxtaglomerular cells of the afferent arterioles of the kidneys detect a drop in blood pressure, they secrete an enzyme called **renin**. Renin interacts with a plasma protein called **angiotensinogen**, producing **angiotensin I**. As angiotensin I enters the capillaries of the lungs, it is acted on by another enzyme that converts it to **angiotensin II**. This hormone raises blood pressure by promoting vasoconstriction and stimulating the adrenal cortex to release **aldosterone**. Aldosterone increases the reabsorption of sodium, which increases water reabsorption, causing the blood volume and pressure to increase.

OSMOREGULATION

Osmoregulation describes the regulation of water and solute concentrations of body fluids. The primary organ involved in this process is the kidney. Dehydration or excessive salt intake will raise the osmolality of the blood. (Plasma osmolality is determined mainly by the concentrations of electrolytes, such as Na^+, Cl^-, and K^+.) When osmoreceptors in the hypothalamus detect an increase in osmolality, signals are sent to the pituitary gland to release ADH. ADH causes the collecting ducts in the kidneys to be more permeable to water, and water crosses the epithelium from the urine into the interstitium where it is returned to the blood. As a result, the blood osmolality decreases, and urine osmolality increases.

Aldosterone also plays a role in osmoregulation. When blood pressure is low, this hormone is secreted by the adrenal cortex. Aldosterone increases sodium reabsorption, which causes more water to leave the collecting tubule, thus raising blood osmolality. It also regulates the concentrations of other ions, such as potassium and chloride.

ACID–BASE BALANCE

The kidneys are key players in the maintenance of blood pH, which must be kept within a narrow range of 7.35 and 7.45. This is achieved by regulating the ratio of hydrogen ions to bicarbonate ions. (The higher the concentration of H^+ ions, the lower the pH.) Buffer systems in the body such as the phosphate, protein, and bicarbonate systems are in place to resist changes in H^+ concentration. Recall that the respiratory system helps to control pH through the bicarbonate buffer system. When carbon dioxide combines with water, carbonic acid (H_2CO_3) is formed, before dissociating into bicarbonate ions (HCO_3^-) and H^+. (Reaction: $CO_2 + H_2O \leftrightarrow H_2CO_3 \leftrightarrow HCO_3^- + H^+$.) Increasing the rate of respiration decreases the concentration of H^+, which increases pH. The reverse is true when the rate of respiration decreases. The response from the *kidneys* is slower, but lasts longer. As blood pH decreases, H^+ ions are excreted by the renal tubules via urine (which is now more acidic) and bicarbonate ions are retained. The intercalated cells of the late distal tubule and collecting duct can also generate new bicarbonate ions. The kidneys lower pH by reabsorbing H^+ ions and secreting bicarbonate ions.

REMOVAL OF SOLUBLE NITROGENOUS WASTE

Nitrogen-containing wastes such as ammonia, urea, uric acid, and creatinine are excreted in urine. **Ammonia** is a toxic base that is formed during the breakdown of amino acids. Enzymes in the liver convert it to a less toxic form called **urea**. There is a high concentration of urea in the medulla because the collecting ducts are permeable to it. Much of the urea enters the interstitium, and it is then reabsorbed into the descending loop of Henle. Urea is the most abundant nitrogenous waste product in the urine, but since most of it is recycled, only a small amount is eliminated in urine. The high concentration of urea in the interstitium is helpful because it promotes the reabsorption of water. **Uric acid** is another nitrogenous waste that is excreted in the urine. It is formed as a byproduct of the catabolism of purine nucleotides, and most of it is reabsorbed in the proximal tubule by active transport. Like urea, only a small percentage is excreted. **Creatinine** is produced in the muscles as byproduct of the metabolism of creatine phosphate. It is filtered by the kidneys and excreted. Unlike urea and uric acid, creatinine is not reabsorbed by the tubules.

KIDNEY STRUCTURE

The kidneys are bean-shaped organs located in the lumbar region of the body that function in the filtering of blood and the excretion of wastes. Each kidney is surrounded by three protective layers of connective tissue: the **renal fascia**, the **adipose capsule**, and the innermost **renal capsule**. The capsule surrounds the outer region of the kidney called the **renal cortex**. The cortex contains many filtration units called **nephrons**, which have tubules that dip into the interior region called the **medulla**. The tubules in the medulla run parallel to each other and form striped cone-shaped masses of tissue called **medullary pyramids**. A cavity called the **renal sinus** contains the basin-like **renal pelvis**, which funnels the urine into the ureter. The **hilum** is the concave region of the kidney where the blood vessels and nerves enter and leave. Blood enters the kidney through the renal artery, which branches into smaller and smaller arteries until the blood reaches a tuft of capillaries called the **glomerulus**. Here, the blood is filtered before leaving the kidney through a network of veins that merge into the renal vein.

Frontal section through the Kidney

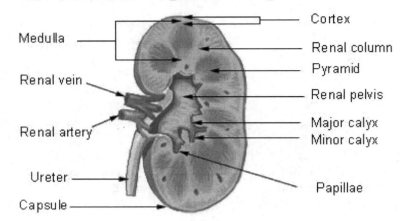

CORTEX

The renal cortex is the outer portion of the kidney, and it is the site of **ultrafiltration**: the nonspecific filtration of blood under high pressure. It is also responsible for the majority of reabsorption of water. The cortex is very vascular, and has a granular appearance due to the presence of nephrons. The renal corpuscles and the convoluted tubules of the nephrons are within the cortex (forming the **cortical labyrinth**), but the loops of Henle extend into the adjacent region known as the renal medulla. The thick, straight portions of the proximal and distal tubules, as well as the collecting ducts, form **medullary rays** that begin in the cortex and run perpendicular to the capsule. About 85% of nephrons (cortical nephrons) have short loops of Henle that extend only slightly into the medulla. The remaining 15% (juxtamedullary nephrons) have longer loops that extend deeper. Extensions of the cortex called **renal columns** dip down in between the renal pyramids of the medulla.

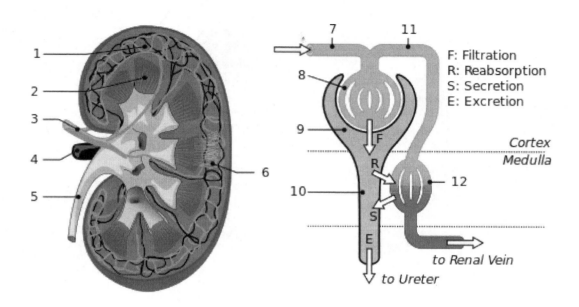

1: Renal cortex. 2: Medulla. 3: Renal artery. 4: Renal vein. 5: Ureter. 6: Nephrons. 7: Afferent arteriole. 8: Glomerulus. 9: Bowman's capsule. 10: Renal tubule. 11: Efferent arteriole. 12: Peritubular capillaries.

MEDULLA

The adrenal medulla is the inner part of the kidney, and it continues the reabsorption of water and salts that began in the cortex. These substances enter the peritubular capillaries that are associated with the nephrons. Any filtrate that is not reclaimed by the circulatory system will leave as urine.

The medulla contains cone-shaped regions of tissue called **renal pyramids** that are separated by **renal columns**. The tips of the pyramids are oriented toward the pelvis of the kidney, and the bases face the cortex. The renal pyramids contain tubules that transport renal filtrate from the renal cortex to the apex of the pyramids. At the apex is a structure called the **renal papilla** that contains ducts that allow the processed filtrate (now called urine) to pass out of the medulla to collecting chambers called **calyces**. From here the urine passes through the renal pelvis, through the ureter, and finally into the bladder.

NEPHRON STRUCTURE

The nephron is the functional unit of the kidney. Each kidney has over a million of these microscopic structures, and each one consists of two main parts: the **renal corpuscle** (which filters the blood) and the **renal tubule** (which collects and concentrates the filtrate). The renal corpuscle consists of a cup-shaped structure called **Bowman's capsule** that wraps partially around a cluster of capillaries called the **glomerulus**. The renal tubule is a looping canal that is continuous with Bowman's capsule. It consists of different regions that differ in structure and function. The **proximal convoluted tubule** begins at Bowman's capsule and then plunges into the medulla, forming a u-shape called the **loop of Henle**. It then becomes the **distal convoluted tubule**, which is continuous with the **collecting duct**. The collecting duct is typically considered as a separate structure, and not part of the nephron.

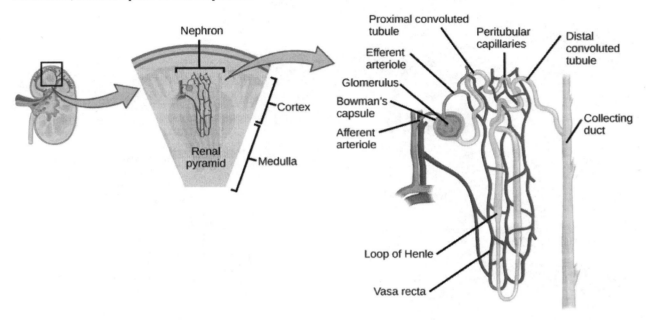

GLOMERULUS AND BOWMAN'S CAPSULE

Each renal corpuscle consists of a **glomerulus** and a **Bowman's capsule**. The glomerulus is a tangled network of blood capillaries that occupies Bowman's capsule. These fenestrated capillaries are lined with a thin layer of epithelial cells. An **afferent arteriole** takes blood to the glomerulus and an **efferent arteriole** takes it away. The smaller diameter of the efferent arteriole increases the pressure within the glomerulus, which is required for ultrafiltration. **Mesangial cells** contract to regulate blood flow, and also support the capillary network.

Bowman's capsule is a cup-like structure at the closed end of the renal tubule that encloses the glomerulus. It has an outer layer of epithelial cells that form the parietal layer, and a visceral layer of **podocytes** with processes called **pedicels** that wrap around the capillaries. Gaps between the pedicels (filtration slits) allow the passage of tiny molecules and ions. Together, the endothelial cells of the capillaries, the basement membrane, and the pedicels make up the **filtration membrane**. Fluid from the blood leaves the fenestrated capillaries and passes through the filtration membrane and collects in **Bowman's space** (the cavity between the two layers of Bowman's capsule). From here, the filtrate enters the renal tubule.

PROXIMAL TUBULE, LOOP OF HENLE, AND DISTAL TUBULE

The renal tubule is divided into three continuous regions: the proximal convoluted tubule, the loop of Henle, and the distal convoluted tubule. The **proximal convoluted tubule** extends from Bowman's capsule, and this coiled tube is characterized by cuboidal cells with dense microvilli that aid in reabsorption and secretion. There are only sparse microvilli in the rest of the tubule. The middle, hairpin-shaped portion of the renal tubule is called the **loop of Henle**, and it maintains a relatively high solute concentration in the medulla, which in turn assists in the reabsorption of water. The loop consists of a descending limb (which reabsorbs water) that plunges into the medulla, a U-turn that curves back toward the cortex, and an ascending limb (which reabsorbs ions). The ascending limb widens into a thick portion composed of larger epithelial cells. The loop is lined with simple squamous epithelial cells, with the exception of the thick ascending limb which is lined with simple cuboidal cells. This limb becomes the **distal convoluted tubule** (also lined with cuboidal cells), which is involved in absorption and secretion, but not to the extent of the proximal convoluted tubule. It is also shorter in length.

COLLECTING DUCT

The collecting duct is the final site of reabsorption in the kidney, and it is shared by multiple nephrons. The distal tubule empties filtrate into the collecting tubule, which merges with other collecting tubules to form the collecting duct. Collecting tubules are lined with simple cuboidal epithelium, but these cells elongate to form columnar cells as they get closer to the duct. Some of these cells are **principal cells**, which reabsorb sodium ions and water (under ADH and aldosterone control). Other cells are **intercalated cells**, and they play an important role in acid-base balance and the reabsorption of sodium ions. Both these types of cells can also be found toward the end part of the distal tubule, but there are fewer microvilli than in the collecting duct. The filtrate that passes through the collecting duct enters the minor calyces at the apex of a medullary pyramid.

FORMATION OF URINE

GLOMERULAR FILTRATION

The formation of urine begins with glomerular filtration. This nonspecific filtration is driven by the hydrostatic pressure of the blood. This pressure is higher than in other capillaries because the efferent arterioles that exit the glomerulus have a smaller diameter than the afferent arterioles that enter. Water and small solutes from the blood are forced through fenestrations in the capillaries, leaving behind larger particles. The fluid must pass through the 3-layered filtration membrane before entering Bowman's space as renal filtrate. The first layer is the endothelial lining of the capillaries. Fenestrations in the capillaries prevent the passage of blood cells. The second layer is the basement membrane, which excludes plasma proteins such as albumin. The third layer is the visceral lining of Bowman's capsule. Small filtration slits between the podocytes allow only the smallest of particles to pass. The concentration of a solute in the glomerular filtrate is the same as the concentration in the blood. On average, about 1/5 of the blood is filtered, but this varies depending on the pressure.

SECRETION AND REABSORPTION OF SOLUTES

Secretion removes solutes from the blood and adds them to the filtrate, while reabsorption removes solutes from the filtrate and returns them to the blood. Solutes are moved by either primary active transport, secondary active transport, or diffusion, and water is reabsorbed by osmosis. The functions of each region of the renal tubule and collecting duct are summarized in the table below:

Region	Role in Secretion	Role in Reabsorption
Proximal convoluted tubule	H^+, creatinine, NH_4^+, drugs, toxins - active transport	Main site of reabsorption in the kidney; 60–70% of the volume of filtrate is reclaimed in the PCT. Glucose, amino acids, vitamins, Na^+, Cl^-, K^+, Ca^{2+}, Mg^{2+}, bicarbonate, phosphate, water, urea
Loop of Henle - Descending limb	Urea	Water
Loop of Henle - Ascending limb		Na^+, Cl^-, K^+, Mg^{2+}, Ca^{2+}
Distal convoluted tubule	K^+, H^+	Cl^-, Ca^{2+}, Na^+, Water (variable permeability - opening of Na^+ channels is dependent on aldosterone)
Collecting duct	K^+, H^+	Urea, bicarbonate, Na^+, Water (variable permeability - dependent on aldosterone and ADH)

CONCENTRATION OF URINE

The concentration of urine is influenced by the high solute concentration of the medulla, and the hormones that control the permeability of the distal convoluted tubule and collecting duct.

The **countercurrent mechanism** describes the use of active transport to move solutes out of the ascending loop of Henle (which is impermeable to water) into the medullary interstitium. The osmotic gradient that is created causes water diffuse out of the descending limb (which *is* permeable to water), concentrating the filtrate. The recycling of urea also helps to maintain a high medullary osmolarity. The descending loop of Henle and the collecting duct are both permeable to urea, but the descending limb and the distal tubule are not. Urea enters the descending loop from the interstitium, and travels through the renal tubule to the collecting duct, where it reenters the interstitium.

The concentration of urine is also regulated by hormones. The permeability of the distal convoluted tubule to sodium is dependent on aldosterone. Aldosterone promotes the reabsorption of Na^+, and since water follows the sodium, the urine becomes more concentrated. The permeability of the collecting duct is dependent on both aldosterone and ADH. ADH increases the duct's permeability by water by inserting aquaporins that allow the passage of water.

COUNTERCURRENT MULTIPLIER MECHANISM

A countercurrent system in the loop of Henle is responsible for the generation of an osmotic gradient in the medulla that promotes the reabsorption of water. The descending limb is permeable to water, but not solutes. The ascending limb is permeable to solutes, but not water. Na^+, Cl^-, and other ions are actively transported from the ascending limb into the medullary interstitium. The concentration gradient causes water to leave the descending limb by osmosis, which increases the concentration of the filtrate in the descending limb. As the filtrate moves up the ascending limb, ions are actively absorbed, raising the solute concentration in the medulla. This positive feedback loop is known as the countercurrent *multiplier* mechanism because it multiplies the concentration of the interstitial fluid as a result of the functional differences between the two limbs.

The countercurrent multiplier system is distinguished from the countercurrent *exchange* system, in which the hypertonicity of the medulla is *maintained* (not generated) by the countercurrent flow of blood in the vasa recta. As blood in the *descending* part of the vasa recta passes the *ascending* limb, it picks up ions that left the filtrate. As blood in the *ascending* vasa recta passes the *descending* limb, most of the ions diffuse back into the medulla.

STORAGE AND ELIMINATION: URETER, BLADDER, URETHRA

A **ureter** is a tubular organ that delivers urine from the kidney to the bladder for storage. The collecting ducts (the final sites of reabsorption) empty urine into the ureter, and both gravity and peristalsis move the urine into the bladder. The bladder is a bag-like organ that can store up to 600 ml of urine (though the desire to urinate begins at around 150 ml). The ureters, bladder, and superior portion of the urethra are lined with transitional epithelial tissue that allows expansion. When the organ becomes distended, the stretched epithelium appears to have fewer cell layers.

Urine is stored in the bladder until contraction of the **detrusor muscle** (the smooth muscle within the bladder wall) forces urine into the urethra. Contraction of the bladder is controlled by the parasympathetic nervous system. Stretch receptors in the bladder send impulses to the sacral region of the spinal cord. Impulses are then sent along efferent neurons to the bladder, telling it to contract. A circular smooth muscle called the internal urethral sphincter relaxes, and (if the timing is appropriate) the voluntary external urethral sphincter relaxes as well. Urine flows from the bladder, through the urethra, and out of the body in a process called micturition.

MUSCULAR CONTROL: SPHINCTER MUSCLE

There are two sphincters of the urethra that delay the emptying of the bladder. The **internal urethral sphincter** (IUS) is found between the bladder and the urethra. It consists of smooth muscle and is continuous with the smooth muscle of the bladder (the detrusor muscle). The sympathetic nervous system keeps the IUS contracted until the micturition reflex is triggered. The IUS relaxes as a result of sympathetic inhibition, allowing urine to pass through. The second sphincter that controls the elimination of urine is the **external urethral sphincter** (EUS), which is made of skeletal muscle, and under the control of the somatic nervous system. A conscious decision can be made to relax the EUS under appropriate circumstances. Involuntary contraction of the detrusor forces urine out of the body, and the voluntary contraction of abdominal muscles can increase the rate of flow by compressing the bladder.

Immune System

INNATE (NON-SPECIFIC) VS. ADAPTIVE (SPECIFIC) IMMUNITY

Innate immunity refers to the nonspecific first line of defense against pathogens that is present at birth. There is no potential for this system to "learn" from previous pathogens or adapt to new threats. The first barriers to infection include mechanical barriers such as the skin and mucous membranes. Chemical barriers include the low pH of gastric juice, interferons that block viral replication, lysozyme in tears, and other antimicrobial proteins such as defensins, collectins, and complements. Pathogens can also be engulfed by phagocytes, or by the destruction of the infected cell by natural killer cells. Fever and inflammation can offer nonspecific protection as well. **Adaptive immunity** develops over time. It may be slow to act initially, but the "memory" of the first encounter with an **antigen** (a toxin or a molecule on the surface of a pathogen that triggers an immune response) allows for faster responses in subsequent exposures to that same antigen. The antigen is recognized as foreign, and the appropriate type of cell is selected to combat the pathogen with which it is associated. These cells are primarily lymphocytes. Depending on the type of lymphocyte, they respond to infection by producing antibodies, killing infected cells, or directing other immune responses.

ADAPTIVE IMMUNE SYSTEM CELLS

There are two main types of lymphocytes that are involved in adaptive immune responses: T-lymphocytes (T cells) and B-lymphocytes (B cells).

T cells mature in the thymus, and are involved in cell-mediated immunity. The initial activation of T cells occurs when they encounter their specific antigen on the surface of an antigen-presenting cell (or APC). When they bind to these APCs, they proliferate and differentiate into various types of T cells. **Cytotoxic T cells** are specialized to kill infected or abnormal cells. Some cytotoxic T cells produce **memory T cells** that respond to subsequent infections. **Helper T cells** secrete cytokines that stimulate the division of T and B cells, while alerting other types of WBCs. **Regulatory (suppressor) T cells** inhibit T and B cells to stop the immune response.

B cells mature in the bone marrow, and are involved in humoral-mediated immunity. The initial activation of B cells occurs when they encounter freely circulating antigens. (Many B cells require co-stimulation by a helper T cell.) After binding to specific antigens, B cells differentiate into plasma cells and memory B cells. **Plasma cells** secrete antibodies that bind to antigens. **Memory B cells** also produce antibodies, but only during a subsequent infection.

INNATE IMMUNE SYSTEM CELLS

There are various types of cells involved in innate immunity, many of which are phagocytes. **Neutrophils** account for most of the white blood cells in the bloodstream. These phagocytes are usually the first to arrive at the site of infection and they chase pathogens using chemotaxis. **Eosinophils** regulate inflammatory responses and release chemicals that kill foreign invaders - often parasitic worms. **Mast cells** (found in connective tissues) and **basophils** (which circulate in the blood before entering tissues) both release histamine to promote inflammation and heparin to inhibit clotting. **Macrophages** (derived from monocytes, the largest leukocytes) are large WBCs that engulf debris and pathogenic microorganisms, and function as antigen presenters to effector T cells. **Dendritic cells** function in much the same way, except they activate "naive" T cells (T cells that have not yet encountered their antigen). **Natural killer cells** are not phagocytes; they destroy cells that have been infected with a pathogen by binding to them and releasing granzymes that trigger apoptosis.

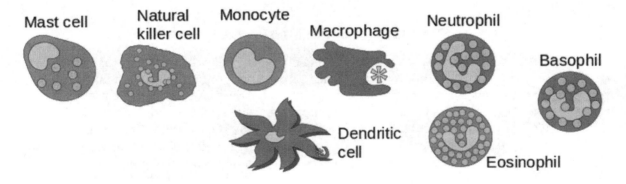

Tissues

The functions of the major tissues and organs that play a role in the immune system:

Tissue of the Immune System	Function
Bone Marrow	Produces hematopoietic stem cells that give rise to all types of blood cells, including lymphocytes. Site of B cell differentiation
Thymus	Site of T cell differentiation
Spleen	Splenic cords of the red pulp contain an abundance of macrophages and lymphocytes that help to filter aged blood cells, pathogens, and debris from the blood The white pulp is a lymphatic tissue that consists almost entirely of B and T cells, and provides a place for these lymphocytes to proliferate
Lymph nodes	Provide a place for lymphocytes and other WBCs to proliferate (cortex contains B cells and macrophages, medulla contains T cells) Filter the lymph of microorganisms, toxins, and wastes B cells produce antibodies that assist in the immune response
MALT	Mucosa-associated lymphoid tissue refers to the small clusters of lymphatic cells that are found in the tonsils, appendix, and Peyer's patches of the small intestine. T cells, B cells, and macrophages provide protection against pathogens

Structure of Lymphatic System

The lymphatic system includes the thymus, bone marrow, tonsils, spleen, lymphatic vessels, lymph nodes, and lymph. Lymph is a clear liquid similar in composition to plasma. It is transported in one direction (toward the neck) where it is emptied into the subclavian veins. Lymph consists of white blood cells and the fluid that leaks out of the blood capillaries. Lymphatic vessels are similar in structure to veins; they have thin walls, and also have valves to prevent backflow. Their walls are more porous, however, allowing the lymph to drain into them for circulation. Lymph is moved by contractions of both smooth and skeletal muscle. Lymphatic vessels are found nearly everywhere in the body except the central nervous system and avascular tissues. The vessels are interrupted by oval-shaped masses of tissue called lymph nodes that contain lymphocytes and filter out foreign substances. The primary organs of the lymphatic system (bone marrow and thymus) produce mature lymphocytes. There are also secondary organs (such as the spleen and tonsils) that house lymphocytes. These specialized white blood cells destroy disease-causing microorganisms.

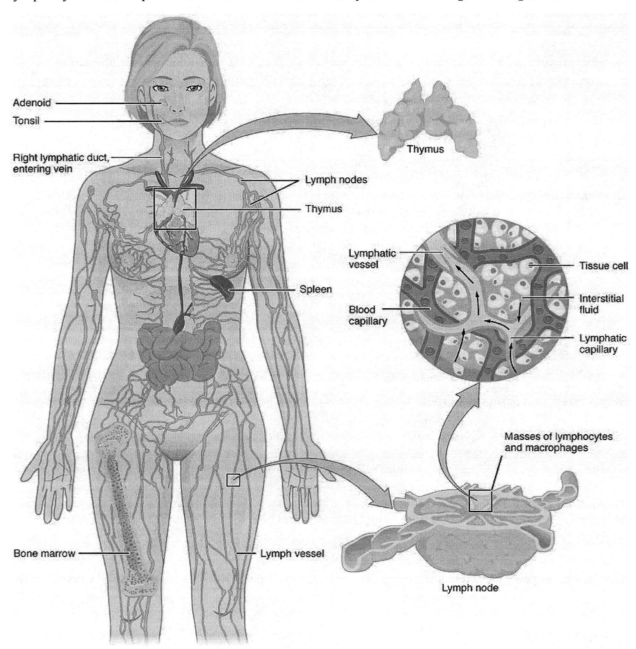

CONCEPT OF ANTIGEN AND ANTIBODY

An **antigen** is a substance that elicits a response from the immune system. Antigens are usually large biomolecules (often proteins) that are identified as foreign or non-self. They can be found on the surfaces of antigenic substances such as viruses, bacteria, fungi, and pollen grains. **Foreign antigens** originate outside the body, and include the examples listed above. **Self-antigens** are produced by the body and rarely initiate an immune response. They often trigger a response in other people, as seen in the rejection of transplanted tissues or organs.

Antibodies (also called immunoglobulins) are products of B cells that bind to specific antigens. The binding of an antibody to an antigen can disarm the pathogen in a variety of ways. In some cases, the pathogens **agglutinate** (clump together) before being destroyed. Antibodies can also **neutralize** the antigen by blocking its ability to attach to cells, or cause it to become insoluble and **precipitate** out of solution. Sometimes, they activate **complement** - a system of proteins that enhances the effectiveness of the immune response. Other cells of the immune system can be called to action, and phagocytosis can be enhanced in a process called **opsonization**. Antibodies also promote **inflammation** to help slow the spread of infection.

EQUALIZATION OF FLUID DISTRIBUTION AND TRANSPORT OF PROTEINS AND LARGE GLYCERIDES

One key function of the immune system is the equalization of fluid between the blood and tissues. Greater hydrostatic pressure in the blood vessels (as compared to the interstitial fluid) causes fluid to leak out of the vessels into the surrounding tissues. Porous lymphatic capillaries collect excess interstitial fluid (now called lymph) for delivery to the right and left subclavian veins. As it travels through the lymphatic system, the lymph passes through lymph nodes where it is filtered and cleansed. Eventually, it reaches either the right lymphatic duct (which drains into the right subclavian vein) or the thoracic duct (which drains into the left subclavian vein), returning fluid back into the blood. If pressure is too great in the lymphatic vessels, edema will occur as fluid leaks back into the tissues.

The lymphatic system also helps to transport certain biomolecules. The villi of the small intestine harbor specialized lymph capillaries called **lacteals** that absorb fats. These fats are transported in the form of **chylomicrons**, which give the lymph (called **chyle**) a whitish appearance. The lymphatic system is also used to return plasma proteins or cells that leaked out of the blood vessels back into the bloodstream.

PRODUCTION OF LYMPHOCYTES INVOLVED IN IMMUNE REACTIONS

The bone marrow and thymus are the "primary" lymphatic organs because they are the sites of lymphocyte production. Stem cells in the red bone marrow called **hemocytoblasts** give rise to immature lymphocytes. Lymphocytes that stay in the bone marrow differentiate into **B cells** and **natural killer (NK) cells**, and other immature lymphocytes migrate to the thymus where they differentiate into **T cells**. Lymphocytes use the bloodstream to migrate from these primary lymphatic organs to "secondary" lymphatic organs, such as the lymph nodes, spleen, and tonsils. When they make contact with antigens, the lymphocytes are activated and mature into effector cells that can participate in immune reactions.

CYCLE OF INFECTION

The cycle of infection starts with the presence of a pathogen (a disease-causing organism) and an environment that allows it to grow and multiply. Aside from being able to grow and multiply, the conditions must allow it to be passed on (transmission) from one organism (host) to another. Transmission can be either direct or indirect. Direct transmission occurs when the infection is passed from one infected host to another. There are several different possible modes of indirect transmission. An object can become contaminated and a person becomes infected when they touch the contaminated object (called a fomite). A vector can be employed by the pathogen, infecting an intermediate host where it can multiply and develop before being passed on to a new host. The pathogen can become airborne before finding a new host to infect. In any mode of transmission, there must be a way for the pathogen to enter the new host and the host must be susceptible to the infection.

RESERVOIR

Medical professionals must understand all five components of the cycle of infection to prevent the spread of disease. All of these factors must be present for an infection to transpire. They are a reservoir host, exit mode, method of transmission, route of entrance, and a susceptible host. The first aspect takes place when a microorganism (pathogen) latches onto a living host. This living host is referred to as a reservoir host and may be a human, an insect, or even an animal. A reservoir's body will offer the proper nourishment for the pathogen for it to live and/or proliferate. When humans serve as the reservoir hosts, they become carriers of the disease but are often oblivious that they have been infected and can easily transmit the disease to other people. When there is evidence of a disease in a reservoir host, one may be more aware of hand washing and other methods to prevent the spread of disease.

PORTAL OF EXIT

The second step that must take place for an infection to occur is that the reservoir host provides a portal of exit. This describes the method in which the microorganism leaves the reservoir host to continue on to infect another organism, known as the susceptible host. The most prevalent avenues for exiting the body are via the mouth, nose, blood, urine, vaginal or seminal fluid, feces, and even the eyes. Often the portal of exit is the exact same as the entrance portals, which is the fourth step in the cycle of infection.

MODE OF TRANSMISSION: DROPLET

Droplet (mucous) particles may be transmitted when the reservoir host sneezes or coughs. It is known that the reservoir host does not need to be in close proximity to the susceptible host as droplet particles can travel several feet in the air. Respiratory diseases such as influenza and tuberculosis may be transmitted via a direct airborne method when the susceptible host inhales the droplets of the infected person. These types of infections may sweep through a population rapidly, so it is important to practice proper techniques to prevent airborne transmission. This includes coughing or sneezing into a tissue when possible. If a tissue is not available, one should sneeze or cough into the crook of the elbow and then perform proper hand washing. Often, patients who have a respiratory infection are asked to wear a mask to prevent the spread of infected droplets.

MODE OF TRANSMISSION: DIRECT CONTACT

Bloodborne transmission may occur by direct mode if blood from the infected reservoir host comes into contact with the susceptible host's mucous membranes or when the integrity of the skin is compromised. Health-care workers must always practice universal precautions and utilize personal protective equipment (PPE) such as gloves, gowns, masks, eye protection, and face shields to prevent blood from reaching these mucous membranes or from getting into any cut in the skin. The most common bloodborne pathogens that may be transmitted in a health-care setting are hepatitis B (HBV), hepatitis C (HCV), and the human immunodeficiency virus (HIV). Health-care professionals should assume and treat all bodily fluids as if they are contaminated, and any PPE should be managed and disposed of properly. Another example of direct transmission is when a pregnant female passes on a sexually transmitted infection (STI) onto her baby via the placenta or during a vaginal delivery, such as gonorrhea, herpes, or syphilis.

MODE OF TRANSMISSION: AIRBORNE

The spread of microorganisms can take place when particles are dispersed from the respiratory system of the reservoir host and inhaled by another individual. This is known as airborne transmission. An example of airborne transmission is inhaling droplets when an infected individual coughs or sneezes. It is known that people do not need to be located right next to each other as these droplets are capable of traveling several feet following a cough or sneeze. This is a common method in which influenza, tuberculosis, or even chickenpox is spread. People may also become ill after the inhalation of bacteria or fungi within water that is contaminated. One example of this type of airborne infection is Legionnaires' disease. This is not spread from person to person but rather when somebody inhales water droplets that contain the bacteria. This is often heard of in contaminated water supplies such as in hotels, resorts, or air-conditioning systems of apartment complexes.

MODE OF TRANSMISSION: VEHICLE-BORNE FOMITE

A fomite is referred to any inanimate object that can spread a pathogen from one person to the next. Common examples of fomites that aid in the transmission of disease are doorknobs, drinking fountains, water glasses, pens, toys, books, and shopping carts. With these examples, it is easy to see why schools or child-care centers can readily spread germs among individuals. Note that this transmission is carried out in an indirect fashion as body membranes do not need to touch each other. Examples of vehicle-borne fomites in the medical industry could be instruments used in clinical care settings such as tools used for surgical procedures or patient care. Other examples of a vehicle-borne fomite in the medical field could be blood, biopsy specimens, or organs and tissues used for transplants or grafting material.

MODE OF TRANSMISSION: VECTOR-BORNE MECHANICAL OR BIOLOGICAL

A vector-borne method of transmission occurs when pathogens are spread from one living organism to another. Vectors are commonly insects that act as couriers that transport bacteria and other common pathogens from one individual to the next. Examples of vectors are mosquitoes, flies, ticks, and fleas. Mosquitoes are known for spreading West Nile virus. Flies can mechanically transmit disease as they continuously land on food and people. Infected ticks are widely known for spreading Lyme disease when they bite a person. Another disease that ticks may spread is Rocky Mountain spotted fever, which may be deadly if not diagnosed correctly. Fleas are the culprits in transferring pathogens that allow people and animals to contract the plague. Mosquitoes, ticks, and fleas tend to fall under the biological mode of transmission as they tend to become infected because they feed on the blood of their hosts.

PORTAL OF ENTRY

A portal of entrance is the fourth step that must take place for an infection to occur known as the cycle of infection. As the microorganism exits the reservoir host, it must have an entrance portal to infect the susceptible host. Examples of entrance portals are similar to exit routes and include any mucous membrane such as the nose, mouth, rectum, or vagina. These pathogens can also enter via the integumentary system when the skin is no longer intact. The eyes are yet another entrance portal, and conjunctivitis is a very contagious disease that is spread via this entrance method. Urinary tract infections are another common infection seen, especially in females. This occurs as bacteria from the rectum are transferred to the urethra because of the close proximity of these structures. It is important to practice proper hygiene whether it is wiping after using the toilet or hand washing to prevent the transfer of bacteria and other pathogens.

SUSCEPTIBLE HOST

A susceptible host is the fifth and final component in the cycle of infection. A susceptible host is an individual that is unable to fight off an infection and will enable the cycle to continue when this individual passes the pathogen onto another person. There are many factors that determine whether the susceptible host will become infected. These may include the strength of the immune system, overall health, and level of nourishment. Age is another important factor as infants and the elderly are more susceptible to certain diseases. Hygiene practices as well as living conditions are yet another determining factor that may induce an infection. For example, perhaps the host employs great hand-washing techniques but is forced to wash with water that is contaminated while living in a house with rodents and insects. Sometimes the susceptible host, regardless of how healthy he or she is, may be infected with a microorganism so potent that the host is unable to fight it off even with a strong immune system.

BACTERIA

Clinical classification of bacteria takes into account those characteristics that are helpful in identifying infectious processes:

- *Gram-positive or Gram-negative status: Most* bacteria are Gram-negative stains (red) or Gram-positive (purple) although a few cannot be identified by staining. While Gram stain isn't used to identify bacteria, it's frequently referred to clinically.
- *Taxonomic status:* Taxonomy is based on the genera and species of a bacterium, but this can be confusing because some names have changed or two names are used. Genome sequencing should standardize identification.
- *Anaerobic/aerobic status:* Some bacteria are strictly anaerobic, but very few are strictly aerobic. Those that have flexibility and can grow in either aerobic or anaerobic conditions are called *facultative.*
- *Usual environment:* Bacteria are classified according to where they usually reside as flora or where they usually cause infection.
- *Virulence factor:* Bacteria vary widely in virulence. Some are actively invasive but others only cause opportunistic infections.

GRAM-NEGATIVE BACTERIA

The cell walls of Gram-negative bacteria are characterized by red staining. The cell wall is thinner than that of Gram-positive bacteria; however, there are two separate layers to the wall: a thin inner layer of peptidoglycan (carbohydrate polymers bound by proteins), an intervening periplasmic space, and the outer membranous layer (the lipopolysaccharide layer), which produces endotoxins, making Gram-negative bacteria extremely pathogenic. A component of the outer layer is called the S-layer; it aids in adherence and protection from pathogens. The outer layer serves to protect Gram-negative organisms from antibiotics or detergents that would disrupt the inner peptidoglycan layer and provides resistance to penicillin and other compounds. Ampicillin is able to penetrate the exterior wall although many bacteria have become resistant.

Common Gram-negative cocci (round) bacteria include:

- Neisseria gonorrhoeae
- Neisseria meningitides
- Moraxella catarrhalis

Common Gram-negative bacilli (rods) include:

- Haemophilus influenzae
- Legionella pneumophila
- Pseudomonas aeruginosa
- Escherichia coli
- Helicobacter pylori

GRAM-POSITIVE BACTERIA

Gram-positive bacteria are characterized by purple staining; the cell walls tend to be thicker than those of Gram-negative bacteria. About 90% of the cell wall of Gram-positive bacteria is made of peptidoglycan (carbohydrate polymers bound by proteins). The number of peptidoglycan layers varies, but can be more than 20, making a thick-walled cell. An S-layer is attached to the peptidoglycan layer to protect the cell and aid in adherence. Gram-positive organisms tend to be easier to kill than Gram-negative because they lack the outer wall of Gram-negative organisms, and they are more sensitive to penicillin although there are resistant strains. Peptidoglycan does not occur naturally in the human body, so it is easily recognized by the immune system as an invading organism.

Common Gram-positive cocci bacteria include:

- Streptococcus pneumoniae
- Staphylococcus aureus
- Enterococcus

Common Gram-positive bacilli bacteria include:

- Corynbacterium diphtheriae
- Listeria monocytogenes
- Bacillus anthracis.

BACTERIAL GROWTH

Bacterial growth generally proceeds through a series of four phases:

- Lag phase: time for microorganisms to become accustomed to their new environment. There is little or no growth during this phase.
- Log phase: bacteria logarithmic, or exponential, growth begins; the rate of multiplication is the most rapid and constant.
- Stationary phase: the rate of multiplication slows down due to lack of nutrients and build-up of toxins. At the same time, bacteria are constantly dying so the numbers actually remain constant.
- Death phase: cell numbers decrease as growth stops and existing cells die off.

VIRUSES

Viruses (virions) are sub-microscopic and generally considered non-living because they lack cell structures. Viruses consist of nucleic acid, single or double-strand DNA and/or RNA (the genome), encapsulated in a protein coating called a capsid. Some have a lipid envelope about the capsid with glycoprotein spikes. The purpose of viruses is to reproduce, but they require a host cell with a protein receptor to which a virus must bind to penetrate the cell membrane. The viral genome carries encoding that allows it to use the cell to replicate in a *lytic* or *lysogenic* cycle. In the lytic cycle, the virus forces the cell to manufacture proteins and new genomes. After new viral particles form, the cell ruptures, releasing the viruses. In a lysogenic cycle, the virus integrates the DNA of the host and as the cell replicates, the virus replicates with it. The virus remains dormant until it activates and begins a lytic cycle. Viruses that infect bacteria are *bacteriophages* (or *phages).*

> **Review Video: Viruses**
> Visit mometrix.com/academy and enter code: 984455

GENERALIZED PHAGE AND ANIMAL VIRUS LIFE CYCLES

For a virus to attach to a host cell (a process called **adsorption**), it must bind to receptor proteins. The pathway for entry of the viral genome after adsorption varies according to the type of virus, and the type of host cell. Some viruses (particularly bacteriophages) use tail fibers to attach to the host cell's receptors before injecting their genome using the tail sheath. Viruses that infect eukaryotic cells tend to enter either by receptor-mediated endocytosis or by membrane fusion. In receptor-mediated endocytosis, attachment sites on the surface of the virus bind to cell surface receptors, and cell membrane invaginates around the virus, pinching off to forming a vacuole that enters the cytoplasm. Some cells mistake the virus for a desired resource, like nutrients. Enveloped viruses typically gain entry when proteins within their lipid envelope bind to receptor proteins on the cell membrane, and the envelope and membrane fuse. The virus enters, and the protein coat is degraded. If the cell does not have the specific receptor proteins used by a particular virus, then that cell cannot be infected.

Viruses depend on the biosynthetic machinery of the cell to replicate. They cannot copy their own genome, nor can they produce the proteins needed for the capsid. The host cell provides ATP, nucleotides, transfer RNA, amino acids, and most of the enzymes required for viral replication (though some viral genomes contain genes that are translated into enzymes). The cell's ribosomes are redirected to translate viral proteins that are used in the assembly of progeny. The cell can no longer perform its own functions, and has essentially become a virus factory.

PRIONS AND VIROIDS: SUBVIRAL PARTICLES

Prions and viroids are tiny, non-living infectious particles that are much smaller than viruses. In fact, these pathogens are nothing more than proteins and RNA molecules, respectively.

Prions are misfolded variations of normal proteins that incubate for many years before symptoms of disease begin to show. They do not replicate, but rather prompt the misfolding of other proteins, though the mechanism is not well understood. The misfolded proteins group together, triggering the formation of even more prions. The cell cannot function normally under these conditions, and animal diseases such as mad cow disease and Creutzfeldt-Jakob disease result.

Viroids are short circular molecules (approximately 250–400 nucleobases) of ssRNA that are not translated into proteins, but replicate in host plant cells. Replication requires the enzyme RNA polymerase II, and occurs either in the nucleus or in chloroplasts. Viroids cause a number of plant diseases by silencing the normal RNA of the plant, and therefore interfering with gene expression. The human disease hepatitis D is caused by a viroid-like pathogen.

FUNGI

Fungi were originally classified as plants, but they do not produce their own food through photosynthesis and must, like animals, get the food from another source. Fungi vary widely, from one-celled microorganisms to multi-celled chains that are miles long. Fungi are used to make antibiotics, but they can also cause infection and disease. Two common classifications of fungi are molds (including mushrooms) and yeast. Fungi are not motile, but some produce spores, which can be inhaled. Some, such as the yeast *Candida albicans*, are part of the normal flora of the skin but can overgrow in an opportunistic infection. As microorganisms, fungal infections can invade the sinuses, the mouth, the respiratory system, and the vagina. Antibiotics may affect the balance between bacteria and yeast, causing infection. Fungal infections include histoplasmosis, blastomycosis, and coccidioidomycosis. Fungal infections, such as *Pneumocystis jiroveci (*formerly *carinii)* pose a serious problem for the immunocompromised. Antifungal drugs are available, but systemic fungal infections are difficult to treat.

PARASITES

PROTISTS/PROTOZOA

Types/Classifications	Description
Intestinal flagellates: *Giardia lamblia, Trichomonas vaginalis, Dientamoeba fragilis.* **Hemoflagellates:** *Trypanosoma, Leishmania, Trypanosoma cruzi*	Contain one or more flagella (whip-like tails), and some have undulating membrane.
Intestinal amoebas: *Entamoeba histolytica, Balantidium coli*	Have 3 stages: amoeba, inactive cyst, and intermediate precyst. Move with pseudopodia.
Blood apicomplexa/sporozoa: *Plasmodium vivax, ovale, malariae,* and *falciparum; Isospora belli; Babesia microti, sarcocystis spp.; Cryptosporidium spp; Toxoplasma gondii*	Spore-forming with organelle to penetrate host cell.
Microsporida: *Encephalitozoon hellum, Enterocytozoon bieneusi, encephalitozoon intestinalis*	One-celled spore with tubular polar filament to inject sporoplasm into host where it develops.
Ciliates: *Balantidium coli*	Organism with cilia in rows/patches and 2 kinds of nuclei.

ECTOPARASITES

Ectoparasites, parasites that that live on the outside of a host, include such "bugs" as lice, fleas, ticks, mites, and scabies. Common sources are household pets whose vermin can be controlled with pesticides known to be safe to animals and humans. Precautions can be taken against encounters with ectoparasites such as ticks which carry Lyme Disease – they can be kept at bay by protectively covering the body from the waist down when walking in wooded areas. Infestations of head lice, body lice, scabies, and chiggers are common causes of rash and pruritus in children. Head lice are an annoyance, but body lice are a vector of human diseases, including typhus, relapsing fever, and trench fever. They are transmitted through infested clothing; the best way to control outbreaks is by changing and laundering clothes and linens.

HELMINTH PARASITES

Helminths are parasitic worms that live in humans, primarily in the intestines. There are a variety of helminths, including roundworms, tapeworms, pinworms, flukes, and the worm Trichinella spiralis, which is responsible for causing trichinosis. Eggs from helminths can contaminate a variety of things, including feces, pets and other animals, water, air, food, and surfaces like toilet seats. Eggs of helminths usually enter a human via the anus, the nose, or the mouth, and they then travel to the intestines, where they hatch, grow, and multiply. The presence of helminths can be determined in most cases by examining stool samples of suspected infected individuals. Drugs known as vermifuges can be used to treat infections from helminth worms. To prevent infection from helminths, thoroughly cook meats, keep a clean kitchen and bathroom, and wash hands frequently.

MEDICAL ASEPSIS

In order to prevent or control the spread of infection, the cycle of infection must be broken. The cycle of infection refers to the conditions that allow infection to spread. These conditions (presence of pathogen, growth and reproduction, transmission to host, susceptibility of host) must all be present in order for an infection to exist. Medical asepsis (also called clean or aseptic technique) refers to cleanliness practices in a non-sterile environment. The point is to remove as many pathogens as possible from the environment and prevent the spread of those that do exist. The biggest thing that can be done in medical asepsis is the washing of hands. The basic technique of hand washing is the use of warm water, antiseptic cleaner, the removal of jewelry, and specific cleaning of fingernails. Hands should be washed before and after contact with a patient, after contact with organic materials or contaminated equipment, after removing sterile or non-sterile gloves.

SURGICAL ASEPSIS

In order to prevent or control the spread of infection, the cycle of infection must be broken. The cycle of infection refers to the conditions that allow infection to spread. These conditions (presence of pathogen, growth and reproduction, transmission to host, susceptibility of host) must all be present in order for an infection to exist. Surgical asepsis (also called sterile technique) is a strict process of keeping an area sterile by removing any microorganisms from objects in the environment. This is done with the use of an autoclave, gas sterilization, or chemical cleaning solution. The area is them kept sterile by protecting it from contamination with the use of sterile draping, masks, caps, gowns, and gloves. Surgical asepsis should be used any time a patient is cut open for a procedure, if there is damaged skin (burns, cuts), or if a medical device is being inserted into a patient.

There are basic principles that govern surgical asepsis. They are in place to help keep an environment sterile, thus preventing and controlling the spread of infection. The most important (and basic) principle is that sterile objects remain sterile only when they come into contact with other sterile objects. No matter how clean the object it comes into contact with is, if it is not sterile, it should be considered a contaminant. If you are not sure if an object is sterile, or if the object is out of your field of view, it should be treated as contaminated.

UNIVERSAL/STANDARD PRECAUTIONS FOR PREVENTION AND CONTROL OF INFECTION

Universal (also called standard) precautions were developed in 1991 when, to help prevent and control the spread of infection, OSHA (Occupational Health Administration) and the CDC (Centers for Disease Control) mandated that every patient and specimen be treated as if it is contaminated. These precautions apply to all blood and bodily fluids (including peritoneal, amniotic, vaginal, seminal, cerebrospinal, synovial and saliva, pleural and pericardial fluids). Care should be taken when handling any of these fluids, or items contaminated with these fluids. Personal protective equipment (PPE), hand washing, and preventative measures should be employed.

Skeletal System

FUNCTIONS

STRUCTURAL RIGIDITY AND SUPPORT

The skeletal system provides a framework for the body that consists of bones, ligaments, tendons, cartilage, and other tissues. This system is essential in the support and physical protection of the body. Bones support the weight of the body, give shape to body parts, and help to keep internal organs in place. Bones also serve as attachment points for muscles, allowing for body movement. Skeletal muscles connect to bones via tendons, and bones attach to each other via ligaments. Cartilage is more flexible, and supports body parts such as the ear, the nose, the trachea, and various joints. The skeletal system also protects vital organs. The skull encloses the brain, the vertebrae surround the spinal cord, the thoracic cage protects the heart and lungs, and the pelvic girdle protects the inferior portion of the digestive system, the bladder, and the internal reproductive organs. Delicate bone marrow is also protected within the hollow spaces of certain bones.

CALCIUM STORAGE

Bone is a reservoir for calcium. The bone cells produce a hard acellular **matrix** composed of about 35% collagen and 65% inorganic material. Most of the inorganic matter is a type of **calcium phosphate** known as **hydroxyapatite**. Calcium is required for a number of processes, including the contraction of muscles, the conduction of a nerve impulse, and the clotting of blood. The body takes in calcium in the diet, and about 99% of absorbed calcium is stored in bones and teeth. When calcium levels are high, bone-forming cells called **osteoblasts** remove calcium from the blood and deposit it into the bone along with other components of the matrix. Eventually, these cells become surrounded by the hard, calcium-rich secretion and differentiate into mature bone cells called **osteocytes**. If blood calcium is low, cells called **osteoclasts** can break down bone and put calcium back into the blood. In a healthy individual, there is a balance between the amount of calcium deposited and the amount removed. Homeostatic imbalances result in hypercalcemia or hypocalcemia.

SKELETAL STRUCTURE

Bones can be classified as long, short, flat, irregular, and sesamoid. **Long bones** function primarily in movement and supporting body weight. They are rod shaped, and are longer than they are wide. The extremities of a long bone (**epiphyses**) are covered in articular cartilage, and they are wider than the shaft (**diaphysis**). Most of the bones of the upper and lower limbs are long bones, as are the collar bones. **Short bones** are roundish or cube-shaped. They have little to no role in movement, and instead function in support and stability. Examples of short bones include the carpals and tarsals of the wrist and ankle, respectively. **Flat bones** are flattened, thin bones that are usually curved. Their broad shape is suited for protection, as well as muscle attachment. The scapulae, sternum, ribs, ilia of the pelvic girdle, and certain cranial bones are all flat bones. **Irregular bones** have complex shapes that do not fit the classifications above, and their form is suited to their function. Examples of irregular bones include the vertebrae and many facial bones. **Sesamoid bones**, such as the kneecap, are found embedded in tendons where there is considerable mechanical stress.

ADULT HUMAN SKELETON

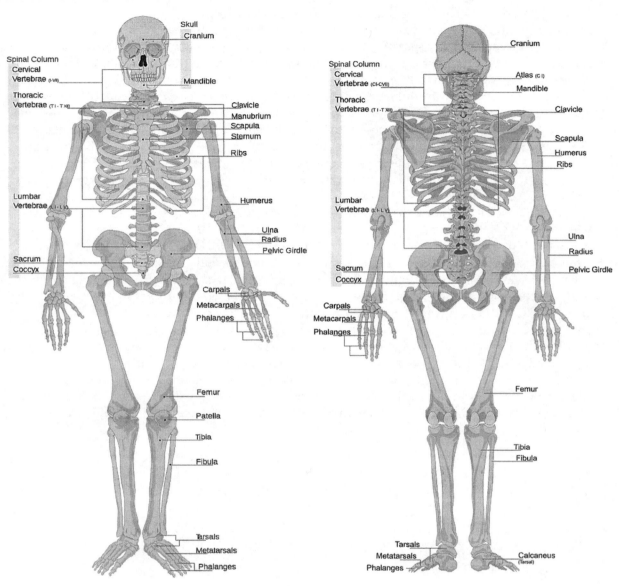

JOINT CLASSIFICATION

Joints are the locations where two or more elements of the skeleton connect. They can be classified according to range of motion, as well as the material that holds the joint together.

Functional classification		
Type of Joint	**Description / Range of Motion**	**Examples**
Synarthrosis	Immovable - either fibrous or cartilaginous	Skull sutures, teeth/mandible
Amphiarthrosis	Slight range of motion - either fibrous or cartilaginous	Intervertebral discs, distal tibiofibular joint
Diarthrosis	Moves freely - always synovial	Wrist, knee, shoulder

Structural classification		
Type of Joint	**Description / Material**	**Types / Examples**
Fibrous	Held together by fibrous connective tissue	Suture: immovable, ex: skull Gomphosis: immovable, ex: teeth/mandible Syndesmosis: slightly movable, ex: distal tibiofibular joint
Cartilaginous	Held together by cartilage	Synchondrosis: hyaline cartilage, nearly immovable, ex: first rib/sternum Symphysis: fibrocartilage, slightly movable, ex: intervertebral discs, pubic symphysis
Synovial	The most common type of joint; characterized by a joint cavity filled with synovial fluid	Pivot: allows rotation, ex: atlantoaxial joint Hinge: allows movement in one plane, ex: knee Saddle: allows pivoting in two planes and axial rotation, ex: first metacarpal/trapezium Gliding: allows sliding, ex: carpals Condyloid: allows pivoting in two planes but no axial rotation, ex: radiocarpal joint Ball and socket: have the highest range of motion, ex: hip

BONE STRUCTURE

Compact (or cortical) bone is the hard, dense tissue that forms the outer surfaces of bones, as well as the shafts of long bones. It consists of cylindrical structures called **osteons**, also called Haversian systems. Each osteon consists of a central **Haversian canal** that contains nerve fibers and blood vessels, and these canals connect to each other via **perforating canals** (or **Volkmann's canals**). The Haversian canal is surrounded by concentric layers of calcified **lamellae** with small spaces called **lacunae**, each of which contains an **osteocyte**. Tiny channels called **canaliculi** connect the lacunae to allow oxygen and nutrients to reach the osteocytes, and wastes to be removed.

Spongy (or cancellous) bone is the porous tissue found at the ends of long bones and inside the vertebrae and flat bones. It is not as strong or abundant as compact bone, and does not contain osteons. Instead, it consists of flattened, interconnected plates called **trabeculae**. Within the spaces of the trabeculae is the **red bone marrow** that produces blood cells. There are no central canals, but osteocytes do reside in lacunae that are connected by canaliculi.

Compact Bone & Spongy (Cancellous Bone)

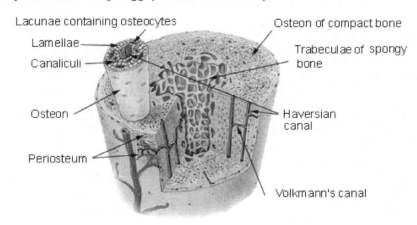

CELLULAR COMPOSITION OF BONE

Bone consists of an extracellular matrix that surrounds bone cells and functions much like reinforced concrete. The matrix consists of about 2/3 inorganic matter; mostly calcium phosphate (hydroxyapatite) with calcium carbonate and other minerals. The organic portion makes up about 1/3 of the matrix. It consists mainly of collagen, which adds strength and flexibility to the matrix, as well as ground substance proteins such as glycosaminoglycans (GAGs).

There are three types of bone cells. **Osteoblasts** (derived from osteoprogenitor cells) take calcium from the blood, and produce the matrix (including collagen fibers) that forms bone. When it is completely encased in matrix, the osteoblast differentiates into a mature bone cell called an **osteocyte**. Osteocytes are the most abundant bone cells, and they maintain the matrix by recycling calcium salts. **Osteoclasts** are large multinucleate cells that are formed by the fusion of monocytes (large white blood cells). They reside on bone surfaces and secrete acid and digestive enzymes that break down bone and return calcium to the blood.

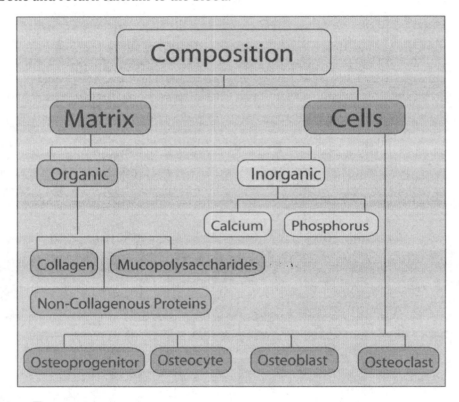

TYPES OF BONE FRACTURES

A bone fracture is caused when the force against the bone is greater than the bone can sustain causing it to splinter, fracture, or break. There are multiple classifications of fractures. A **closed fracture** is when the bone breaks but does not puncture through the skin and protrude through to the outside. An **open fracture** is when the bone breaks and punctures the skin protruding to the outside of the body. A **comminuted fracture** is when the bone breaks in multiple areas. This is often seen in a trauma such as a car accident or in competitive sports. A **greenstick fracture** is when part of the bone bends and does not fully break. This is often seen in young children because the bones are flexible, softer, and still developing. A **spiral fracture** is when the bone is twisted or rotated like a corkscrew. An **avulsion fracture** is when a tendon or ligament is taxed and pulled too hard causing it to pull away and break the bone. An **oblique fracture** is a break at an angle caused by the outside force coming at a right angle to the bone. A **transverse fracture** is when the fracture is perpendicular to the shaft of the bone. A **pathological fracture** is caused by disease making the bone weak, and the bone can break without warning simply by putting minimal pressure on it.

CARTILAGE: STRUCTURE AND FUNCTION

Cartilage is a connective tissue with a matrix that is flexible yet resistant to stretching. Cartilage is not innervated, nor does it have a blood supply, except for the **perichondrium** that forms the surfaces of nearly all cartilage. The immature cartilage cells that secrete the matrix are called **chondroblasts**. Chondroblasts give rise to mature cells called **chondrocytes** that reside in lacunae.

There are three types of cartilage: hyaline, elastic, and fibrocartilage. **Hyaline cartilage** is the most common cartilage in the body. It consists of evenly distributed collagen fibrils that explain its glassy appearance. It is found in locations that require strong support with some pliability, such as the ribs, nose, trachea, and articular surfaces. **Elastic cartilage** is similar to hyaline cartilage but is more flexible due to the presence of elastic fibers. It is found in the epiglottis and external ear. **Fibrocartilage** has collagen arranged into thick fibers, which allows it to withstand tension and compression. It is found in the jaw, in the knee, and between the vertebrae.

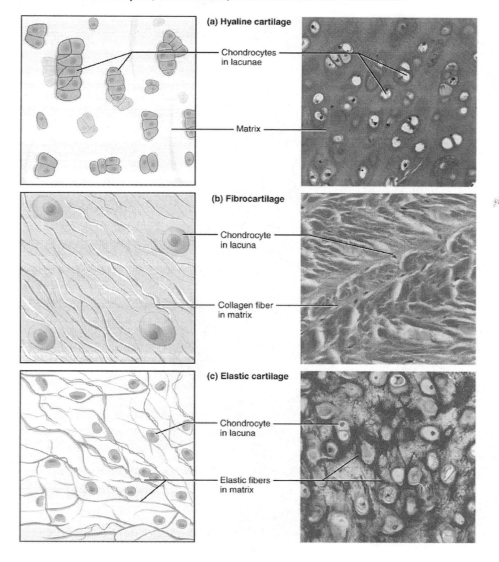

(a) Hyaline cartilage
- Chondrocytes in lacunae
- Matrix

(b) Fibrocartilage
- Chondrocyte in lacuna
- Collagen fiber in matrix

(c) Elastic cartilage
- Chondrocyte in lacuna
- Elastic fibers in matrix

LIGAMENTS, TENDONS

Ligaments connect bones to bones, and help to stabilize joints. **Tendons** connect muscles to bones or other structures such as the eyeballs, and facilitate movement. They are both composed of **dense regular connective tissue**, which consists of bundles of collagen fibers as well as elastic fibers. This gives them strength and resistance to stretching. The collagen fibers of tendons are more densely packed than those of ligaments. They are also arranged in parallel bundles, while the fibers of many ligaments are not. Tendons are tougher, but ligaments are more elastic. The yellowish color of certain ligaments results from the protein elastin.

ENDOCRINE CONTROL

The calcium-regulating hormones of the endocrine system are responsible for breaking down and reabsorbing bone tissue. The kidneys produce 1,25-hydroxyvitamin D, a biologically active form of vitamin D also known as **calcitriol**. This hormone regulates levels of calcium by promoting the absorption of dietary calcium in the intestines, which increases the level of calcium in the blood. Calcitriol also stimulates osteoclasts to break down bone, which moves calcium into the blood. When blood calcium is high, the peptide hormone **calcitonin** is secreted by the parafollicular cells of the thyroid gland. Calcitonin inhibits the activity of osteoclasts, and stimulates the activity of bone-forming osteoblasts. When blood calcium is low, parathyroid glands secrete a peptide hormone known as **parathyroid hormone (PTH)**. This increases the quantity and also the activity of osteoclasts.

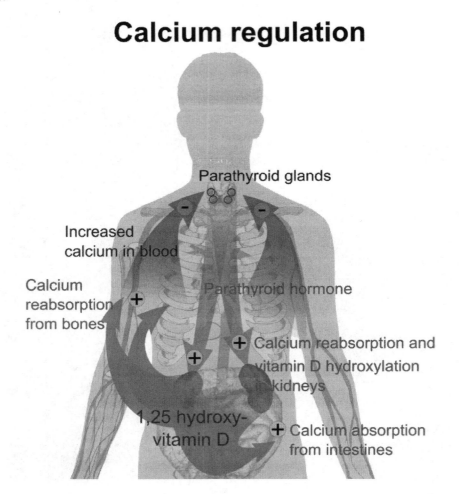

Calcium regulation

Parathyroid glands

Increased calcium in blood

Calcium reabsorption from bones

Parathyroid hormone

Calcium reabsorption and vitamin D hydroxylation in kidneys

1,25 hydroxy-vitamin D

Calcium absorption from intestines

Life and Physical Sciences

MACROMOLECULES

Macromolecules are large and complex, and play an important role in cell structure and function. The four basic organic macromolecules produced by anabolic reactions are **carbohydrates** (polysaccharides), **nucleic acids**, **proteins**, and **lipids**. The four basic building blocks involved in catabolic reactions are **monosaccharides** (glucose), **amino acids**, **fatty acids** (glycerol), and **nucleotides**.

An **anabolic reaction** is one that builds larger and more complex molecules (macromolecules) from smaller ones. **Catabolic reactions** are the opposite. Larger molecules are broken down into smaller, simpler molecules. Catabolic reactions *release energy*, while anabolic ones *require energy*.

Endothermic reactions are chemical reactions that *absorb* heat and **exothermic reactions** are chemical reactions that *release* heat.

CARBOHYDRATE

Carbohydrates are the primary source of energy and are responsible for providing energy as they can be easily converted to **glucose**. It is the oxidation of carbohydrates that provides the cells with most of their energy. Glucose can be further broken down by respiration or fermentation by **glycolysis**. They are involved in the metabolic energy cycles of photosynthesis and respiration.

Structurally, carbohydrates usually take the form of some variation of CH_2O as they are made of carbon, hydrogen, and oxygen. Carbohydrates (**polysaccharides**) are broken down into sugars or glucose.

The simple sugars can be grouped into monosaccharides (glucose, fructose, and galactose) and disaccharides. These are both types of carbohydrates. Monosaccharides have one monomer of sugar and disaccharides have two. Monosaccharides (CH_2O) have one carbon for every water molecule.

A **monomer** is a small molecule. It is a single compound that forms chemical bonds with other monomers to make a polymer. A **polymer** is a compound of large molecules formed by repeating monomers. Carbohydrates, proteins, and nucleic acids are groups of macromolecules that are polymers.

LIPIDS

Lipids are molecules that are soluble in nonpolar solvents, but are hydrophobic, meaning they do not bond well with water or mix well with water solutions. Lipids have numerous **C–H bonds**. In this way, they are similar to **hydrocarbons** (substances consisting only of carbon and hydrogen). The major roles of lipids include *energy storage and structural functions*. Examples of lipids include fats, phospholipids, steroids, and waxes. **Fats** (which are triglycerides) are made of long chains of fatty acids (three fatty acids bound to a glycerol). **Fatty acids** are chains with reduced carbon at one end and a carboxylic acid group at the other. An example is soap, which contains the sodium salts of free fatty acids. **Phospholipids** are lipids that have a phosphate group rather than a fatty acid. **Glycerides** are another type of lipid. Examples of glycerides are fat and oil. Glycerides are formed from fatty acids and glycerol (a type of alcohol).

Review Video: Lipids
Visit mometrix.com/academy and enter code: 269746

PROTEINS

Proteins are macromolecules formed from amino acids. They are **polypeptides**, which consist of many (10 to 100) peptides linked together. The peptide connections are the result of condensation reactions. A **condensation reaction** results in a loss of water when two molecules are joined together. A **hydrolysis reaction** is the opposite of a condensation reaction. During hydrolysis, water is added. –H is added to one of the smaller molecules and OH is added to another molecule being formed. A **peptide** is a compound of two or more amino acids. **Amino acids** are formed by the partial hydrolysis of protein, which forms an **amide bond**. This partial hydrolysis involves an amine group and a carboxylic acid. In the carbon chain of amino acids, there is a **carboxylic acid group** (–COOH), an **amine group** (–NH$_2$), a **central carbon atom** between them with an attached hydrogen, and an attached **"R" group** (side chain), which is different for different amino acids. It is the "R" group that determines the properties of the protein.

> **Review Video: Proteins**
> Visit mometrix.com/academy and enter code: 903713

ENZYMES

Enzymes are proteins with strong **catalytic** power. They greatly accelerate the speed at which specific reactions approach equilibrium. Although enzymes do not start chemical reactions that would not eventually occur by themselves, they do make these reactions happen *faster and more often*. This acceleration can be substantial, sometimes making reactions happen a million times faster. Each type of enzyme deals with **reactants**, also called **substrates**. Each enzyme is highly selective, only interacting with substrates that are a match for it at an active site on the enzyme. This is the "key in the lock" analogy: a certain enzyme only fits with certain substrates. Even with a matching substrate, sometimes an enzyme must reshape itself to fit well with the substrate, forming a strong bond that aids in catalyzing a reaction before it returns to its original shape. An unusual quality of enzymes is that they are not permanently consumed in the reactions they speed up. They can be used again and again, providing a constant source of energy accelerants for cells. This allows for a tremendous increase in the number and rate of reactions in cells.

NUCLEIC ACIDS

Nucleic acids are macromolecules that are composed of **nucleotides**. **Hydrolysis** is a reaction in which water is broken down into **hydrogen cations** (H or H$^+$) and **hydroxide anions** (OH or OH$^-$). This is part of the process by which nucleic acids are broken down by enzymes to produce shorter strings of RNA and DNA (oligonucleotides). **Oligonucleotides** are broken down into smaller sugar nitrogenous units called **nucleosides**. These can be digested by cells since the sugar is divided from the nitrogenous base. This, in turn, leads to the formation of the five types of nitrogenous bases, sugars, and the preliminary substances involved in the synthesis of new RNA and DNA. DNA and RNA have a helix shape.

Macromolecular nucleic acid polymers, such as RNA and DNA, are formed from nucleotides, which are monomeric units joined by **phosphodiester bonds**. Cells require energy in the form of ATP to synthesize proteins from amino acids and replicate DNA. **Nitrogen fixation** is used to synthesize nucleotides for DNA and amino acids for proteins. Nitrogen fixation uses the enzyme nitrogenase in the reduction of dinitrogen gas (N$_2$) to ammonia (NH$_3$).

Nucleic acids store information and energy and are also important catalysts. It is the **RNA** that catalyzes the transfer of **DNA genetic information** into protein coded information. ATP is an RNA nucleotide. **Nucleotides** are used to form the nucleic acids. Nucleotides are made of a five-carbon sugar, such as ribose or deoxyribose, a nitrogenous base, and one or more phosphates. Nucleotides consisting of more than one phosphate can also store energy in their bonds.

> **Review Video: Nucleic Acids**
> Visit mometrix.com/academy and enter code: 503931

DNA

Chromosomes consist of **genes**, which are single units of genetic information. Genes are made up of deoxyribonucleic acid (DNA). DNA is a nucleic acid located in the cell nucleus. There is also DNA in the **mitochondria**. DNA replicates to pass on genetic information. The DNA in almost all cells is the same. It is also involved in the biosynthesis of proteins.

The model or structure of DNA is described as a **double helix**. A helix is a curve, and a double helix is two congruent curves connected by horizontal members. The model can be likened to a spiral staircase. It is right-handed. The British scientist Rosalind Elsie Franklin is credited with taking the x-ray diffraction image in 1952 that was used by Francis Crick and James Watson to formulate the double-helix model of DNA and speculate about its important role in carrying and transferring genetic information.

> **Review Video: DNA**
> Visit mometrix.com/academy and enter code: 639552

DNA STRUCTURE

DNA has a double helix shape, resembles a twisted ladder, and is compact. It consists of **nucleotides**. Nucleotides consist of a **five-carbon sugar** (pentose), a **phosphate group**, and a **nitrogenous base**. Two bases pair up to form the rungs of the ladder. The "side rails" or backbone consists of the covalently bonded sugar and phosphate. The bases are attached to each other with hydrogen bonds, which are easily dismantled so replication can occur. Each base is attached to a phosphate and to a sugar. There are four types of nitrogenous bases: **adenine** (A), **guanine** (G), **cytosine** (C), and **thymine** (T). There are about 3 billion bases in human DNA. The bases are mostly the same in everybody, but their order is different. It is the order of these bases that creates diversity in people. *Adenine (A) pairs with thymine (T)*, and *cytosine (C) pairs with guanine (G)*.

PURINES AND PYRIMIDINES

The five bases in DNA and RNA can be categorized as either pyrimidine or purine according to their structure. The **pyrimidine bases** include *cytosine, thymine, and uracil*. They are six-sided and have a single ring shape. The **purine bases** are *adenine and guanine*, which consist of two attached rings. One ring has five sides and the other has six. When combined with a sugar, any of the five bases become **nucleosides**. Nucleosides formed from purine bases end in "osine" and those formed from pyrimidine bases end in "idine." **Adenosine** and **thymidine** are examples of nucleosides. Bases are the most basic components, followed by nucleosides, nucleotides, and then DNA or RNA.

CODONS

Codons are groups of three nucleotides on the messenger RNA, and can be visualized as three rungs of a ladder. A **codon** has the code for a single amino acid. There are 64 codons but 20 amino acids. More than one combination, or triplet, can be used to synthesize the necessary amino acids. For example, AAA (adenine-adenine-adenine) or AAG (adenine-adenine-guanine) can serve as codons for lysine. These groups of three occur in strings, and might be thought of as frames. For example, AAAUCUUCGU, if read in groups of three from the beginning, would be AAA, UCU, UCG, which are codons for lysine, serine, and serine, respectively. If the same sequence was read in groups of three starting from the second position, the groups would be AAU (asparagine), CUU (proline), and so on. The resulting amino acids would be completely different. For this reason, there are **start and stop codons** that indicate the beginning and ending of a sequence (or frame). **AUG** (methionine) is the start codon. **UAA, UGA,** and **UAG**, also known as ocher, opal, and amber, respectively, are stop codons.

> **Review Video: <u>Codons</u>**
> Visit mometrix.com/academy and enter code: 978172

DNA REPLICATION

Pairs of chromosomes are composed of DNA, which is tightly wound to conserve space. When replication starts, it unwinds. The steps in **DNA replication** are controlled by enzymes. The enzyme **helicase** instigates the deforming of hydrogen bonds between the bases to split the two strands. The splitting starts at the A-T bases (adenine and thymine) as there are only two hydrogen bonds. The cytosine-guanine base pair has three bonds. The term "**origin of replication**" is used to refer to where the splitting starts. The portion of the DNA that is unwound to be replicated is called the **replication fork**. Each strand of DNA is transcribed by an mRNA. It copies the DNA onto itself, base by base, in a complementary manner. The exception is that uracil replaces thymine.

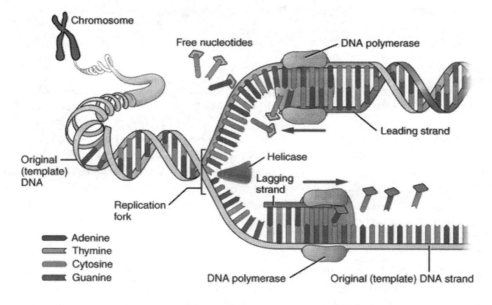

RNA

TYPES OF RNA

RNA acts as a *helper* to DNA and carries out a number of other functions. Types of RNA include ribosomal RNA (rRNA), transfer RNA (tRNA), and messenger RNA (mRNA). Viruses can use RNA to carry their genetic material to DNA. **Ribosomal RNA** is not believed to have changed much over time. For this reason, it can be used to study relationships in organisms. **Messenger RNA** carries a copy of a strand of DNA and transports it from the nucleus to the cytoplasm. **Transcription** is the process in which RNA polymerase copies DNA into RNA. DNA unwinds itself and serves as a template while RNA is being assembled. The DNA molecules are copied to RNA. **Translation** is the process whereby ribosomes use transcribed RNA to put together the needed protein. **Transfer RNA** is a molecule that helps in the translation process, and is found in the cytoplasm.

DIFFERENCES BETWEEN RNA AND DNA

RNA and DNA differ in terms of structure and function. RNA has a different sugar than DNA. It has **ribose** rather than **deoxyribose** sugar. The RNA nitrogenous bases are adenine (A), guanine (G), cytosine (C), and uracil (U). **Uracil** is found only in RNA and **thymine** in found only in DNA. RNA consists of a single strand and DNA has two strands. If straightened out, DNA has two side rails. RNA only has one "backbone," or strand of sugar and phosphate group components. RNA uses the fully hydroxylated sugar **pentose**, which includes an extra oxygen compared to deoxyribose, which is the sugar used by DNA. RNA supports the functions carried out by DNA. It aids in gene expression, replication, and transportation.

MENDEL'S LAWS

Mendel's laws are the law of segregation (the first law) and the law of independent assortment (the second law). The **law of segregation** states that there are two **alleles** and that half of the total number of alleles are contributed by each parent organism. The **law of independent assortment** states that traits are passed on randomly and are not influenced by other traits. The exception to this is linked traits. A **Punnett square** can illustrate how alleles combine from the contributing genes to form various **phenotypes**. One set of a parent's genes are put in columns, while the genes from the other parent are placed in rows. The allele combinations are shown in each cell. When two different alleles are present in a pair, the **dominant** one is expressed. A Punnett square can be used to predict the outcome of crosses.

GENE, GENOTYPE, PHENOTYPE, AND ALLELE

A gene is a portion of DNA that identifies how traits are expressed and passed on in an organism. A gene is part of the **genetic code**. Collectively, all genes form the **genotype** of an individual. The genotype includes genes that may not be expressed, such as **recessive genes**. The **phenotype** is the physical, visual manifestation of genes. It is determined by the basic genetic information and how genes have been affected by their environment.

An **allele** is a variation of a gene. Also known as a trait, it determines the manifestation of a gene. This manifestation results in a specific physical appearance of some facet of an organism, such as eye color or height. For example, the genetic information for eye color is a gene. The gene variations responsible for blue, green, brown, or black eyes are called alleles. **Locus** (pl. loci) refers to the location of a gene or alleles.

DOMINANT AND RECESSIVE

Gene traits are represented in pairs with an uppercase letter for the dominant trait (A) and a lowercase letter for the recessive trait (a). Genes occur in pairs (AA, Aa, or aa). There is one gene on each chromosome half supplied by each parent organism. Since half the genetic material is from each parent, the offspring's traits are represented as a combination of these. A **dominant trait** only requires one gene of a gene pair for it to be expressed in a **phenotype**, whereas a **recessive** requires both genes in order to be manifested. For example, if the mother's genotype is Dd and the father's is dd, the possible combinations are Dd and dd. The dominant trait will be manifested if the genotype is DD or Dd. The recessive trait will be manifested if the genotype is dd. Both DD and dd are **homozygous** pairs. Dd is **heterozygous**.

MONOHYBRID AND HYBRID CROSSES

Genetic crosses are the possible combinations of alleles, and can be represented using Punnett squares. A **monohybrid cross** refers to a cross involving only one trait. Typically, the ratio is 3:1 (DD, Dd, Dd, dd), which is the ratio of dominant gene manifestation to recessive gene manifestation. This ratio occurs when both parents have a pair of dominant and recessive genes. If one parent has a pair of dominant genes (DD) and the other has a pair of recessive (dd) genes, the recessive trait cannot be expressed in the next generation because the resulting crosses all have the Dd genotype.

A **dihybrid cross** refers to one involving more than one trait, which means more combinations are possible. The ratio of genotypes for a dihybrid cross is 9:3:3:1 when the traits are not linked. The ratio for incomplete dominance is 1:2:1, which corresponds to dominant, mixed, and recessive phenotypes.

MONOHYBRID CROSS EXAMPLE

A monohybrid cross is a genetic cross for a single trait that has two alleles. A monohybrid cross can be used to show which allele is **dominant** for a single trait. The first monohybrid cross typically occurs between two **homozygous** parents. Each parent is homozygous for a separate allele for a particular trait. For example, in pea plants, green pods (G) are dominant over yellow pods (g). In a genetic cross of two pea plants that are homozygous for pod color, the F_1 generation will be 100% heterozygous green pods.

	g	g
G	Gg	Gg
G	Gg	Gg

If the plants with the heterozygous green pods are crossed, the F_2 generation should be 50% heterozygous green, 25% homozygous green, and 25% homozygous yellow.

	G	g
G	GG	Gg
g	Gg	gg

DIHYBRID CROSS EXAMPLE

A dihybrid cross is a genetic cross for **two traits** that each have two alleles. For example, in pea plants, green pods (G) are dominant over yellow pods (g), and yellow seeds (Y) are dominant over green seeds (y). In a genetic cross of two pea plants that are homozygous for pod color and seed color, the F_1 generation will be 100% heterozygous green pods and yellow seeds (GgYy). If these F_1 plants are crossed, the resulting F_2 generation is shown below. There are nine genotypes for green-pod, yellow-seed plants: one GGYY, two GGYy, two GgYY, and four GgYy. There are three genotypes for green-pod, green-seed plants: one GGyy and two Ggyy. There are three genotypes for yellow-pod, yellow-seed plants: one ggYY and two ggYy. There is only one genotype for yellow-pod, green-seed plants: ggyy. This cross has a 9:3:3:1 ratio.

	GY	Gy	gY	gy
GY	GGYY	GGYy	GgYY	GgYy
Gy	GGYy	GGyy	GgYy	Ggyy
gY	GgYY	GgYy	ggYY	ggYy
gy	GgYy	Ggyy	ggYy	ggyy

NON-MENDELIAN CONCEPTS

CO-DOMINANCE

Co-dominance refers to the expression of *both alleles* so that both traits are shown. Cows, for example, can have hair colors of red, white, or red and white (not pink). In the latter color, both traits are fully expressed. The ABO human blood typing system is also co-dominant.

> **Review Video: Mendelian & Non-Mendelian Concepts (Co-Dominance, Incomplete Dominance, Polygenic Inheritance, and Multiple Alleles)**
> Visit mometrix.com/academy and enter code: 113159

INCOMPLETE DOMINANCE

Incomplete dominance is when both the **dominant** and **recessive** genes are expressed, resulting in a phenotype that is a mixture of the two. The fact that snapdragons can be red, white, or pink is a good example. The dominant red gene (RR) results in a red flower because of large amounts of red pigment. White (rr) occurs because both genes call for no pigment. Pink (Rr) occurs because one gene is for red and one is for no pigment. The colors blend to produce pink flowers. A cross of pink flowers (Rr) can result in red (RR), white (rr), or pink (Rr) flowers.

POLYGENIC INHERITANCE

Polygenic inheritance goes beyond the simplistic Mendelian concept that one gene influences one trait. It refers to traits that are influenced by *more than one gene*, and takes into account environmental influences on development.

MULTIPLE ALLELES

Each gene is made up of only two alleles, but in some cases, there are more than two possibilities for what those two alleles might be. For example, in blood typing, there are three alleles (A, B, O), but each person has only two of them. A gene with more than two possible alleles is known as a multiple allele. A gene that can result in two or more possible forms or expressions is known as a polymorphic gene.

BASIC ATOMIC STRUCTURE

PIECES OF AN ATOM

All matter consists of atoms. Atoms consist of a **nucleus** and **electrons**. The nucleus consists of **protons** and **neutrons**. The properties of these are measurable; they have mass and an electrical charge. The nucleus is **positively charged** due to the presence of protons. Electrons are **negatively charged** and orbit the nucleus. The nucleus has considerably more mass than the surrounding electrons. Atoms can bond together to make **molecules**. Atoms that have an equal number of protons and electrons are electrically **neutral**. If the number of protons and electrons in an atom is not equal, the atom has a positive or negative charge and is an **ion**.

> **Review Video: Structure of Atoms**
> Visit mometrix.com/academy and enter code: 905932

MODELS OF ATOMS

Atoms are extremely small. A hydrogen atom is about 5×10^{-8} mm in diameter. According to some estimates, five trillion hydrogen atoms could fit on the head of a pin. **Atomic radius** refers to the average distance between the nucleus and the outermost electron. Models of atoms that include the proton, nucleus, and electrons typically show the electrons very close to the nucleus and revolving around it, similar to how the Earth orbits the sun. However, another model relates the Earth as the nucleus and its atmosphere as electrons, which is the basis of the term "**electron cloud**." Another description is that electrons swarm around the nucleus. It should be noted that these atomic models are not to scale. A more accurate representation would be a nucleus with a diameter of about 2 cm in a stadium. The electrons would be in the bleachers. This model is similar to the not-to-scale solar system model.

ATOMIC NUMBER

The atomic number of an element refers to the **number of protons** in the nucleus of an atom. It is a unique identifier. It can be represented as Z. Atoms with a neutral charge have an atomic number that is equal to the **number of electrons**.

ATOMIC MASS

Atomic mass is also known as the **mass number**. The atomic mass is the *total number of protons and neutrons* in the nucleus of an atom. It is referred to as "A." The atomic mass (A) is equal to the number of protons (Z) plus the number of neutrons (N). This can be represented by the equation A = Z + N. The mass of electrons in an atom is basically insignificant because it is so small. Atomic weight may sometimes be referred to as "**relative atomic mass**," but should not be confused with atomic mass. Atomic weight is the ratio of the average mass per atom of a sample (which can include various isotopes of an element) to 1/12 of the mass of an atom of carbon-12.

> **Review Video: Isotopes**
> Visit mometrix.com/academy and enter code: 294271

ISOTOPES

Isotopes are denoted by the element symbol, preceded in superscript and subscript by the mass number and atomic number, respectively. For instance, the notations for protium, deuterium, and tritium are, respectively: ^1_1H, ^2_1H, and ^3_1H.

Isotopes that have not been observed to decay are **stable**, or non-radioactive, isotopes. It is not known whether some stable isotopes may have such long decay times that observing decay is not possible. Currently, 80 elements have one or more stable isotopes. There are 256 known stable isotopes in total. Carbon, for example, has three isotopes. Two (carbon-12 and carbon-13) are stable and one (carbon-14) is radioactive. **Radioactive isotopes** have unstable nuclei and can undergo spontaneous nuclear reactions, which results in particles or radiation being emitted. It cannot be predicted when a specific nucleus will decay, but large groups of identical nuclei decay at predictable rates. Knowledge about rates of decay can be used to *estimate the age of materials* that contain radioactive isotopes.

ELECTRONS

Electrons are subatomic particles that orbit the nucleus at various levels commonly referred to as **layers**, **shells**, or **clouds**. The orbiting electron or electrons account for only a fraction of the atom's mass. They are much smaller than the nucleus, are negatively charged, and exhibit wave-like characteristics. Electrons are part of the **lepton** family of elementary particles. Electrons can occupy orbits that are varying distances away from the nucleus, and tend to occupy the lowest energy level they can. If an atom has all its electrons in the lowest available positions, it has a **stable** electron arrangement. The outermost electron shell of an atom in its uncombined state is known as the **valence shell**. The electrons there are called **valence electrons**, and it is their number that determines **bonding behavior**. Atoms tend to react in a manner that will allow them to fill or empty their valence shells.

CHEMICAL BONDS AND ELECTRON SHELLS

Chemical bonds involve a negative-positive attraction between an electron or electrons and the nucleus of an atom or nuclei of more than one atom. The attraction keeps the atom cohesive, but also enables the formation of bonds among other atoms and molecules. Each of the four **energy levels** (or shells) of an atom has a maximum number of electrons they can contain. Each level must be completely filled before electrons can be added to the **valence level**. The farther away from the nucleus an electron is, the more energy it has. The first shell, or K-shell, can hold a maximum of 2 electrons; the second, the L-shell, can hold 8; the third, the M-shell, can hold 18; the fourth, the N-shell, can hold 32. The shells can also have **subshells**. Chemical bonds form and break between atoms when atoms gain, lose, or share an electron in the outer valence shell. **Polar bond** refers to a covalent type of bond with a separation of charge. One end is negative and the other is positive. The hydrogen-oxygen bond in water is one example of a polar bond.

IONS

Most atoms are **neutral** since the positive charge of the protons in the nucleus is balanced by the negative charge of the surrounding electrons. Electrons are transferred between atoms when they come into contact with each other. This creates a molecule or atom in which the number of electrons does not equal the number of protons, which gives it a positive or negative charge. A **negative ion** is created when an atom gains electrons, while a **positive ion** is created when an atom loses electrons. An **ionic bond** is formed between ions with opposite charges. The resulting compound is neutral. **Ionization** refers to the process by which neutral particles are ionized into charged particles. Gases and plasmas can be partially or fully ionized through ionization.

CHEMICAL BONDS BETWEEN ATOMS

Atoms of the same element may bond together to form **molecules** or **crystalline solids**. When two or more different types of atoms bind together chemically, a **compound** is made. The physical properties of compounds reflect the nature of the interactions among their molecules. These interactions are determined by the structure of the molecule, including the atoms they consist of and the distances and angles between them.

A union between the electron structures of atoms is called **chemical bonding**. An atom may gain, surrender, or share its electrons with another atom it bonds with. Listed below are three types of chemical bonding.

- **Ionic bonding** – When an atom gains or loses electrons it becomes negatively or positively charged, turning it into an ion. An ionic bond is a relationship between two *oppositely charged ions*.
- **Covalent bonding** – Atoms that share electrons have what is called a covalent bond. Electrons shared equally have a *non-polar bond*, while electrons shared unequally have a *polar bond*.
- **Hydrogen bonding** – The atom of a molecule interacts with a hydrogen atom in the same area. Hydrogen bonds can also form between two different parts of the same molecule, as in the structure of DNA and other large molecules.

A **cation** or positive ion is formed when an atom loses one or more electrons. An **anion** or negative ion is formed when an atom gains one or more electrons.

IONIC BONDING

The transfer of electrons from one atom to another is called **ionic bonding**. Atoms that lose or gain electrons are referred to as **ions**. The gain or loss of electrons will result in an ion having a positive or negative charge. Here is an example:

Take an atom of sodium (Na) and an atom of chlorine (Cl). The sodium atom has a total of 11 electrons (including one electron in its outer shell). The chlorine has 17 electrons (including 7 electrons in its outer shell). From this, the atomic number, or number of protons, of sodium can be calculated as 11 because the number of protons equals the number of electrons in an atom. When sodium chloride (NaCl) is formed, one electron from sodium transfers to chlorine. Ions have charges. They are written with a plus (+) or minus (–) symbol. Ions in a compound are attracted to each other because they have *opposite charges*.

$$Na \cdot + \overset{\times \times}{\underset{\times \times}{\times Cl \times}} \longrightarrow [Na]^+ [\overset{\times \times}{\underset{\times \times}{\cdot Cl \times}}]^-$$

electron transer from
sodium to chlorine

COVALENT BONDING

Covalent bonding is characterized by the sharing of one or more pairs of electrons between two atoms or between an atom and another **covalent bond**. This produces an attraction to repulsion stability that holds these molecules together.

Atoms have the tendency to share electrons with each other so that all outer electron shells are filled. The resultant bonds are always stronger than the **intermolecular hydrogen bond** and are similar in strength to ionic bonds.

Covalent bonding occurs most frequently between atoms with similar **electronegativities**. **Nonmetals** are more likely to form covalent bonds than metals since it is more difficult for nonmetals to liberate an electron. **Electron sharing** takes place when one species encounters another species with similar electronegativity. Covalent bonding of metals is important in both *process chemistry* and *industrial catalysis*.

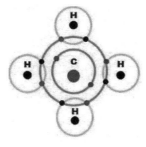

ELECTRONEGATIVITY

Electronegativity is a measure of how capable an atom is of attracting a pair of bonding electrons. It refers to the fact that one atom exerts slightly more force in a bond than another, creating a **dipole**. If the electronegative difference between two atoms is small, the atoms will form a **polar covalent**

bond. If the difference is large, the atoms will form an **ionic bond**. When there is no electronegativity, a **pure nonpolar covalent bond** is formed.

> **Review Video: Electronegativity**
> Visit mometrix.com/academy and enter code: 823348

COMPOUNDS

An **element** is the most basic type of matter. It has unique properties and cannot be broken down into other elements. The smallest unit of an element is the **atom**. A chemical combination of two or more types of elements is called a **compound**.

Compounds often have properties that are very different from those of their constituent elements. The smallest independent unit of an element or compound is known as a **molecule**. Most elements are found somewhere in nature in single-atom form, but a few elements only exist naturally in pairs. These are called **diatomic elements**, of which some of the most common are hydrogen, nitrogen, and oxygen.

Elements and compounds are represented by **chemical symbols**, one or two letters, most often the first in the element name. More than one atom of the same element in a compound is represented with a subscript number designating how many atoms of that element are present. Water, for instance, contains two hydrogens and one oxygen. Thus, the chemical formula is H_2O. Methane contains one carbon and four hydrogens, so its formula is CH_4.

PERIODIC TABLE

1 IA																	18 VIIIA
1 **H** 1.01	2 IIA											13 IIIA	14 IVA	15 VA	16 VIA	17 VIIA	2 **He** 4.00
3 **Li** 6.94	4 **Be** 9.01											5 **B** 10.81	6 **C** 12.01	7 **N** 14.01	8 **O** 16.00	9 **F** 19.00	10 **Ne** 20.18
11 **Na** 22.99	12 **Mg** 24.31	3 IIIB	4 IVB	5 VB	6 VIB	7 VIIB	8	9 VIIIB	10	11 IB	12 IIB	13 **Al** 26.98	14 **Si** 28.09	15 **P** 30.97	16 **S** 32.07	17 **Cl** 35.45	18 **Ar** 39.95
19 **K** 39.1	20 **Ca** 40.08	21 **Sc** 44.96	22 **Ti** 47.88	23 **V** 50.94	24 **Cr** 52.00	25 **Mn** 54.94	26 **Fe** 55.85	27 **Co** 58.93	28 **Ni** 58.69	29 **Cu** 63.55	30 **Zn** 65.39	31 **Ga** 69.72	32 **Ge** 72.61	33 **As** 74.92	34 **Se** 78.96	35 **Br** 79.90	36 **Kr** 83.80
37 **Rb** 85.47	38 **Sr** 87.62	39 **Y** 88.91	40 **Zr** 91.22	41 **Nb** 92.91	42 **Mo** 95.94	43 **Tc** (98)	44 **Ru** 101.07	45 **Rh** 102.91	46 **Pd** 106.42	47 **Ag** 107.87	48 **Cd** 112.41	49 **In** 114.82	50 **Sn** 118.71	51 **Sb** 121.76	52 **Te** 127.6	53 **I** 126.9	54 **Xe** 131.29
55 **Cs** 132.9	56 **Ba** 137.3	57 **La*** 138.9	72 **Hf** 178.5	73 **Ta** 180.9	74 **W** 183.9	75 **Re** 186.2	76 **Os** 190.2	77 **Ir** 192.2	78 **Pt** 195.1	79 **Au** 197.0	80 **Hg** 200.6	81 **Tl** 204.4	82 **Pb** 207.2	83 **Bi** 209	84 **Po** (209)	85 **At** (210)	86 **Rn** (222)
87 **Fr** (223)	88 **Ra** (226)	89 **Ac^** (227)	104 **Rf** (261)	105 **Db** (262)	106 **Sg** (263)	107 **Bh** (264)	108 **Hs** (265)	109 **Mt** (268)	110 **Ds** (271)	111 **Rg** (272)							

	58 **Ce** 140.1	59 **Pr** 140.9	60 **Nd** 144.2	61 **Pm** (145)	62 **Sm** 150.4	63 **Eu** 152.0	64 **Gd** 157.3	65 **Tb** 158.9	66 **Dy** 162.5	67 **Ho** 164.9	68 **Er** 167.3	69 **Tm** 168.9	70 **Yb** 173.0	71 **Lu** 175.0
*	58 **Ce** 140.1	59 **Pr** 140.9	60 **Nd** 144.2	61 **Pm** (145)	62 **Sm** 150.4	63 **Eu** 152.0	64 **Gd** 157.3	65 **Tb** 158.9	66 **Dy** 162.5	67 **Ho** 164.9	68 **Er** 167.3	69 **Tm** 168.9	70 **Yb** 173.0	71 **Lu** 175.0
^	90 **Th** 232.0	91 **Pa** (231)	92 **U** 238.0	93 **Np** (237)	94 **Pu** (244)	95 **Am** (243)	96 **Cm** (247)	97 **Bk** (247)	98 **Cf** (251)	99 **Es** (252)	100 **Fm** (257)	101 **Md** (258)	102 **No** (259)	103 **Lr** (260)

The **periodic table** is a tabular arrangement of the elements and is organized according to **periodic law**. The properties of the elements depend on their **atomic structure** and vary with **atomic number**. It shows periodic trends of physical and chemical properties and identifies families of elements with similar properties. In the periodic table, the elements are arranged by atomic number in horizontal rows called **periods** and vertical columns called **groups** or **families**. They are further categorized as metals, metalloids, or nonmetals. The majority of known elements are metals; there are seventeen nonmetals and eight metalloids. **Metals** are situated at the left end of the periodic table, **nonmetals** to the right and **metalloids** between the two.

A typical periodic table shows the elements' symbols and atomic number, the number of protons in the atomic nucleus. Some more detailed tables also list **atomic mass, electronegativity**, and other data. The position of an element in the table reveals its group, its block, and whether it is a representative, transition, or inner transition element. Its position also shows the element as a metal, nonmetal, or metalloid.

For the representative elements, the last digit of the **group number** reveals the number of outer-level electrons. Roman numerals for the A groups also reveal the number of outer level electrons within the group. The position of the element in the table reveals its **electronic configuration** and how it differs in atomic size from neighbors in its period or group. In this example, Boron has an atomic number of 5 and an atomic weight of 10.811. It is found in group 13, in which all atoms of the group have 3 valence electrons; the group's Roman numeral representation is IIIA.

IMPORTANT FEATURES AND STRUCTURE

The most important feature of the table is its arrangement according to **periodicity**, or the predictable trends observable in atoms. The arrangement enables classification, organization, and prediction of important elemental properties.

The table is organized in horizontal rows called **Periods**, and vertical columns called **Groups** or **Families**. Groups of elements share predictable characteristics, the most important of which is that their outer energy levels have the same configuration of electrons. For example, the highest group is group 18, the noble gases. Each element in this group has a full complement of electrons in its outer level, making the reactivity low. Elements in periods also share some common properties, but most classifications rely more heavily on groups.

CHEMICAL REACTIVITY

Reactivity refers to the tendency of a substance to engage in **chemical reactions**. If that tendency is high, the substance is said to be highly reactive, or to have **high reactivity**. Because the basis of a chemical reaction is the transfer of electrons, reactivity depends upon the presence of uncommitted electrons which are available for transfer. **Periodicity** allows us to predict an element's reactivity based on its position on the periodic table. High numbered groups on the right side of the table have a fuller complement of electrons in their outer levels, making them less likely to react. Noble gases, on the far right of the table, each have eight electrons in the outer level, with the exception of He, which has two. Because atoms tend to lose or gain electrons to reach an ideal of eight in the outer level, these elements have very low reactivity.

GROUPS AND PERIODS IN TERMS OF REACTIVITY

Reading left to right within a period, each element contains one more electron than the one preceding it. (Note that H and He are in the same period, though nothing is between them and they are in different groups.) As electrons are added, their attraction to the nucleus increases, meaning that as we read to the right in a period, each atom's electrons are more densely compacted, more strongly bound to the nucleus, and less likely to be pulled away in reactions. As we read down a group, each successive atom's outer electrons are less tightly bound to the nucleus, thus increasing their reactivity, because the principal energy levels are increasingly full as we move downward within the group. **Principal energy levels** shield the outer energy levels from nuclear attraction, allowing the valence electrons to react. For this reason, noble gases farther down the group can react under certain circumstances.

METALS, NONMETALS, AND METALLOIDS IN THE PERIODIC TABLE

The metals are located on the left side and center of the periodic table, and the nonmetals are located on the right side of the periodic table. The metalloids or semimetals form a zigzag line between the metals and nonmetals. Metals include the **alkali metals** such as lithium, sodium, and potassium and the **alkaline earth metals** such as beryllium, magnesium, and calcium. Metals also include the **transition metals** such as iron, copper, and nickel and the **inner transition metals** such as thorium, uranium, and plutonium. **Nonmetals** include the **chalcogens** such as oxygen and sulfur, the **halogens** such as fluorine and chlorine, and the **noble gases** such as helium and argon. Carbon, nitrogen, and phosphorus are also nonmetals. **Metalloids** or **semimetals** include boron, silicon, germanium, antimony, and polonium.

CHARACTERISTIC PROPERTIES OF SUBSTANCES

INTENSIVE AND EXTENSIVE PROPERTIES

Physical properties are categorized as either intensive or extensive. **Intensive properties** *do not* depend on the amount of matter or quantity of the sample. This means that intensive properties will not change if the sample size is increased or decreased. Intensive properties include color, hardness, melting point, boiling point, density, ductility, malleability, specific heat, temperature, concentration, and magnetization.

Extensive properties *do* depend on the amount of matter or quantity of the sample. Therefore, extensive properties do change if the sample size is increased or decreased. If the sample size is increased, the property increases. If the sample size is decreased, the property decreases. Extensive properties include volume, mass, weight, energy, entropy, number of moles, and electrical charge.

PHYSICAL PROPERTIES OF MATTER

Physical properties are any property of matter that can be **observed** or **measured**. These include properties such as color, elasticity, mass, volume, and temperature. **Mass** is a measure of the amount of substance in an object. **Weight** is a measure of the gravitational pull of Earth on an object. **Volume** is a measure of the amount of space occupied. There are many formulas to determine volume. For example, the volume of a cube is the length of one side cubed (a^3) and the volume of a rectangular prism is length times width times height ($l \times w \times h$). The volume of an irregular shape can be determined by how much water it displaces. **Density** is a measure of the amount of mass per unit volume. The formula to find density is mass divided by volume ($D=m/V$). It is expressed in terms of mass per cubic unit, such as grams per cubic centimeter (g/cm^3). **Specific gravity** is a measure of the ratio of a substance's density compared to the density of water.

DENSITY

The density of an object is equal to its *mass divided by its volume* ($d = m/v$). It is important to note the difference between an *object's density* and a *material's density*. Water has a density of one gram per cubic centimeter, while steel has a density approximately eight times that. Despite having a much higher material density, an object made of steel may still float. A hollow steel sphere, for instance, will float easily because the density of the object includes the air contained within the sphere.

SPECIFIC HEAT CAPACITY

Specific heat capacity, also known as **specific heat**, is the *heat capacity per unit mass*. Each element and compound has its own specific heat. For example, it takes different amounts of heat energy to raise the temperature of the same amounts of magnesium and lead by one degree. The equation for relating heat energy to specific heat capacity is $Q = mc\Delta T$, where m represents the mass of the object, and c represents its specific heat capacity.

Review Video: Specific Heat Capacity
Visit mometrix.com/academy and enter code: 736791

CONDUCTION

Heat always flows from a region of higher temperature to a region of lower temperature. If two regions are at the same temperature, there is a **thermal equilibrium** between them and there will be **no net heat transfer** between them. **Conduction** is a form of heat transfer that requires contact. Since heat is a measure of kinetic energy, most commonly vibration, at the atomic level, it may be transferred from one location to another or one object to another by contact.

CHEMICAL PROPERTIES OF MATTER

If a chemical change must be carried out in order to observe and measure a property, then the property is a **chemical property**. For example, when hydrogen gas is burned in oxygen, it forms water. This is a chemical property of hydrogen because after burning, a different chemical substance – water – is all that remains. The hydrogen cannot be recovered from the water by means of a physical change such as freezing or boiling.

PROPERTIES OF WATER

The important properties of water (H_2O) are *high polarity, hydrogen bonding, cohesiveness, adhesiveness, high specific heat, high latent heat, and high heat of vaporization*. It is **essential to life** as we know it, as water is one of the main if not the main constituent of many living things. Water is a liquid at room temperature. The high specific heat of water means it resists the breaking of its hydrogen bonds and resists heat and motion, which is why it has a relatively high boiling point and high vaporization point. It also resists temperature change. In its solid state, water floats. (Most substances are heavier in their solid forms.) Water is **cohesive**, which means it is attracted to itself. It is also **adhesive**, which means it readily attracts other molecules. If water tends to adhere to another substance, the substance is said to be **hydrophilic**. Water makes a good **solvent**. Substances, particularly those with polar ions and molecules, readily dissolve in water.

Review Video: Properties of Water
Visit mometrix.com/academy and enter code: 279526

HYDROGEN BONDS

Hydrogen bonds are weaker than covalent and ionic bonds, and refer to the type of attraction in an **electronegative atom** such as oxygen, fluorine, or nitrogen. Hydrogen bonds can form within a single molecule or between molecules. A water molecule is **polar**, meaning it is partially positively charged on one end (the hydrogen end) and partially negatively charged on the other (the oxygen end). This is because the hydrogen atoms are arranged around the oxygen atom in a close tetrahedron. Hydrogen is **oxidized** (its number of electrons is reduced) when it bonds with oxygen to form water. Hydrogen bonds tend not only to be weak, but also short-lived. They also tend to be numerous. Hydrogen bonds give water many of its important properties, including its high specific heat and high heat of vaporization, its solvent qualities, its adhesiveness and cohesiveness, its hydrophobic qualities, and its ability to float in its solid form. Hydrogen bonds are also an important component of *proteins, nucleic acids, and DNA*.

PASSIVE TRANSPORT MECHANISMS: DIFFUSION AND OSMOSIS

Transport mechanisms allow for the movement of substances through membranes. **Passive transport mechanisms** include simple and facilitated diffusion and osmosis. They do not require energy from the cell. **Diffusion** occurs when particles are transported from areas of higher concentration to areas of lower concentration. When equilibrium is reached, diffusion stops. Examples are gas exchange (carbon dioxide and oxygen) during photosynthesis and the transport of oxygen from air to blood and from blood to tissue. **Facilitated diffusion** occurs when specific molecules are transported by a specific carrier protein. **Carrier proteins** vary in terms of size, shape, and charge. Glucose and amino acids are examples of substances transported by carrier proteins.

Osmosis is the diffusion of water through a semi-permeable membrane from an area of lower solute concentration to one of higher solute concentration. Examples of osmosis include the absorption of water by plant roots and the alimentary canal. Plants lose and gain water through osmosis. A plant cell that swells because of water retention is said to be **turgid**.

> **Review Video: Passive Transport: Diffusion and Osmosis**
> Visit mometrix.com/academy and enter code: 642038

STATES OF MATTER

Matter refers to substances that *have mass and occupy space* (or volume). The traditional definition of matter describes it as having three states: solid, liquid, and gas. These different states are caused by differences in the distances and angles between molecules or atoms, which result in differences in the energy that binds them. **Solid** structures are rigid or nearly rigid and have strong bonds. Molecules or atoms of **liquids** move around and have weak bonds, although they are not weak enough to readily break. Molecules or atoms of **gases** move almost independently of each other, are typically far apart, and do not form bonds. The current definition of matter describes it as having four states. The fourth is **plasma**, which is an ionized gas that has some electrons that are described as free because they are not bound to an atom or molecule. However, the TEAS will only be concerned with solids, liquids, and gases.

The table below outlines the characteristic properties of the three states of matter:

State of matter	Volume/shape	Density	Compressibility	Molecular motion
Gas	Assumes volume and shape of its container	Low	High	Very free motion
Liquid	Volume remains constant but it assumes shape of its container	High	Virtually none	Move past each other freely
Solid	Definite volume and shape	High	Virtually none	Vibrate around fixed positions

The three states of matter can be traversed by the addition or removal of **heat**. For example, when a solid is heated to its melting point, it can begin to form a liquid. However, in order to transition from solid to liquid, additional heat must be added at the melting point to overcome the **latent heat of fusion**. Upon further heating to its boiling point, the liquid can begin to form a gas, but again, additional heat must be added at the boiling point to overcome the **latent heat of vaporization**.

In the solid state, water is less dense than in the liquid state. This can be observed quite simply by noting that an ice cube floats at the surface of a glass of water. Were this not the case, ice would not form on the surface of lakes and rivers in those regions of the world where the climate produces temperatures below the freezing point. If water behaved as other substances do, lakes and rivers would freeze from the bottom up, which would be detrimental to many forms of aquatic life.

The lower density of ice occurs because of a combination of the unique structure of the water molecule and hydrogen bonding. In the case of ice, each oxygen atom is bound to four hydrogen atoms, two covalently and two by hydrogen bonds. This forms an ordered roughly **tetrahedral** structure that prevents the molecules from getting close to each other. As such, there are empty spaces in the structure that account for the low density of ice.

> **Review Video: States of Matter**
> Visit mometrix.com/academy and enter code: 742449
>
> **Review Video: Chemical and Physical Properties of Matter**
> Visit mometrix.com/academy and enter code: 717349

CHANGES IN STATES OF MATTER

A substance that is undergoing a change from a solid to a liquid is said to be **melting**. If this change occurs in the opposite direction, from liquid to solid, this change is called **freezing**. A liquid which is being converted to a gas is undergoing **vaporization**. The reverse of this process is known as **condensation**. Direct transitions from gas to solid and solid to gas are much less common in everyday life, but they can occur given the proper conditions. Solid to gas conversion is known as **sublimation**, while the reverse is called **deposition**.

Evaporation: Evaporation is the change of state in a substance from a liquid to a gaseous form at a temperature below its boiling point (the temperature at which all of the molecules in a liquid are changed to gas through vaporization). Some of the molecules at the surface of a liquid always maintain enough **heat energy** to escape the cohesive forces exerted on them by neighboring molecules. At higher temperatures, the molecules in a substance move more rapidly, increasing their number with enough energy to break out of the liquid form. The rate of evaporation is higher when more of the surface area of a liquid is exposed (as in a large water body, such as an ocean). The amount of moisture already in the air also affects the rate of evaporation—if there is a significant amount of water vapor in the air around a liquid, some evaporated molecules will return to the liquid. The speed of the evaporation process is also decreased by increased **atmospheric pressure**.

Condensation: Condensation is the phase change in a substance from a gaseous to liquid form; it is the opposite of evaporation or vaporization. When temperatures decrease in a gas, such as water vapor, the material's component molecules move more slowly. The decreased motion of the molecules enables **intermolecular cohesive forces** to pull the molecules closer together and, in water, establish hydrogen bonds. Condensation can also be caused by an increase in the pressure exerted on a gas, which results in a decrease in the substance's volume (it reduces the distance between particles). In the **hydrologic cycle**, this process is initiated when warm air containing water vapor rises and then cools. This occurs due to convection in the air, meteorological fronts, or lifting over high land formations.

OVERVIEW OF CHEMICAL REACTIONS

Chemical reactions measured in human time can take place quickly or slowly. They can take a fraction of a second or billions of years. The **rates** of chemical reactions are determined by how frequently reacting atoms and molecules interact. Rates are also influenced by the temperature and various properties (such as shape) of the reacting materials. **Catalysts** accelerate chemical reactions, while **inhibitors** decrease reaction rates. Some types of reactions release energy in the form of heat and light. Some types of reactions involve the transfer of either electrons or hydrogen ions between reacting ions, molecules, or atoms. In other reactions, chemical bonds are broken down by heat or light to form **reactive radicals** with electrons that will readily form new bonds. Processes such as the formation of ozone and greenhouse gases in the atmosphere and the burning and processing of fossil fuels are controlled by radical reactions.

READING AND BALANCING CHEMICAL EQUATIONS

Chemical equations describe chemical reactions. The **reactants** are on the left side before the arrow and the **products** are on the right side after the arrow. The arrow indicates the **reaction** or change. The **coefficient**, or stoichiometric coefficient, is the number before the element, and indicates the ratio of reactants to products in terms of moles. The equation for the formation of water from hydrogen and oxygen, for example, is $2H_{2(g)} + O_{2(g)} \rightarrow 2H_2O_{(l)}$. The 2 preceding hydrogen and water is the coefficient, which means there are 2 moles of hydrogen and 2 of water. There is 1 mole of oxygen, which does not have to be indicated with the number 1. In parentheses, g stands for gas, l stands for liquid, s stands for solid, and aq stands for aqueous solution (a substance dissolved in water). **Charges** are shown in superscript for individual ions, but not for ionic compounds. **Polyatomic ions** are separated by parentheses so the ion will not be confused with the number of ions.

An **unbalanced equation** is one that does not follow the **law of conservation of mass**, which states that matter can only be changed, not created. If an equation is unbalanced, the numbers of atoms indicated by the stoichiometric coefficients on each side of the arrow will not be equal. Start by writing the formulas for each species in the reaction. Count the atoms on each side and determine if the number is equal. **Coefficients** must be whole numbers. Fractional amounts, such as half a molecule, are not possible. Equations can be **balanced** by multiplying the coefficients by a constant that will produce the smallest possible whole number coefficient. $H_2 + O_2 \rightarrow H_2O$ is an example of an unbalanced equation. The balanced equation is $2H_2 + O_2 \rightarrow 2H_2O$, which indicates that it takes two moles of hydrogen and one of oxygen to produce two moles of water.

LAW OF CONSERVATION OF MASS

The Law of Conservation of Mass in a chemical reaction is commonly stated as follows:

In a chemical reaction, matter is neither created nor destroyed.

What this means is that there will always be the same **total mass** of material after a reaction as before. This allows for predicting how molecules will combine by balanced equations in which the number of each type of atom is the same on either side of the equation. For example, two hydrogen molecules combine with one oxygen molecule to form water. This is a balanced chemical equation because the number of each type of atom is the same on both sides of the arrow. It has to balance because the reaction obeys the Law of Conservation of Mass.

REACTIONS

BASIC MECHANISMS

Chemical reactions normally occur when electrons are transferred from one atom or molecule to another. Reactions and reactivity depend on the **octet rule**, which describes the tendency of atoms to gain or lose electrons until their outer energy levels contain eight. The changes in a reaction may be in **composition** or **configuration** of a compound or substance, and result in one or more products being generated which were not present in isolation before the reaction occurred. For instance, when oxygen reacts with methane (CH_4), water and carbon dioxide are the products; one set of substances (CH_4 + O) was transformed into a new set of substances (CO_2 + H_2O).

Reactions depend on the presence of a **reactant**, or substance undergoing change, a **reagent**, or partner in the reaction less transformed than the reactant (such as a catalyst), and **products**, or the final result of the reaction. **Reaction conditions**, or environmental factors, are also important components in reactions. These include conditions such as temperature, pressure, concentration, whether the reaction occurs in solution, the type of solution, and presence or absence of catalysts. Chemical reactions are usually written in the following format: Reactants → Products.

FIVE BASIC CHEMICAL REACTIONS

COMBINATION REACTIONS

Combination reactions: In a combination reaction, two or more reactants combine to form a single product (A + B → C). These reactions are also called **synthesis** or **addition reactions**. An example is burning hydrogen in air to produce water. The equation is $2H_2$ (g) + O_2 (g) → $2H_2O$ (l). Another example is when water and sulfur trioxide react to form sulfuric acid. The equation is H_2O + SO_3 → H_2SO_4.

DECOMPOSITION REACTIONS

Decomposition (or *desynthesis, decombination, or deconstruction*) reactions are considered chemical reactions whereby a single compound breaks down into component parts or simpler compounds (A → B + C). When a compound or substance separates into these simpler substances, the **byproducts** are often substances that are different from the original. Decomposition can be viewed as the *opposite* of combination reactions. These reactions are also called analysis reactions. Most decomposition reactions are **endothermic**. Heat needs to be added for the chemical reaction to occur. **Thermal decomposition** is caused by heat. **Electrolytic decomposition** is due to electricity. An example of this type of reaction is the decomposition of water into hydrogen and oxygen gas. The equation is $2H_2O$ → $2H_2$ + O_2. Separation processes can be **mechanical** or **chemical**, and usually involve reorganizing a mixture of substances without changing their chemical nature. The separated products may differ from the original mixture in terms of chemical or physical properties. Types of separation processes include **filtration**, **crystallization**, **distillation**, and **chromatography**. Basically, decomposition *breaks down* one compound into two or more compounds or substances that are different from the original; separation *sorts* the substances from the original mixture into like substances.

SINGLE REPLACEMENT REACTIONS

Single substitution, displacement, or replacement reactions occur when one reactant is displaced by another to form the final product (A + BC → B + AC). Single substitution reactions can be **cationic** or **anionic**. When a piece of copper (Cu) is placed into a solution of silver nitrate ($AgNO_3$), the solution turns blue. The copper appears to be replaced with a silvery-white material. The equation is $2AgNO_3$ + Cu → $Cu(NO_3)_2$ + 2Ag. When this reaction takes place, the copper dissolves and the silver in the silver nitrate solution precipitates (becomes a solid), thus resulting in copper nitrate and silver. Copper and silver have switched places in the nitrate.

DOUBLE REPLACEMENT REACTIONS

Double displacement, double replacement, substitution, metathesis, or ion exchange reactions occur when ions or bonds are exchanged by two compounds to form different compounds (AC + BD → AD + BC). An example of this is that silver nitrate and sodium chloride form two different products (silver chloride and sodium nitrate) when they react. The formula for this reaction is $AgNO_3 + NaCl \rightarrow AgCl + NaNO_3$.

Double replacement reactions are **metathesis reactions**. In a double replacement reaction, the chemical reactants exchange ions but the oxidation state stays the same. One of the indicators of this is the formation of a **solid precipitate**. In acid/base reactions, an **acid** is a compound that can donate a proton, while a **base** is a compound that can accept a proton. In these types of reactions, the acid and base react to form a salt and water. When the proton is donated, the base becomes **water** and the remaining ions form a **salt**. One method of determining whether a reaction is an oxidation/reduction or a metathesis reaction is that the oxidation number of atoms does not change during a metathesis reaction.

COMBUSTION REACTIONS

Combustion, or burning, is a sequence of chemical reactions involving **fuel** and an **oxidant** that produces heat and sometimes light. There are many types of combustion, such as rapid, slow, complete, turbulent, microgravity, and incomplete. Fuels and oxidants determine the **compounds** formed by a combustion reaction. For example, when rocket fuel consisting of hydrogen and oxygen combusts, it results in the formation of water vapor. When air and wood burn, resulting compounds include nitrogen, unburned carbon, and carbon compounds. Combustion is an **exothermic** process, meaning it releases energy. Exothermic energy is commonly released as heat, but can take other forms, such as light, electricity, or sound.

> **Review Video: Combustion**
> Visit mometrix.com/academy and enter code: 592219

CATALYSTS

Catalysts, substances that help *change the rate of reaction* without changing their form, can increase reaction rate by decreasing the number of steps it takes to form products. The **mass** of the catalyst should be the same at the beginning of the reaction as it is at the end. The **activation energy** is the minimum amount required to get a reaction started. Activation energy causes particles to collide with sufficient energy to start the reaction. A **catalyst** enables more particles to react, which lowers the activation energy. Examples of catalysts in reactions are manganese oxide (MnO_2) in the decomposition of hydrogen peroxide, iron in the manufacture of ammonia using the Haber process, and concentrate of sulfuric acid in the nitration of benzene.

pH

The **potential of hydrogen** (pH) is a measurement of the *concentration of hydrogen ions* in a substance in terms of the number of moles of H^+ per liter of solution. All substances fall between 0 and 14 on the pH scale. A lower pH indicates a higher H^+ concentration, while a higher pH indicates a lower H^+ concentration.

Pure water has a **neutral pH**, which is 7. Anything with a pH lower than pure water (<7) is considered **acidic**. Anything with a pH higher than pure water (>7) is a **base**. Drain cleaner, soap, baking soda, ammonia, egg whites, and sea water are common bases. Urine, stomach acid, citric acid, vinegar, hydrochloric acid, and battery acid are acids. A **pH indicator** is a substance that acts as a detector of hydrogen or hydronium ions. It is **halochromic**, meaning it changes color to indicate that hydrogen or hydronium ions have been detected.

> **Review Video: pH**
> Visit mometrix.com/academy and enter code: 187395

BASES

Basic chemicals are usually in aqueous solution and have the following traits: a bitter taste; a soapy or slippery texture to the touch; the capacity to restore the blue color of litmus paper which had previously been turned red by an acid; the ability to produce salts in reaction with acids. The word **alkaline** is used to describe bases.

In contrast to acids, which yield **hydrogen ions** (H^+) when dissolved in solution, bases yield **hydroxide ions** (OH^-); the same models used to describe acids can be inverted and used to describe bases—Arrhenius, Bronsted-Lowry, and Lewis.

Some **nonmetal oxides** (such as Na_2O) are classified as bases even though they do not contain hydroxides in their molecular form. However, these substances easily produce hydroxide ions when reacted with water, which is why they are classified as bases.

ACIDS

Acids are a unique class of compounds characterized by consistent properties. The most significant property of an acid is not readily observable and is what gives acids their unique behaviors: the **ionization of H atoms**, or their tendency to dissociate from their parent molecules and take on an electrical charge. **Carboxylic acids** are also characterized by ionization, but of the O atoms. Some other properties of acids are easy to observe without any experimental apparatus. These properties include the following:

- They have a sour taste
- They change the color of litmus paper to red
- They produce gaseous H_2 in reaction with some metals
- They produce salt precipitates in reaction with bases

Other properties, while no more complex, are less easily observed. For instance, most inorganic acids are easily soluble in water and have high boiling points.

STRONG OR WEAK ACIDS AND BASES

The characteristic properties of acids and bases derive from the tendency of atoms to **ionize** by donating or accepting charged particles. The strength of an acid or base is a reflection of the degree to which its atoms ionize in solution. For example, if all of the atoms in an acid ionize, the acid is said to be **strong**. When only a few of the atoms ionize, the acid is **weak**. Acetic acid ($HC_2H_3O_2$) is a weak acid because only its O_2 atoms ionize in solution. Another way to think of the strength of an acid or base is to consider its **reactivity**. Highly reactive acids and bases are strong because they tend to form and break bonds quickly and most of their atoms ionize in the process.

> **Review Video: Strong and Weak Acids and Bases**
> Visit mometrix.com/academy and enter code: 268930

SALTS

Some properties of **salts** are that they are formed from acid base reactions, are ionic compounds consisting of metallic and nonmetallic ions, dissociate in water, and are comprised of tightly bonded ions. Some common salts are sodium chloride (NaCl), sodium bisulfate, potassium dichromate ($K_2Cr_2O_7$), and calcium chloride ($CaCl_2$). Calcium chloride is used as a drying agent, and may be used to absorb moisture when freezing mixtures. Potassium nitrate (KNO_3) is used to make fertilizer and in the manufacture of explosives. Sodium nitrate ($NaNO_3$) is also used in the making of fertilizer.

Baking soda (sodium bicarbonate) is a salt, as are Epsom salts [magnesium sulfate ($MgSO_4$)]. Salt and water can react to form a base and an acid. This is called a **hydrolysis reaction**.

Scientific Reasoning

METRIC SYSTEM

Using the metric system is generally accepted as the preferred method for taking measurements. Having a universal standard allows individuals to interpret measurements more easily, regardless of where they are located.

The basic units of measurement are: the **meter**, which measures length; the **liter**, which measures volume; and the **gram**, which measures mass. The metric system starts with a **base unit** and increases or decreases in units of 10. The prefix and the base unit combined are used to indicate an amount.

For example, deka is 10 times the base unit. A dekameter is 10 meters; a dekaliter is 10 liters; and a dekagram is 10 grams. The prefix hecto refers to 100 times the base amount; kilo is 1,000 times the base amount. The prefixes that indicate a fraction of the base unit are deci, which is 1/10 of the base unit; centi, which is 1/100 of the base unit; and milli, which is 1/1000 of the base unit.

SI UNITS OF MEASUREMENT

SI uses the **second** (s) to measure time. Fractions of seconds are usually measured in metric terms using prefixes such as millisecond (1/1,000 of a second) or nanosecond (1/1,000,000,000 of a second). Increments of time larger than a second are measured in minutes and hours, which are multiples of 60 and 24. An example of this is a swimmer's time in the 800-meter freestyle being described as 7:32.67, meaning 7 minutes, 32 seconds, and 67 one-hundredths of a second. One second is equal to 1/60 of a minute, 1/3,600 of an hour, and 1/86,400 of a day.

Other SI base units are the **ampere** (A) (used to measure electric current), the **kelvin** (K) (used to measure thermodynamic temperature), the **candela** (cd) (used to measure luminous intensity), and the **mole** (mol) (used to measure the amount of a substance at a molecular level). **Meter** (m) is used to measure length and **kilogram** (kg) is used to measure mass.

METRIC PREFIXES FOR MULTIPLES AND SUBDIVISIONS

The prefixes for multiples are as follows:

- deka (da), 10^1 (deka is the American spelling, but deca is also used)
- hecto (h), 10^2
- kilo (k), 10^3
- mega (M), 10^6
- giga (G), 10^9
- tera (T), 10^{12}

The prefixes for subdivisions are as follows:

- deci (d), 10^{-1}
- centi (c), 10^{-2}
- milli (m), 10^{-3}
- micro (μ), 10^{-6}
- nano (n), 10^{-9}
- pico (p), 10^{-12}

The rule of thumb is that prefixes greater than 10^3 are capitalized when abbreviating. Abbreviations do not need a period after them. A decimeter (dm) is a tenth of a meter, a deciliter (dL) is a tenth of a liter, and a decigram (dg) is a tenth of a gram. Pluralization is understood. For example, when referring to 5 mL of water, no "s" needs to be added to the abbreviation.

LAB GLASSWARE

GRADUATED CYLINDERS AND BURETTES

Graduated cylinders are used for precise measurements and are considered more accurate than flasks or beakers. They are made of either **polypropylene** (which is shatter-resistant and resistant to chemicals but cannot be heated) or **polymethylpentene** (which is known for its clarity). They are lighter to ship and less fragile than glass.

To read a graduated cylinder, it should be placed on a flat surface and read at eye level. The surface of a liquid in a graduated cylinder forms a lens-shaped curve. The measurement should be taken from the bottom of the curve. A ring may be placed at the top of tall, narrow cylinders to help avoid breakage if they are tipped over.

A **burette**, or buret, is a piece of lab glassware used to accurately dispense liquid. It looks similar to a narrow graduated cylinder, but includes a stopcock and tip. It may be filled with a funnel or pipette.

FLASKS, BEAKERS, AND PIPETTES

Two types of flasks commonly used in lab settings are **Erlenmeyer flasks** and **volumetric flasks**, which can also be used to accurately measure liquids. Erlenmeyer flasks and **beakers** can be used for mixing, transporting, and reacting, but are not appropriate for accurate measurements.

A **pipette** can be used to accurately measure small amounts of liquid. Liquid is drawn into the pipette through the bulb and a finger is then quickly placed at the top of the container. The liquid measurement is read exactly at the **meniscus**. Liquid can be released from the pipette by lifting the finger. There are also plastic disposal pipettes. A **repipette** is a hand-operated pump that dispenses solutions.

BALANCES

Unlike laboratory glassware that measures volume, **balances** such as triple-beam balances, spring balances, and electronic balances measure **mass** and **force**. An **electronic balance** is the most accurate, followed by a **triple-beam balance** and then a **spring balance**.

One part of a triple-beam balance is the **plate**, which is where the item to be weighed is placed. There are also three **beams** that have hatch marks indicating amounts and hold the weights that rest in the notches. The front beam measures weights between 0 and 10 grams, the middle beam measures weights in 100-gram increments, and the far beam measures weights in 10-gram increments.

The sum of the weight of each beam is the total weight of the object. A triple-beam balance also includes a **set screw** to calibrate the equipment and a mark indicating the object and counterweights are in balance. Analytical balances are accurate to within 0.0001 g.

REVIEW A SCIENTIFIC EXPLANATION WITH LOGIC AND EVIDENCE

DATA COLLECTION

A valid experiment must be measurable. **Data tables** should be formed, and meticulous, detailed data should be collected for every trial. First, the researcher must determine exactly what data are needed and why those data are needed. The researcher should know in advance what will be done with those data at the end of the experimental research. The data should be *repeatable, reproducible, and accurate*. The researcher should be sure that the procedure for data collection will be reliable and consistent. The researcher should validate the measurement system by performing **practice tests** and making sure that all of the equipment is correctly **calibrated** and periodically retesting the procedure and equipment to ensure that all data being collected are still valid.

SCIENTIFIC PROCESS SKILLS

Perhaps the most important skill in science is that of **observation**. Scientists must be able to take accurate data from their experimental setup or from nature without allowing bias to alter the results. Another important skill is **hypothesizing**. Scientists must be able to combine their knowledge of theory and of other experimental results to logically determine what should occur in their own tests.

The **data-analysis process** requires the twin skills of ordering and categorizing. Gathered data must be arranged in such a way that it is readable and readily shows the key results. A skill that may be integrated with the previous two is comparing. Scientists should be able to **compare** their own results with other published results. They must also be able to **infer**, or draw logical conclusions, from their results. They must be able to **apply** their knowledge of theory and results to create logical experimental designs and determine cases of special behavior.

Lastly, scientists must be able to **communicate** their results and their conclusions. The greatest scientific progress is made when scientists are able to review and test one another's work and offer advice or suggestions.

SCIENTIFIC STATEMENTS

Hypotheses are educated guesses about what is likely to occur, and are made to provide a starting point from which to begin design of the experiment. They may be based on results of previously observed experiments or knowledge of theory, and follow logically forth from these.

Assumptions are statements that are taken to be fact without proof for the purpose of performing a given experiment. They may be entirely true, or they may be true only for a given set of conditions under which the experiment will be conducted. Assumptions are necessary to simplify experiments; indeed, many experiments would be impossible without them.

Scientific models are mathematical statements that describe a physical behavior. Models are only as good as our knowledge of the actual system. Often models will be discarded when new discoveries are made that show the model to be inaccurate. While a model can never perfectly represent an actual system, it is useful for simplifying a system to allow for better understanding of its behavior.

Scientific laws are statements of natural behavior that have stood the test of time and have been found to produce accurate and repeatable results in all testing. A **theory** is a statement of behavior that consolidates all current observations. Theories are similar to laws in that they describe natural behavior, but are more recently developed and are more susceptible to being proved wrong. Theories may eventually become laws if they stand up to scrutiny and testing.

EVENTS AND OBJECTS

EVENTS

A **cause** is an act or event that makes something happen, and an **effect** is the thing that happens as a result of the cause. A cause-and-effect relationship is not always explicit, but there are some terms in English that signal causes, such as *since*, *because*, and *due to*. Terms that signal effects include *consequently, therefore, this lead(s) to*.

A *single* cause can have *multiple* effects (e.g., *Single cause*: Because you left your homework on the table, your dog engulfs the assignment. *Multiple effects*: As a result, you receive a failing grade; your parents do not allow you to visit your friends; you miss out on the new movie and holding the hand of a potential significant other).

A *single* effect can have *multiple* causes (e.g., *Single effect*: Alan has a fever. *Multiple causes*: An unexpected cold front came through the area, and Alan forgot to take his multi-vitamin to avoid being sick.)

An *effect* can in turn be the cause of *another effect*, in what is known as a **cause-and-effect chain**. (e.g., As a result of her disdain for procrastination, Lynn prepared for her exam. This led to her passing her test with high marks. Hence, her resume was accepted and her application was approved.)

SCALE

From the largest objects in outer space to the smallest pieces of the human body, there are objects that can come in many different sizes and shapes. Many of those objects need to be measured in different ways. So, it is important to know which **unit of measurement** is needed to record the length or width and the weight of an object.

An example is taking the measurements of a patient. When measuring the total height of a patient or finding the length of an extremity, the accepted measure is given in meters. However, when one is asked for the diameter of a vein, the accepted measure is given in millimeters. Another example would be measuring the weight of a patient which would be given in kilograms, while the measurement of a human heart would be given in grams. The same idea for scale holds true with time as well. When measuring the lifespan of a patient, the accepted measure is given in days, months, or years. However, when measuring the number of breaths that a patient takes, the accepted measure is given in terms of minutes (e.g., breaths per minute).

SCIENTIFIC INQUIRY

SCIENTIFIC METHOD

The scientific method of inquiry is a general method by which ideas are tested and either confirmed or refuted by experimentation. The first step in the scientific method is **formulating the problem** that is to be addressed. It is essential to define clearly the limits of what is to be observed, since that allows for a more focused analysis.

Once the problem has been defined, it is necessary to form a **hypothesis**. This educated guess should be a possible solution to the problem that was formulated in the first step.

The next step is to test that hypothesis by **experimentation**. This often requires the scientist to design a complete experiment. The key to making the best possible use of an experiment is observation. Observations may be **quantitative**, that is, when a numeric measurement is taken, or they may be **qualitative**, that is, when something is evaluated based on feeling or preference. This measurement data will then be examined to find trends or patterns that are present.

From these trends, the scientist will draw **conclusions** or make **generalizations** about the results, intended to predict future results. If these conclusions support the original hypothesis, the experiment is complete and the scientist will publish his conclusions to allow others to test them by repeating the experiment. If they do not support the hypothesis, the results should then be used to develop a new hypothesis, which can then be verified by a new or redesigned experiment.

EXPERIMENTAL DESIGN

Designing relevant experiments that allow for meaningful results is not a simple task. Every stage of the experiment must be carefully planned to ensure that the right data can be safely and accurately taken.

Ideally, an experiment should be **controlled** so that all of the conditions except the ones being manipulated are held **constant**. This helps to ensure that the results are not skewed by unintended consequences of shifting conditions. A good example of this is a placebo group in a drug trial. All other conditions are the same, but that group is not given the medication.

In addition to proper control, it is important that the experiment be designed with **data collection** in mind. For instance, if the quantity to be measured is temperature, there must be a temperature device such as a thermocouple integrated into the experimental setup. While the data are being collected, they should periodically be checked for obvious errors. If there are data points that are orders of magnitude from the expected value, then it might be a good idea to make sure that no experimental errors are being made, either in data collection or condition control.

Once all the data have been gathered, they must be **analyzed**. The way in which this should be done depends on the type of data and the type of trends observed. It may be useful to fit curves to the data to determine if the trends follow a common mathematical form. It may also be necessary to perform a statistical analysis of the results to determine what effects are significant. Data should be clearly presented.

CONTROLS

A valid experiment must be carefully **controlled**. All variables except the one being tested must be carefully maintained. This means that all conditions must be kept exactly the same except for the independent variable.

Additionally, a set of data is usually needed for a **control group**. The control group represents the "normal" state or condition of the variable being manipulated. Controls can be negative or positive. **Positive controls** are the variables that the researcher expects to have an effect on the outcome of the experiment. A positive control group can be used to verify that an experiment is set up properly. **Negative control groups** are typically thought of as placebos. A negative control group should verify that a variable has no effect on the outcome of the experiment.

The better an experiment is controlled, the more valid the conclusions from that experiment will be. A researcher is more likely to draw a valid conclusion if all variables other than the one being manipulated are being controlled.

VARIABLES

Every experiment has several **variables**; however, only one variable should be purposely changed and tested. This variable is the **manipulated** or **independent variable**. As this variable is manipulated or changed, another variable, called the **responding** or **dependent variable**, is observed and recorded.

All other variables in the experiment must be carefully controlled and are usually referred to as **constants**. For example, when testing the effect of temperature on solubility of a solute, the independent variable is the temperature, and the dependent variable is the solubility. All other factors in the experiment such as pressure, amount of stirring, type of solvent, type of solute, and particle size of the solute are the constants.

English and Language Usage

Conventions of Standard English

SPELLING RULES

WORDS ENDING WITH A CONSONANT

Usually the final consonant is **doubled** on a word before adding a suffix. This is the rule for single syllable words, words ending with one consonant, and multi-syllable words with the last syllable accented. The following are examples:

- *beg* becomes *begging* (single syllable)
- *shop* becomes *shopped* (single syllable)
- *add* becomes *adding* (already ends in double consonant, do not add another *d*)
- *deter* becomes *deterring* (multi-syllable, accent on last syllable)
- *regret* becomes *regrettable* (multi-syllable, accent on last syllable)
- *compost* becomes *composting* (do not add another *t* because the accent is on the first syllable)

WORDS ENDING WITH Y OR C

The general rule for words ending in *y* is to keep the *y* when adding a suffix if the **y is preceded by a vowel**. If the word **ends in a consonant and y** the *y* is changed to an *i* before the suffix is added (unless the suffix itself begins with *i*). The following are examples:

- *pay* becomes *paying* (keep the *y*)
- *bully* becomes *bullied* (change to *i*)
- *bully* becomes *bullying* (keep the *y* because the suffix is –*ing*)

If a word ends with *c* and the suffix begins with an *e, i,* or *y*, the letter *k* is usually added to the end of the word. The following are examples:

- panic becomes panicky
- mimic becomes mimicking

WORDS CONTAINING IE OR EI, AND/OR ENDING WITH E

Most words are spelled with an *i* before *e*, except when they follow the letter *c*, **or** sound like *a*. For example, the following words are spelled correctly according to these rules:

- piece, friend, believe (*i* before *e*)
- receive, ceiling, conceited (except after *c*)
- weight, neighborhood, veil (sounds like *a*)

To add a suffix to words ending with the letter *e*, first determine if the *e* is silent. If it is, the *e* will be kept if the added suffix begins with a consonant. If the suffix begins with a vowel, the *e* is dropped. The following are examples:

- *age* becomes *ageless* (keep the *e*)
- *age* becomes *aging* (drop the *e*)

An exception to this rule occurs when the word ends in *ce* or *ge* and the suffix *able* or *ous* is added; these words will retain the letter *e*. The following are examples:

- courage becomes courageous
- notice becomes noticeable

WORDS ENDING WITH ISE OR IZE

A small number of words end with *ise*. Most of the words in the English language with the same sound end in *ize*. The following are examples:

- advertise, advise, arise, chastise, circumcise, and comprise
- compromise, demise, despise, devise, disguise, enterprise, excise, and exercise
- franchise, improvise, incise, merchandise, premise, reprise, and revise
- supervise, surmise, surprise, and televise

Words that end with *ize* include the following:

- accessorize, agonize, authorize, and brutalize
- capitalize, caramelize, categorize, civilize, and demonize
- downsize, empathize, euthanize, idolize, and immunize
- legalize, metabolize, mobilize, organize, and ostracize
- plagiarize, privatize, utilize, and visualize

(Note that some words may technically be spelled with *ise*, especially in British English, but it is more common to use *ize*. Examples include *symbolize/symbolise* and *baptize/baptise*.)

WORDS ENDING WITH CEED, SEDE, OR CEDE

There are only three words in the English language that end with *ceed*: *exceed, proceed,* and *succeed*. There is only one word in the English language that ends with *sede*: *supersede*. Most other words that sound like *sede* or *ceed* end with *cede*. The following are examples:

- concede, recede, and precede

WORDS ENDING IN ABLE OR IBLE

For words ending in *able* or *ible*, there are no hard and fast rules. The following are examples:

- adjustable, unbeatable, collectable, deliverable, and likeable
- edible, compatible, feasible, sensible, and credible

There are more words ending in *able* than *ible*; this is useful to know if guessing is necessary.

WORDS ENDING IN ANCE OR ENCE

The suffixes *ence, ency,* and *ent* are used in the following cases:

- the suffix is preceded by the letter *c* but sounds like *s* – *innocence*
- the suffix is preceded by the letter *g* but sounds like *j* – *intelligence, negligence*

The suffixes *ance, ancy,* and *ant* are used in the following cases:

- the suffix is preceded by the letter *c* but sounds like *k* – *significant, vacant*
- the suffix is preceded by the letter *g* with a hard sound – *elegant, extravagance*

If the suffix is preceded by other letters, there are no clear rules. For example: *finance, abundance,* and *assistance* use the letter *a,* while *decadence, competence,* and *excellence* use the letter *e.*

WORDS ENDING IN TION, SION, OR CIAN

Words ending in *tion, sion,* or *cian* all sound like *shun* or *zhun.* There are no rules for which ending is used for words. The following are examples:

- action, agitation, caution, fiction, nation, and motion
- admission, expression, mansion, permission, and television
- electrician, magician, musician, optician, and physician (note that these words tend to describe occupations)

WORDS WITH THE AI OR IA COMBINATION

When deciding if *ai* or *ia* is correct, the combination of *ai* usually sounds like one vowel sound, as in *Britain,* while the vowels in *ia* are pronounced separately, as in *guardian.* The following are examples:

- captain, certain, faint, hair, malaise, and praise (*ai* makes one sound)
- bacteria, beneficiary, diamond, humiliation, and nuptial (*ia* makes two sounds)

PLURAL FORMS OF NOUNS

NOUNS ENDING IN CH, SH, S, X, OR Z

When a noun ends in the letters *ch, sh, s, x,* or *z,* an *es* instead of a singular *s* is added to the end of the word to make it plural. The following are examples:

- church becomes churches
- bush becomes bushes
- bass becomes basses
- mix becomes mixes
- buzz becomes buzzes

This is the rule with proper names as well; the Ross family would become the Rosses.

NOUNS ENDING IN Y OR AY/EY/IY/OY/UY

If a noun ends with a **consonant and y**, the plural is formed by replacing the *y* with *ies.* For example, *fly* becomes *flies* and *puppy* becomes *puppies.* If a noun ends with a **vowel and y**, the plural is formed by adding an *s.* For example, *alley* becomes *alleys* and *boy* becomes *boys.*

NOUNS ENDING IN F OR FE

Most nouns ending in *f* or *fe* are pluralized by replacing the *f* with *v* and adding *es.* The following are examples:

- knife becomes knives; self becomes selves; wolf becomes wolves.

An exception to this rule is the word *roof; roof* becomes *roofs.*

NOUNS ENDING IN O

Most nouns ending with a **consonant and o** are pluralized by adding *es*. The following are examples:

- hero becomes heroes; tornado becomes tornadoes; potato becomes potatoes

Most nouns ending with a **vowel and o** are pluralized by adding *s*. The following are examples:

- portfolio becomes portfolios; radio becomes radios; cameo becomes cameos.

An exception to these rules is seen with musical terms ending in *o*. These words are pluralized by adding *s* even if they end in a consonant and *o*. The following are examples: *soprano* becomes *sopranos; banjo* becomes *banjos; piano* becomes *pianos.*

EXCEPTIONS TO THE RULES OF PLURALS

Some words do not fall into any specific category for making the singular form plural. They are **irregular**. Certain words become plural by changing the vowels within the word. The following are examples:

- woman becomes women; goose becomes geese; foot becomes feet

Some words change in unusual ways in the plural form. The following are examples:

- mouse becomes mice; ox becomes oxen; person becomes people

Some words are the same in both the singular and plural forms. The following are examples:

- *Salmon, deer,* and *moose* are the same whether singular or plural.

PLURAL FORMS OF LETTERS, NUMBERS, SYMBOLS, AND COMPOUND NOUNS WITH HYPHENS

Letters and numbers become plural by adding an apostrophe and *s*. The following are examples:

- The *L's* are the people whose names begin with the letter *L*.
- They broke the teams down into groups of *3's*.
- The sorority girls were all *KD's*.

A **compound noun** is a noun that is made up of two or more words; they can be written with hyphens. For example, *mother-in-law* or *court-martial* are compound nouns. To make them plural, an *s* or *es* is added to the noun portion of the word. The following are examples: *mother-in-law* becomes *mothers-in-law; court-martial* becomes *courts-martial.*

HOMOPHONES

Homophones are words that are **pronounced** in the same way, but they have different **spellings** and different **meanings**. It's easy to make a mistake and use the wrong word when writing. So, it's important to make sure you choose the correct word.

EXAMPLES

bare, bear	for, four	knot, not	plain, plane	stair, stare
brake, break	heal, heel	know, no	pour, poor	steal, steel
buy, by	hear, here	mail, male	principal, principle	toe, tow
dear, deer	hole, whole	pair, pear	right, write	wait, weight
flour, flower	hour, our	peace, piece	son, sun	waist, waste

ADDITIONAL EXAMPLES

AFFECT AND EFFECT

Affect can be used as a noun for feeling, emotion, or mood. Effect can be used as a noun that means result. Affect as a verb means to influence. Effect as a verb means to bring about.

> **Affect**: The sunshine affects plants.
> **Effect**: The new rules will effect order in the office.

ITS AND IT'S

Its is a pronoun that shows ownership.

> Example: The guitar is in its case.

It's is a contraction of *it is*.

> Example: It's an honor and a privilege to meet you.

Note: The *h* in honor is silent. So, the sound of the vowel *o* must have the article *an*.

KNEW AND NEW

Knew is the past tense of *know*.

> Example: I knew the answer.

New is an adjective that means something is current, has not been used, or modern.

> Example: This is my new phone.

THERE, THEIR, AND THEY'RE

There can be an adjective, adverb, or pronoun. Often, *there* is used to show a place or to start a sentence.

> Examples: I went there yesterday. | There is something in his pocket.

Their is a pronoun that shows ownership.

> Examples: He is their father. | This is their fourth apology this week.

They're is a contraction of *they are*.

> Example: Did you know that they're in town?

TO, TOO, AND TWO

To can be an adverb or a preposition for showing direction, purpose, and relationship. See your dictionary for the many other ways use *to* in a sentence.

> Examples: I went to the store. | I want to go with you.

Too is an adverb that means *also, as well, very, or more than enough*.

> Examples: I can walk a mile too. | You have eaten too much.

Two is the second number in the series of natural numbers (e.g., one (1), two, (2), three (3)...)

> Example: You have two minutes left.

<u>YOUR AND YOU'RE</u>

Your is an adjective that shows ownership.

> Example: This is your moment to shine.

You're is a contraction of you are.

> Example: Yes, you're correct.

Those are some of the most frequently misused words, but there are many others which you'll run into from time to time. Unfortunately, there are no easy rules you can memorize to help you use the right word every time. You simply have to **memorize** the different spellings and meanings, and practice using them a lot, so it becomes a habit to use the word with the correct meaning.

HOMOGRAPHS

Homographs are words that share the same **spelling**, and they have multiple meanings. To figure out which meaning is being used, you should be looking for **context clues**. The context clues give hints to the meaning of the word. For example, the word *spot* has many meanings. It can mean "a place" or "a stain or blot." In the sentence "After my lunch, I saw a spot on my shirt," the word *spot* means "a stain or blot." The context clues of "After my lunch..." and "on my shirt" guide you to this decision.

EXAMPLES

<u>BANK</u>

> (noun): an establishment where money is held for savings or lending
> (verb): to collect or pile up

<u>CONTENT</u>

> (noun): the topics that will be addressed within a book
> (adjective): pleased or satisfied

<u>FINE</u>

> (noun): an amount of money that acts a penalty for an offense
> (adjective): very small or thin

<u>INCENSE</u>

> (noun): a material that is burned in religious settings and makes a pleasant aroma
> (verb): to frustrate or anger

<u>LEAD</u>

> (noun): the first or highest position
> (verb): to direct a person or group of followers

<u>OBJECT</u>

> (noun): a lifeless item that can be held and observed
> (verb): to disagree

PRODUCE

> (noun): fruits and vegetables
> (verb): to make or create something

REFUSE

> (noun): garbage or debris that has been thrown away
> (verb): to not allow

SUBJECT

> (noun): an area of study
> (verb): to force or subdue

TEAR

> (noun): a fluid secreted by the eyes
> (verb): to separate or pull apart

SPELLING

Commonly Misspelled Words

accidentally	accommodate	accompanied	accompany
achieved	acknowledgment	across	address
aggravate	aisle	ancient	anxiety
apparently	appearance	arctic	argument
arrangement	attendance	auxiliary	awkward
bachelor	barbarian	beggar	beneficiary
biscuit	brilliant	business	cafeteria
calendar	campaign	candidate	ceiling
cemetery	changeable	changing	characteristic
chauffeur	colonel	column	commit
committee	comparative	compel	competent
competition	conceive	congratulations	conqueror
conscious	coolly	correspondent	courtesy
curiosity	cylinder	deceive	deference
deferred	definite	describe	desirable
desperate	develop	diphtheria	disappear
disappoint	disastrous	discipline	discussion
disease	dissatisfied	dissipate	drudgery
ecstasy	efficient	eighth	eligible
embarrass	emphasize	especially	exaggerate
exceed	exhaust	exhilaration	existence
explanation	extraordinary	familiar	fascinate
February	fiery	finally	forehead
foreign	foreigner	foremost	forfeit
ghost	glamorous	government	grammar
grateful	grief	grievous	handkerchief
harass	height	hoping	hurriedly
hygiene	hypocrisy	imminent	incidentally
incredible	independent	indigestible	inevitable
innocence	intelligible	intentionally	intercede
interest	irresistible	judgment	legitimate
liable	library	likelihood	literature

Commonly Misspelled Words

maintenance	maneuver	manual	mathematics
mattress	miniature	mischievous	misspell
momentous	mortgage	neither	nickel
niece	ninety	noticeable	notoriety
obedience	obstacle	occasion	occurrence
omitted	operate	optimistic	organization
outrageous	pageant	pamphlet	parallel
parliament	permissible	perseverance	persuade
physically	physician	possess	possibly
practically	prairie	preceding	prejudice
prevalent	professor	pronunciation	pronouncement
propeller	protein	psychiatrist	psychology
quantity	questionnaire	rally	recede
receive	recognize	recommend	referral
referred	relieve	religious	resistance
restaurant	rhetoric	rhythm	ridiculous
sacrilegious	salary	scarcely	schedule
secretary	sentinel	separate	severely
sheriff	shriek	similar	soliloquy
sophomore	species	strenuous	studying
suffrage	supersede	suppress	surprise
symmetry	temperament	temperature	tendency
tournament	tragedy	transferred	truly
twelfth	tyranny	unanimous	unpleasant
usage	vacuum	valuable	vein
vengeance	vigilance	villain	Wednesday
weird	wholly		

> **Review Video: Spelling Tips**
> Visit mometrix.com/academy and enter code: 138869

THE EIGHT PARTS OF SPEECH

NOUNS

When you talk about a person, place, thing, or idea, you are talking about **nouns**. The two main types of nouns are common and proper nouns. Also, nouns can be abstract (i.e., general) or concrete (i.e., specific).

Common nouns are the class or group of people, places, and things (Note: do not capitalize common nouns). Examples of common nouns:

People: boy, girl, worker, manager
Places: school, bank, library, home
Things: dog, cat, truck, car

Proper nouns are the names of specific persons, places, or things (Note: capitalize all proper nouns). Examples of proper nouns:

> *People*: Abraham Lincoln, George Washington, Martin Luther King, Jr.
> *Places*: Los Angeles, New York, Asia
> *Things*: Statue of Liberty, Earth*, Lincoln Memorial

*Note: When you talk about the planet that we live on, you capitalize *Earth*. When you mean the dirt, rocks, or land, you lowercase *earth*.

General nouns are the names of conditions or ideas. **Specific nouns** name people, places, and things that are understood by using your senses.

General nouns:

> *Condition*: beauty, strength
> *Idea*: truth, peace

Specific nouns:

> *People*: baby, friend, father
> *Places*: town, park, city hall
> *Things*: rainbow, cough, apple, silk, gasoline

Collective nouns are the names for a person, place, or thing that may act as a whole. The following are examples of collective nouns: *class, company, dozen, group, herd, team,* and *public.*

PRONOUNS

Pronouns are words that are used to stand in for a noun. A pronoun may be grouped as *personal, intensive, relative, interrogative, demonstrative, indefinite,* and *reciprocal.*

Personal: Nominative is the case for nouns and pronouns that are the subject of a sentence. **Objective** is the case for nouns and pronouns that are an object in a sentence. **Possessive** is the case for nouns and pronouns that show possession or ownership.

SINGULAR

	Nominative	Objective	Possessive
First Person	I	me	my, mine
Second Person	you	you	your, yours
Third Person	he, she, it	him, her, it	his, her, hers, its

PLURAL

	Nominative	Objective	Possessive
First Person	we	us	our, ours
Second Person	you	you	your, yours
Third Person	they	them	their, theirs

Intensive: I myself, you yourself, he himself, she herself, the (thing) itself, we ourselves, you yourselves, they themselves
Relative: which, who, whom, whose
Interrogative: what, which, who, whom, whose
Demonstrative: this, that, these, those

Indefinite: all, any, each, everyone, either/neither, one, some, several
Reciprocal: each other, one another

Review Video: Nouns and Pronouns
Visit mometrix.com/academy and enter code: 312073

VERBS

If you want to write a sentence, then you need a **verb** in your sentence. Without a verb, you have no sentence. The verb of a sentence explains **action** or **being**. In other words, the verb shows the subject's movement or the movement that has been done to the subject.

TRANSITIVE AND INTRANSITIVE VERBS

A **transitive verb** is a verb whose action (e.g., drive, run, jump) points to a receiver (e.g., car, dog, kangaroo). **Intransitive verbs** do not point to a receiver of an action. In other words, the action of the verb does not point to a subject or object.

> **Transitive**: He plays the piano. | The piano was played by him.
> **Intransitive**: He plays. | John writes well.

A dictionary will let you know whether a verb is transitive or intransitive. Some verbs can be transitive and intransitive.

ACTION VERBS AND LINKING VERBS

An action verb is a verb that shows what the subject is doing in a sentence. In other words, an **action verb** shows action. A sentence can be complete with one word: an action verb. **Linking verbs** are intransitive verbs that show a condition (i.e., the subject is described but does no action).

Linking verbs link the **subject** of a sentence to a **noun or pronoun**, or they link a subject with an **adjective**. You always need a verb if you want a complete sentence. However, linking verbs are not able to complete a sentence.

Common linking verbs include *appear, be, become, feel, grow, look, seem, smell, sound*, and *taste*. However, any verb that shows a condition and has a noun, pronoun, or adjective that describes the subject of a sentence is a linking verb.

> **Action**: He sings. | Run! | Go! | I talk with him every day. | She reads.
> **Linking**: I am John. | I smell roses. | I feel tired.

Note: Some verbs are followed by words that look like prepositions, but they are a part of the verb and a part of the verb's meaning. These are known as **phrasal verbs** and examples include *call off*, *look up*, and *drop off*.

VOICE

Transitive verbs come in active or passive voice. If the subject does an action or receives the action of the verb, then you will know whether a verb is active or passive. When the subject of the sentence is doing the action, the verb is **active voice**. When the subject receives the action, the verb is **passive voice**.

> **Active**: Jon drew the picture. (The subject *Jon* is doing the action of *drawing a picture*.)
> **Passive**: The picture is drawn by Jon. (The subject *picture* is receiving the action from Jon.)

VERB TENSES

A verb tense shows the different form of a verb to point to the time of an action. The **present** and **past tense** are shown by changing the verb's form. An action in the present *I talk* can change form for the past: *I talked*. However, for the other tenses, an **auxiliary** (i.e., helping) verb is needed to show the change in form. These helping verbs include *am, are, is | have, has, had | was, were, will* (or *shall*).

Present: I talk	Present perfect: I have talked
Past: I talked	Past perfect: I had talked
Future: I will talk	Future perfect: I will have talked

Present: The action happens at the current time.

> Example: He *walks* to the store every morning.

To show that something is happening right now, use the progressive present tense: I *am walking*.

Past: The action happened in the past.

> Example: He *walked* to the store an hour ago.

Future: The action is going to happen later.

> Example: I *will walk* to the store tomorrow.

Present perfect: The action started in the past and continues into the present.

> Example: I *have walked* to the store three times today.

Past perfect: The second action happened in the past. The first action came before the second.

> Example: Before I walked to the store (Action 2), I *had walked* to the library (Action 1).

Future perfect: An action that uses the past and the future. In other words, the action is complete before a future moment.

> Example: When she comes for the supplies (future moment), I *will have walked* to the store (action completed in the past).

> **Review Video: Present Perfect, Past Perfect, and Future Perfect Verb Tenses**
> Visit mometrix.com/academy and enter code: 269472

CONJUGATING VERBS

When you need to change the form of a verb, you are **conjugating** a verb. The key parts of a verb are **first person singular, present tense** (dream); **first person singular, past tense** (dreamed); and the **past participle** (dreamed). Note: the past participle needs a helping verb to make a verb tense. For example, I *have dreamed* of this day. | I *am dreaming* of this day.

PRESENT TENSE: ACTIVE VOICE

	Singular	Plural
First Person	I dream	We dream
Second Person	You dream	You dream
Third Person	He, she, it dreams	They dream

MOOD

There are three moods in English: the indicative, the imperative, and the subjunctive.

The **indicative mood** is used for facts, opinions, and questions.

> **Fact**: You can do this.
> **Opinion**: I think that you can do this.
> **Question**: Do you know that you can do this?

The **imperative** is used for orders or requests.

> **Order**: You are going to do this!
> **Request**: Will you do this for me?

The **subjunctive mood** is for wishes and statements that go against fact.

> **Wish**: I wish that I were going to do this.
> **Statement against fact**: If I were you, I would do this. (This goes against fact because I am not you. You have the chance to do this, and I do not have the chance.)

The mood that causes trouble for most people is the subjunctive mood. If you have trouble with any of the moods, then be sure to practice.

ADJECTIVES

An adjective is a word that is used to **modify** a noun or pronoun. An adjective answers a question: *Which one?*, *What kind of?*, or *How many?*. Usually, adjectives come before the words that they modify.

> **Which one**: The *third* suit is my favorite.
> **How many**: Can I look over the *four* neckties for the suit?

ARTICLES

Articles are adjectives that are used to **mark nouns**. There are only three: the definite (i.e., limited or fixed amount) article *the*, and the indefinite (i.e., no limit or fixed amount) articles *a* and *an*. Note: *An* comes before words that start with a vowel sound (i.e., vowels include *a*, *e*, *i*, *o*, *u*, and *y*). For example, Are you going to get an **u**mbrella?

> **Definite**: I lost *the* bottle that belongs to me.
> **Indefinite**: Does anyone have *a* bottle to share?

COMPARISON WITH ADJECTIVES

Some adjectives are relative and other adjectives are absolute. Adjectives that are **relative** can show the comparison between things. Adjectives that are **absolute** can show comparison. However, they show comparison in a different way. Let's say that you are reading two books. You think that one book is perfect, and the other book is not exactly perfect. It is <u>not</u> possible for the book to be more perfect than the other. Either you think that the book is perfect, or you think that the book is not perfect.

The adjectives that are relative will show the different **degrees** of something or someone to something else or someone else. The three degrees of adjectives include positive, comparative, and superlative.

The **positive degree** is the normal form of an adjective.

> Example: This work is *difficult*. | She is *smart*.

The **comparative degree** compares one person or thing to another person or thing.

> Example: This work is *more difficult* than your work. | She is *smarter* than me.

The **superlative degree** compares more than two people or things.

> Example: This is the *most difficult* work of my life. | She is the *smartest* lady in school.

> **Review Video: <u>What is an Adjective?</u>**
> Visit mometrix.com/academy and enter code: 470154

ADVERBS

An adverb is a word that is used to **modify** a verb, adjective, or another adverb. Usually, adverbs answer one of these questions: *When?*, *Where?*, *How?*, and *Why?* . The negatives *not* and *never* are known as adverbs. Adverbs that modify adjectives or other adverbs strengthen or weaken the words that they modify.

Examples:

> He walks quickly through the crowd.
> The water flows smoothly on the rocks.

Note: While many adverbs end in *-ly*, you need to remember that not all adverbs end in *-ly*. Also, some words that end in *-ly* are adjectives, not adverbs. Some examples include: *early, friendly, holy, lonely, silly*, and *ugly*. To know if a word that ends in *-ly* is an adjective or adverb, you can check whether it answers one of the adjective questions or one of the adverb questions.

Examples:

> He is *never* angry.
> You talk *too* loudly.

COMPARISON WITH ADVERBS

The rules for comparing adverbs are the same as the rules for adjectives.

The **positive degree** is the standard form of an adverb.

> Example: He arrives soon. | She speaks softly to her friends.

The **comparative degree** compares one person or thing to another person or thing.

> Example: He arrives sooner than Sarah. | She speaks more softly than him.

The **superlative degree** compares more than two people or things.

> Example: He arrives soonest of the group. | She speaks most softly of any of her friends.

> **Review Video: <u>Adverbs</u>**
> Visit mometrix.com/academy and enter code: 713951

PREPOSITIONS

A preposition is a word placed before a noun or pronoun that shows the *relationship between an object and another word* in the sentence.

Common Prepositions:

about	before	during	on	under
after	beneath	for	over	until
against	between	from	past	up
among	beyond	in	through	with
around	by	of	to	within
at	down	off	toward	without

Examples:

> The napkin is *in* the drawer.
> The Earth rotates *around* the Sun.
> The needle is *beneath* the haystack.
> Can you find me *among* the words?

> **Review Video: What is a Preposition?**
> Visit mometrix.com/academy and enter code: 946763

CONJUNCTIONS

Conjunctions **join** words, phrases, or clauses, and they show the connection between the joined pieces. There are **coordinating conjunctions** that connect equal parts of sentences. **Correlative conjunctions** show the connection between pairs. **Subordinating conjunctions** join subordinate (i.e., dependent) clauses with independent clauses.

COORDINATING CONJUNCTIONS

The coordinating conjunctions include: *and, but, yet, or, nor, for,* and *so*

Examples:

> The rock was small, but it was heavy.
> She drove in the night, and he drove in the day.

CORRELATIVE CONJUNCTIONS

The correlative conjunctions are: either...or | neither...nor | not only... but also

Examples:

> Either you are coming, or you are staying.
> He not only ran three miles, but also swam 200 yards.

> **Review Video: Coordinating and Correlative Conjunctions**
> Visit mometrix.com/academy and enter code: 390329

SUBORDINATING CONJUNCTIONS

Common subordinating conjunctions include:

after	since	whenever
although	so that	where
because	unless	wherever
before	until	whether
in order that	when	while

Examples:

I am hungry *because* I did not eat breakfast.
He went home *when* everyone left.

Review Video: Subordinating Conjunctions
Visit mometrix.com/academy and enter code: 958913

INTERJECTIONS

An interjection is a word for **exclamation** (i.e., great amount of feeling) that is used alone or as a piece to a sentence. Often, they are used at the beginning of a sentence for an **introduction**. Sometimes, they can be used in the middle of a sentence to show a **change** in thought or attitude.

Common Interjections: Hey! | Oh, ... | Ouch! | Please! | Wow!

Punctuation

END PUNCTUATION

PERIODS

Use a period to end all sentences except direct questions, exclamations, and questions.

DECLARATIVE SENTENCE

A declarative sentence gives information or makes a statement.

> Examples: I can fly a kite. | The plane left two hours ago.

IMPERATIVE SENTENCE

An imperative sentence gives an order or command.

> Examples: You are coming with me. | Bring me that note.

QUESTION MARKS

Question marks should be used following a direct question. A polite request can be followed by a period instead of a question mark.

> *Direct Question*: What is for lunch today? | How are you? | Why is that the answer?
> *Polite Requests*: Can you please send me the item tomorrow. | Will you please walk with me.

EXCLAMATION MARKS

Exclamation marks are used after a word group or sentence that shows much feeling or has special importance. Exclamation marks should not be overused. They are saved for proper **exclamatory interjections**.

> Examples: We're going to the finals! | You have a beautiful car! | That's crazy!

SPECIAL NOTE

PERIODS FOR ABBREVIATIONS

An abbreviation is a shortened form of a word or phrase.

> Examples: 3 P.M. | 2 A.M. | Mr. Jones | Mrs. Stevens | Dr. Smith | Bill Jr. | Pennsylvania Ave.

COMMAS

The comma is a punctuation mark that can help you understand **connections** in a sentence. Not every sentence needs a comma. However, if a sentence needs a comma, you need to put it in the right place. A comma in the wrong place (or an absent comma) will make a sentence's meaning unclear. These are some of the rules for commas:

Use a comma before a **coordinating conjunction** joining independent clauses

> Example: *Bob caught three fish, and I caught two fish.*

Use a comma **after an introductory phrase** or **adverbial clause**

Examples:

> *After the final out,* we went to a restaurant to celebrate.
> *Studying the stars,* I was surprised at the beauty of the sky.

Use a comma **between items in a series**

> Example: I will bring *the turkey, the pie, and the coffee.*

Use a comma between **coordinate adjectives** not joined with *and*

> Incorrect: The kind, brown dog followed me home.
> Correct: The *kind, loyal* dog followed me home.

Not all adjectives are coordinate (i.e., equal or parallel). There are two simple ways to know if your adjectives are coordinate. One, you can join the adjectives with *and*: *The kind and loyal dog.* Two, you can change the order of the adjectives: *The loyal, kind dog.*

Use commas for **interjections** and **after** *yes* **and** *no* **responses**

Examples:

> **Interjection**: Oh, I had no idea. | Wow, you know how to play this game.
> **Yes and No**: *Yes,* I heard you. | *No,* I cannot come tomorrow.

Use commas to **separate nonessential modifiers** and **nonessential appositives**

Examples:

> **Nonessential Modifier**: John Frank, who is coaching the team, was promoted today.
> **Nonessential Appositive**: Thomas Edison, an American inventor, was born in Ohio.

Use commas to **set off nouns of direct address**, **interrogative tags**, and **contrast**

Examples:

> **Direct Address**: You, *John,* are my only hope in this moment.
> **Interrogative Tag**: This is the last time, *correct*?
> **Contrast**: You are my friend, *not my enemy.*

Use commas with **dates**, **addresses**, **geographical names**, and **titles**

Examples:

> **Date**: *July 4, 1776,* is an important date to remember.
> **Address**: He is meeting me at *456 Delaware Avenue, Washington, D.C.,* tomorrow morning.
> **Geographical Name**: *Paris, France,* is my favorite city.
> **Title**: John Smith, *Ph.D.,* will be visiting your class today.

Use commas to separate **expressions like *he said*** and ***she said*** if they come between a sentence of a quote

Examples:

> "I want you to know," he began, "that I always wanted the best for you."
> "You can start," Jane said, "with an apology."

> **Review Video: Commas**
> Visit mometrix.com/academy and enter code: 786797

SEMICOLONS

The semicolon is used to connect major sentence pieces of equal value. Some rules for semicolons include:

Use a semicolon **between closely connected independent clauses** that are not connected with a coordinating conjunction.

Examples:

> She is outside; we are inside.
> You are right; we should go with your plan.

Use a semicolon **between independent clauses linked with a transitional word**.

Examples:

> I think that we can agree on this*; however,* I am not sure about my friends.
> You are looking in the wrong places*; therefore,* you will not find what you need.

Use a semicolon **between items in a series that has internal punctuation**.

> Example: I have visited *New York, New York; Augusta, Maine; and Baltimore, Maryland.*

> **Review Video: Semicolon Usage**
> Visit mometrix.com/academy and enter code: 370605

COLONS

The colon is used to call attention to the words that follow it. A colon must come after an **independent clause**. The rules for colons are as follows:

Use a colon **after an independent clause** to make a list

> Example: I want to learn many languages: Spanish, French, German, and Italian.

Use a colon **for elaboration** or to **give a quote**

Examples:

> **Quote**: The man started with an idea: "We are able to do more than we imagine."
> **Elaboration**: There is one thing that stands out on your resume: responsibility.

Use a colon **after the greeting in a formal letter**, to **show hours and minutes**, and to **separate a title and subtitle**

Examples:

> **Greeting in a formal letter**: Dear Sir: | To Whom It May Concern:
> **Time**: It is 3:14 P.M.
> **Title**: The essay is titled "America: A Short Introduction to a Modern Country"

PARENTHESES

Parentheses are used for additional information. Also, they can be used to put labels for letters or numbers in a series. Parentheses should not be used very often. If they are overused, parentheses can be a distraction instead of a help.

Examples:

> **Extra Information**: The rattlesnake (see Image 2) is a dangerous snake of North and South America.
> **Series**: Include in the email (1) your name, (2) your address, and (3) your question for the author.

QUOTATION MARKS

Use quotation marks to close off **direct quotations** of a person's spoken or written words. Do not use quotation marks around indirect quotations. An indirect quotation gives someone's message without using the person's exact words. Use **single quotation marks** to close off a quotation inside a quotation.

> **Direct Quote**: Nancy said, "I am waiting for Henry to arrive."
> **Indirect Quote**: Henry said that he is going to be late to the meeting.
> **Quote inside a Quote**: The teacher asked, "Has everyone read 'The Gift of the Magi'?"

Quotation marks should be used around the titles of **short works**: newspaper and magazine articles, poems, short stories, songs, television episodes, radio programs, and subdivisions of books or web sites.

Examples:

> "Rip van Winkle" (short story by Washington Irving)
> "O Captain! My Captain!" (poem by Walt Whitman)

Quotation marks may be used to set off words that are being used in a different way from a dictionary definition. Also, they can be used to highlight irony.

Examples:

> The boss warned Frank that he was walking on "thin ice."
> (Frank is not walking on real ice. Instead, Frank is being warned to avoid mistakes.)
>
> The teacher thanked the young man for his "honesty."
> (Honesty and truth are not always the same thing. In this example, the quotation marks around *honesty* show that the teacher does not believe the young man's explanation.)

> **Review Video: Quotation Marks**
> Visit mometrix.com/academy and enter code: 884918

Note: Periods and commas are put *inside* quotation marks. Colons and semicolons are put *outside* the quotation marks. Question marks and exclamation points are placed *inside* quotation marks when they are part of a quote. When the question or exclamation mark goes with the whole sentence, the mark is left *outside* of the quotation marks.

Examples:

> *Period and comma*: We read "The Gift of the Magi," "The Skylight Room," and "The Cactus."
> *Semicolon*: The class read "The Legend of Sleepy Hollow"; then they watched the movie adaptation.
> *Exclamation mark that is a part of a quote*: The crowd cheered, "Victory!"
> *Question mark that goes with the whole sentence*: Is your favorite short story "The Tell-Tale Heart"?

APOSTROPHES

An apostrophe is used to show **possession** or the deletion of letters in **contractions**. An apostrophe is not needed with the possessive pronouns *his, hers, its, ours, theirs, whose,* and *yours.*

> **Singular Nouns**: David's car | a book's theme | my brother's board game
> **Plural Nouns with -s**: the scissors' handle | boys' basketball
> **Plural Nouns without -s**: Men's department | the people's adventure

> **Review Video: Apostrophes**
> Visit mometrix.com/academy and enter code: 213068

HYPHEN

The hyphen is used in **compound words**. The following are the rules for hyphens:

Written-out numbers between 21 and 99 are written with a hyphen

> Correct: *twenty-five* | one hundred *fifty-one* | *ninety-four* thousand
> Incorrect: *seven-hundred* | *five-thousand* | *nine-teen*

Fractions need a hyphen if they are used as adjectives

> Correct: The recipe says that we need a *three-fourths* cup of butter.
> Incorrect: *One-fourth* of the road is under construction.

Compound words used as adjectives that come before a noun need a hyphen

> Correct: The *well-fed* dog took a nap.
> Incorrect: The dog was *well-fed* for his nap.

To **avoid confusion** with some words, use a hyphen

> Examples: semi-irresponsible | Re-collect |Re-claim

Note: This is not a complete set of the rules for hyphens. A dictionary is the best tool for knowing if a compound word needs a hyphen.

DASHES

Dashes are used to show a **break** or a **change in thought** in a sentence or to act as parentheses in a sentence. When typing, use two hyphens to make a dash. Do not put a space before or after the dash. The following are the rules for dashes:

To set off **parenthetical statements** or an **appositive with internal punctuation**

> Example: The three trees—oak, pine, and magnolia—are coming on a truck tomorrow.

To show a **break or change in tone or thought**

> Example: The first question—how silly of me—does not have a correct answer.

ELLIPSIS MARKS

The ellipsis mark has three periods (...) to show when **words have been removed** from a quotation. If a full sentence or more is removed from a quoted passage, you need to use four periods to show the removed text and the end punctuation mark. The ellipsis mark should not be used at the beginning of a quotation. Also, the ellipsis should not be used at the end of a quotation. The exception is when some words have been deleted from the end of the final sentence.

Example:

> "Then he picked up the groceries...paid for them...later he went home."

BRACKETS

There are two main reasons to use brackets:

When **placing parentheses inside of parentheses**

> Example: The hero of this story, Paul Revere (a silversmith and industrialist [see Ch. 4]), rode through towns of Massachusetts to warn of advancing British troops.

When **adding explanation or details that are not part of a quote**

> Example: The father explained, "My children are planning to attend my alma mater [State University]."

Improving Sentences

CAPITALIZATION

The rules for capitalization are:

Capitalize the **first word of a sentence** and the **first word in a direct quotation**

Examples:

> **Sentence**: *Football* is my favorite sport.
> **Direct Quote**: She asked, "*What* is your name?"

Capitalize **proper nouns** and **adjectives that come from proper nouns**

Examples:

> **Proper Noun**: My parents are from *Europe*.
> **Adjective from Proper Noun**: My father is *British*, and my mother is *Italian*.

Capitalize the names of **days**, **months**, and **holidays**

Examples:

> **Day**: Everyone needs to be here on *Wednesday*.
> **Month**: I am so excited for *December*.
> **Holiday**: *Independence Day* comes every July.

Capitalize directional names (north, east, south, west) **when they refer to specific areas**, but *not* **when they refer to the direction**

Examples:

> **Specific Area**: James is from the *West*.
> **Direction**: After three miles, turn *south* toward the highway.

Capitalize **all important words in a title** (articles, short prepositions, and short conjunctions are not capitalized unless they are the first or last word of the title)

Examples:

> **Correct**: <u>*Romeo and Juliet*</u> is a beautiful drama on love.
> **Incorrect**: <u>*The Taming Of The Shrew*</u> is my favorite. (Remember that internal prepositions and articles are not capitalized.)

Note: Books, movies, plays (more than one act), newspapers, magazines, and long musical pieces are put in italics. The two examples of Shakespeare's plays are underlined to show their use as an example.

Capitalize **kinship names** only if they are used as a **part or whole of a proper noun**. When using a kinship name descriptively, *do not* capitalize it.

Examples:

> **Kinship name as proper noun:** Uncle Mark is coming over later tonight.
> **Kinship name as proper noun:** Did you ask Mom if you could eat a cookie?
> **Descriptive kinship name:** Sally 's uncle Jimbo is a ship captain.

SUBJECTS AND PREDICATES

SUBJECTS

The subject of a sentence names who or what the sentence is about. The complete subject is composed of the **simple subject** and all of its **modifiers**.

To find the complete subject, ask *Who* or *What* and insert the verb to complete the question. The answer is the **complete subject**. To find the simple subject, remove all of the modifiers in the complete subject.

> **Review Video: Subjects**
> Visit mometrix.com/academy and enter code: 444771

Examples:

> The small red car is the one that he wants for Christmas.
> (The complete subject is *the small red car*.)

> The young artist is coming over for dinner.
> (The complete subject is *the young artist*.)

In **imperative sentences**, the verb's subject is understood, but not actually present in the sentence. Although the subject ordinarily comes before the verb, in sentences that begin with *There are* or *There was*, the subject follows the verb. The ability to recognize the subject of a sentence helps in editing a variety of problems, such as sentence fragments and subject-verb agreement, as well as the using the correct pronouns.

Direct:

> John knows the way to the park.
> (Who knows the way to the park? Answer: John)

> The cookies need ten more minutes.
> (What needs ten minutes? Answer: The cookies)

> By five o' clock, Bill will need to leave.
> (Who needs to leave? Answer: Bill)

Remember: The subject can come after the verb.

> There are five letters on the table for him.
> (What is on the table? Answer: Five letters)

> There were coffee and doughnuts in the house.
> (What was in the house? Answer: Coffee and doughnuts)

Implied:

> Go to the post office for me.
> (Who is going to the post office? Answer: You are.)

> Come and sit with me, please?
> (Who needs to come and sit? Answer: You do.)

PREDICATES

In a sentence, you always have a predicate and a subject. A **predicate** is what remains when you have found the subject. The **subject** tells what the sentence is about, and the predicate explains or describes the subject.

Think about the sentence: *He sings.* In this sentence, we have a subject (He) and a predicate (sings). This is all that is needed for a sentence to be complete. Would we like more information? Of course, we would like to know more. However, if this all the information that you are given, you have a complete sentence.

Now, let's look at another sentence:

> *John and Jane sing on Tuesday nights at the dance hall.*

What is the subject of this sentence?
Answer: John and Jane.

What is the predicate of this sentence?
Answer: Everything else in the sentence besides John and Jane.

SUBJECT-VERB AGREEMENT

Verbs agree with their subjects in **number**. In other words, singular subjects need singular verbs. Plural subjects need plural verbs. **Singular** is for one person, place, or thing. **Plural** is for more than one person, place, or thing. Subjects and verbs must also agree in person: first, second, or third. The present tense ending *-s* is used on a verb if its subject is third person singular; otherwise, the verb takes no ending.

> **Review Video: Subject Verb Agreement**
> Visit mometrix.com/academy and enter code: 479190

NUMBER AGREEMENT EXAMPLES:

Single Subject and Verb: *Dan calls home.*
(Dan is one person. So, the singular verb *calls* is needed.)

Plural Subject and Verb: *Dan and Bob call home.*
(More than one person needs the plural verb *call*.)

PERSON AGREEMENT EXAMPLES:

First Person: I *am* walking.
Second Person: You *are* walking.
Third Person: He *is* walking.

PROBLEMS WITH SUBJECT-VERB AGREEMENT

WORDS BETWEEN SUBJECT AND VERB

The joy of my life returns home tonight.
(**Singular Subject**: joy. **Singular Verb**: returns)
The phrase *of my life* does not influence the verb *returns*.

The question that still remains unanswered is "Who are you?"
(**Singular Subject**: question. **Singular Verb**: is)
Don't let the phrase "*that still remains…*" trouble you. The subject *question* goes with *is*.

COMPOUND SUBJECTS

You and Jon are invited to come to my house.
(**Plural Subject**: You and Jon. **Plural Verb**: are)

The pencil and paper belong to me.
(**Plural Subject**: pencil and paper. **Plural Verb**: belong)

SUBJECTS JOINED BY OR AND NOR

Today or tomorrow is the day.
(**Subject**: Today / tomorrow. **Verb**: is)

Stan or Phil wants to read the book.
(**Subject**: Stan / Phil. **Verb**: wants)

Neither the books nor the *pen is* on the desk.
(**Subject**: Books / Pen. **Verb**: is)

Either the blanket or *pillows arrive* this afternoon.
(**Subject**: Blanket / Pillows. **Verb**: arrive)

Note: Singular subjects that are joined with the conjunction *or* need a singular verb. However, when one subject is singular and another is plural, you make the verb agree with the **closer subject**. The example about books and the pen has a singular verb because the pen (singular subject) is closer to the verb.

INDEFINITE PRONOUNS: EITHER, NEITHER, AND EACH

Is either of you ready for the game?
(**Singular Subject**: Either. **Singular Verb**: is)

Each man, woman, and child is unique.
(**Singular Subject**: Each. **Singular Verb**: is)

THE ADJECTIVE EVERY AND COMPOUNDS: EVERYBODY, EVERYONE, ANYBODY, ANYONE

Every day passes faster than the last.
(**Singular Subject**: Every day. **Singular Verb**: passes)

Anybody is welcome to bring a tent.
(**Singular Subject**: Anybody. **Singular Verb**: is)

COLLECTIVE NOUNS

The family eats at the restaurant every Friday night.
(The members of the family are one at the restaurant.)

The team are leaving for their homes after the game.
(The members of the team are leaving as individuals to go to their own homes.)

WHO, WHICH, AND THAT AS SUBJECT

This is the man *who* is helping me today.
He is a good man *who* serves others before himself.
This painting *that* is hung over the couch is very beautiful.

PLURAL FORM AND SINGULAR MEANING

Some nouns are singular in meaning but plural in form: news, mathematics, physics, and economics

> The news is coming on now.
> Mathematics is my favorite class.

Some nouns are plural in meaning: athletics, gymnastics, scissors, and pants

> Do these pants come with a shirt?
> The scissors are for my project.

Note: Look to your dictionary for help when you aren't sure whether a noun with a plural form has a singular or plural meaning.

Addition, Multiplication, Subtraction, and Division are normally singular.

> One plus one is two.
> Three times three is nine.

COMPLEMENTS

A complement is a noun, pronoun, or adjective that is used to give more information about the verb in the sentence.

DIRECT OBJECTS

A direct object is a noun that takes or receives the **action** of a verb. Remember: a complete sentence does not need a direct object. A sentence needs only a subject and a verb. When you are looking for a direct object, find the verb and ask *who* or *what*.

Examples:

> I took the blanket. (Who or what did I take? *The blanket*)
> Jane read books. (Who or what does Jane read? *Books*)

INDIRECT OBJECTS

An indirect object is a word or group of words that show how an action had an **influence** on someone or something. If there is an indirect object in a sentence, then you always have a direct object in the sentence. When you are looking for the indirect object, find the verb and ask *to/for whom or what.*

Examples:

> We taught the old dog a new trick.
> (To/For Whom or What was taught? *The old dog*)

> I gave them a math lesson.
> (To/For Whom or What was given? *Them*)

Predicate nouns are nouns that *modify the subject and finish linking verbs.*

> Example: My father is a lawyer. (*Father* is the subject. *Lawyer* is the predicate noun.)

Predicate adjectives are adjectives that *modify the subject and finish linking verbs.*

> Example: Your mother is patient. (*Mother* is the subject. *Patient* is the predicate adjective.)

PRONOUN USAGE

AGREEMENT

The **antecedent** is the noun that has been replaced by a pronoun. A pronoun and the antecedent agree when they have matching number and gender.

Singular agreement:

> *John* came into town, and *he* played for us.
> (The word *He* replaces *John*.)

Plural agreement:

> *John and Rick* came into town, and *they* played for us.
> (The word *They* replaces *John* and *Rick*.)

CASE

To determine the correct pronoun to use in a compound subject or object, try each pronoun separately in the sentence. Your knowledge of pronouns will tell you which one is correct.

> Example: Bob and (I, me) will be going.
> (Answer: Bob and I will be going.)

Test: (1) *I will be going* or (2) *Me will be going*. The second choice cannot be correct because *me* is not used as a subject of a sentence. Instead, *me* is used as an object.

When a pronoun is used with a noun immediately following (as in "we boys"), try the sentence without the added noun.

> Example: (We/Us) boys played football last year.
> (Answer: We boys played football last year.)

Test: (1) *We* played football last year or (2) *Us* played football last year. Again, the second choice cannot be correct because *us* is not used as a subject of a sentence. Instead, *us* is used as an object.

> **Review Video: Pronoun Usage**
> Visit mometrix.com/academy and enter code: 666500

REFERENCE

A pronoun should point clearly to the **antecedent**. Here is how a pronoun reference can be unhelpful if it is not directly stated or puzzling.

> **Unhelpful**: Ron and Jim went to the store, and he bought soda.
> (Who bought soda? Ron or Jim?)

> **Helpful**: Jim went to the store, and he bought soda.
> (The sentence is clear. Jim bought the soda.)

CHANGING FORMS

Some pronouns change their form by their placement in a sentence. A pronoun that is a subject in a sentence comes in the **subjective case**. Pronouns that serve as objects appear in the **objective case**. Finally, the pronouns that are used as possessives appear in the **possessive case**.

> **Subjective case**: *He* is coming to the show.
> (The pronoun *He* is the subject of the sentence.)

> **Objective case**: Josh drove *him* to the airport.
> (The pronoun *him* is the object of the sentence.)

> **Possessive case**: The flowers are *mine*.
> (The pronoun *mine* shows ownership of the flowers.)

WHO OR WHOM

Who, a subjective-case pronoun, can be used as a subject. *Whom*, an objective case pronoun, can be used as an object. The words *who* and *whom* are common in **subordinate clauses** or in **questions**.

> **Subject**: He knows *who* wants to come.
> (*Who* is the subject of the verb *wants*.)

> **Object**: He knows *whom* we want at the party.
> (*Whom* is the object of *we want*.)

CLAUSES

There are two types of clauses: independent and dependent. Unlike phrases, a **clause** has a subject and a verb. So, what is the difference between a clause that is independent and one that is dependent? An **independent clause** gives a complete thought. A **dependent clause** does not share a complete thought. Instead, a dependent clause has a subject and a verb, but it needs an independent clause. **Subordinate** (i.e., dependent) clauses look like sentences. They may have a subject, a verb, and objects or complements. They are used within sentences as adverbs, adjectives, or nouns.

> **Independent Clause**: I am running outside. (Subject is *I* and verb is *am running*.)
> **Dependent Clause**: I am running <u>because I want to stay in shape</u>.

The clause *I am running* is an independent clause. The underlined clause is dependent. Remember: a dependent clause does not give a complete thought. Think about the dependent clause: *because I want to stay in shape*.

Without any other information, you think: So, you want to stay in shape. What are you are doing to stay in shape? Answer: *I am running*.

TYPES OF DEPENDENT CLAUSES

An **adjective clause** is a dependent clause that modifies nouns and pronouns. Adjective clauses begin with a **relative pronoun** (*who, whose, whom, which,* and *that*) or a **relative adverb** (*where, when,* and *why*). Also, adjective clauses come after the noun that the clause needs to explain or rename. This is done to have a clear connection to the independent clause.

Examples:

> I learned the reason why I won the award.
> This is the place where I started my first job.

An adjective clause can be an essential or nonessential clause. An **essential clause** is very important to the sentence. Essential clauses explain or define a person or thing. **Nonessential clauses** give more information about a person or thing. However, they are not necessary to the sentence.

Examples:

> **Essential**: A person *who works hard at first* can rest later in life.
> **Nonessential**: Neil Armstrong, *who walked on the moon*, is my hero.

An **adverb clause** is a dependent clause that modifies verbs, adjectives, and other adverbs. To show a clear connection to the independent clause, put the adverb clause immediately before or after the independent clause. An adverb clause can start with *after, although, as, as if, before, because, if, since, so, so that, unless, when, where,* or *while*.

Examples:

> *When you walked outside*, I called the manager.
> I want to go with you *unless you want to stay*.

A **noun clause** is a dependent clause that can be used as a subject, object, or complement. Noun clauses can begin with *how, that, what, whether, which, who,* or *why*. These words can also come with an adjective clause. Remember that the entire clause makes a noun or an adjective clause, not the word that starts a clause. So, be sure to look for more than the word that begins the clause. To show a clear connection to the independent clause, be sure that a noun clause comes after the verb. The exception is when the noun clause is the subject of the sentence.

Examples:

> The fact that you were alone alarms me.
> What you learn from each other depends on your honesty with others.

PHRASES

A phrase is not a complete sentence; it cannot be a statement and cannot give a complete thought. Instead, a phrase is a group of words that can be used as a noun, adjective, or adverb in a sentence. Phrases strengthen sentences by *adding explanation or renaming something*.

PREPOSITIONAL PHRASES

A phrase that can be found in many sentences is the **prepositional phrase**. A prepositional phrase begins with a preposition and ends with a noun or pronoun that is used as an object. Normally, the prepositional phrase works as an adjective or an adverb.

Examples:

> The picnic is *on the blanket.*
> I am sick *with a fever* today.
> *Among the many flowers,* a four-leaf clover was found by John.

VERBALS AND VERBAL PHRASES

A verbal looks like a verb, but it is not used as a verb. Instead, a **verbal** is used as a noun, adjective, or adverb. Be careful with verbals. They do not replace a verb in a sentence.

> **Correct**: Walk a mile daily.
> (*Walk* is the verb of this sentence. As in, "*You* walk a mile daily.")
>
> **Incorrect**: To walk a mile.
> (*To walk* is a type of verbal. But, verbals cannot be a verb for a sentence.)

A **verbal phrase** is a verb form that does not function as the verb of a clause. There are three major types of verbal phrases: participial, gerund, and infinitive phrases.

PARTICIPLES

A participle is a verbal that is used as an adjective. The **present participle** always ends with *-ing*. **Past participles** end with *-d, -ed, -n,* or *-t.*

Examples: Verb: *dance* | Present Participle: *dancing* | Past Participle: *danced*

Participial phrases are made of a participle and any complements or modifiers. Often, they come right after the noun or pronoun that they modify.

Examples:

> *Shipwrecked on an island,* the boys started to fish for food.
> *Having been seated for five hours,* we got out of the car to stretch our legs.
> *Praised for their work,* the group accepted the first-place trophy.

GERUNDS

A **gerund** is a verbal that is used as a noun. Gerunds can be found by looking for their *-ing* endings. However, you need to be careful that you have found a gerund, not a present participle. Since gerunds are nouns, they can be used as a subject of a sentence and the object of a verb or preposition.

Gerund phrases are built around present participles (i.e., *-ing* endings to verbs) and they are always used as nouns. The gerund phrase has a gerund and any complements or modifiers.

Examples:

> We want to be known for *teaching the poor.* (Object of Preposition)
> *Coaching this team* is the best job of my life. (Subject)
> We like *practicing our songs* in the basement. (Object of the verb: *like*)

INFINITIVES

An infinitive is a verbal that can be used as a noun, an adjective, or an adverb. An infinitive is made of the basic form of a verb with the word *to* coming before the verb.

Infinitive phrases are made of an infinitive and all complements and modifiers. They are used as nouns, adjectives, or adverbs.

Examples:

> *To join the team* is my goal in life. (Noun)
> The animals have enough food *to eat for the night*. (Adjective)
> People lift weights *to exercise their muscles*. (Adverb)

APPOSITIVE PHRASES

An appositive is a word or phrase that is used to explain or rename nouns or pronouns. In a sentence they can be noun phrases, prepositional phrases, gerund phrases, or infinitive phrases.

Examples:

> Terriers, *hunters at heart*, have been dressed up to look like lap dogs.
> (The phrase *hunters at heart* renames the noun *terriers*.)
>
> His plan, *to save and invest his money*, was proven as a safe approach.
> (The italicized infinitive phrase renames the plan.)

Appositive phrases can be essential or nonessential. An appositive phrase is **essential** if the person, place, or thing being described or renamed is too general.

> **Essential**: Two Founding Fathers George Washington and Thomas Jefferson served as presidents.
> **Nonessential**: George Washington and Thomas Jefferson, two Founding Fathers, served as presidents.

ABSOLUTE PHRASES

An absolute phrase is a phrase with a participle that comes after a noun. The absolute phrase is never the subject of a sentence. Also, the phrase does not explain or add to the meaning of a word in a sentence. Absolute phrases are used *independently* from the rest of the sentence. However, they are still phrases, and a phrase cannot give a complete thought.

Examples:

> *The alarm ringing*, he pushed the snooze button.
> *The music paused*, she continued to dance through the crowd.

Note: Appositive and absolute phrases can be confusing in sentences. So, don't be discouraged if you have a difficult time with them.

MODES OF SENTENCE PATTERNS

Sentence patterns fall into five common modes with some exceptions. They are:

- Subject + linking verb + subject complement
- Subject + transitive verb + direct object
- Subject + transitive verb + indirect object + direct object
- Subject + transitive verb + direct object + object complement
- Subject + intransitive verb

Common exceptions to these patterns are questions and commands, sentences with delayed subjects, and passive transformations.

TYPES OF SENTENCES

For a sentence to be complete, it must have a subject and a verb or **predicate**. A complete sentence will express a complete thought, otherwise it is known as a **fragment**. An example of a fragment is: *As the clock struck midnight.* A complete sentence would be: *As the clock struck midnight, she ran home.* The types of sentences are declarative, imperative, interrogative, and exclamatory.

A **declarative sentence** states a fact and ends with a period.

> Example: The football game starts at seven o'clock.

An **imperative sentence** tells someone to do something and ends with a period.

> Example: Go to the store and buy milk.

An **interrogative sentence** asks a question and ends with a question mark.

> Example: Are you going to the game on Friday?

An **exclamatory sentence** shows strong emotion and ends with an exclamation point.

> Example: I can't believe we won the game!

SENTENCE STRUCTURES

There are four major types of sentences: simple, compound, complex, and compound-complex.

Simple Sentences – Simple sentences have one independent clause with no subordinate clauses. A simple sentence can have **compound elements** (e.g., a compound subject or verb).

Examples:

> Judy *watered* the lawn. (single subject, single *verb*)
> Judy and Alan *watered* the lawn. (compound subject, single *verb*)
> Judy *watered* the lawn and *pulled* weeds. (single subject, compound *verb*)
> Judy and Alan *watered* the lawn and *pulled* weeds. (compound subject, compound *verb*)

Compound Sentences – Compound sentences have two or more *independent clauses* with no dependent clauses. Usually, the independent clauses are joined with a comma and coordinating conjunction or with a semicolon.

Examples:

> *The time has come*, and *we are ready.*
> *I woke up at dawn*; then *I went outside to watch the sun rise.*

Complex Sentences – A complex sentence has one *independent clause* and one or more dependent clauses.

Examples:

> Although he had the flu, *Harry went to work.*
> *Marcia got married* after she finished college.

Compound-Complex Sentences – A compound-complex sentence has at least two *independent clauses* and at least one <u>dependent clause</u>.

Examples:

> *John is my friend* <u>who went to India</u>, and *he brought souvenirs for us.*
> *You may not know*, but *we heard the music* <u>that you played last night</u>.

> **Review Video: <u>Sentence Structure</u>**
> Visit mometrix.com/academy and enter code: 700478

SENTENCE FRAGMENTS

A part of a sentence should not be treated like a complete sentence. A sentence must be made of at least one **independent clause**. An independent clause has a subject and a verb. Remember that the independent clause can stand alone as a sentence. Some fragments are independent clauses that begin with a subordinating word (e.g., as, because, so, etc.). Other fragments may not have a subject, a verb, or both.

A **sentence fragment** can be repaired in several ways. One way is to put the fragment with a neighbor sentence. Another way is to be sure that punctuation is not needed. You can also turn the fragment into a sentence by adding any missing pieces. Sentence fragments are allowed for writers who want to show off their art. However, for your exam, sentence fragments are not allowed.

> **Fragment**: Because he wanted to sail for Rome.
> **Sentence**: He dreamed of Europe because he wanted to sail for Rome.

RUN-ON SENTENCES

Run-on sentences consist of multiple independent clauses that have not been joined properly. Run-on sentences can be corrected in a variety of ways:

Joining the two independent clauses: Depending on how they are related, this could be done with a comma and coordinating conjunction, a semicolon, or a dash.

> **Incorrect**: I went on the trip I had a good time.
> **Correct**: I went on the trip, and I had a good time.

Changing one independent clause into a dependent clause: This is most easily done by simply adding a subordinating conjunction to the less important clause.

> **Incorrect**: I went to the store I bought some eggs.
> **Correct**: I went to the store where I bought some eggs.

Separating each independent clause into its own sentence: This correction is most effective when both independent clauses are long, or are not closely related. This can also be used when one sentence is a question and one is not.

> **Incorrect**: I had pancakes for breakfast this morning they're my favorite.
> **Correct**: I had pancakes for breakfast this morning. They're my favorite.

Reorganizing the thoughts in the sentence: This is often the best correction but requires the most work.

> **Incorrect**: The drive to New York takes ten hours it makes me very tired.
> **Correct**: During the ten-hour drive to New York, I get very tired.

> **Review Video: <u>Fragments and Run-on Sentences</u>**
> Visit mometrix.com/academy and enter code: 541989

DANGLING AND MISPLACED MODIFIERS

DANGLING MODIFIERS

A dangling modifier is a verbal phrase that does not have a clear connection to a word. A dangling modifier can also be a dependent clause (the subject and/or verb are not included) that does not have a clear connection to a word.

Examples:

> **Dangling**: *Reading each magazine article*, the stories caught my attention.
> **Corrected**: Reading each magazine article, *I* was entertained by the stories.

In this example, the word *stories* cannot be modified by *Reading each magazine article*. People can read, but stories cannot read. So, the pronoun *I* is needed for the modifying phrase *Reading each magazine article*.

> **Dangling**: Since childhood, my grandparents have visited me for Christmas.
> **Corrected**: Since childhood, I have been visited by my grandparents for Christmas.

In this example, the dependent adverb clause *Since childhood* cannot modify grandparents. So, the pronoun *I* is needed for the modifying adverb clause.

MISPLACED MODIFIERS

In some sentences, a **modifier** can be put in more than one place. However, you need to be sure that there is no confusion about which word is being explained or given more detail.

> **Incorrect**: He read the book to a crowd that was filled with beautiful pictures.
> **Correct**: He read the book that was filled with beautiful pictures to a crowd.

The book was filled with beautiful pictures, not the crowd.

> **Incorrect**: Derek saw a bus nearly hit a man on his way to work.
> **Correct**: On his way to work, Derek saw a bus nearly hit a man.

Derek was on his way to work, not the other man.

SPLIT INFINITIVES

A split infinitive occurs when a modifying word comes between the word *to* and the verb that pairs with *to*.

> Example: To *clearly* explain vs. *To explain* clearly | To *softly* sing vs. *To sing* softly

Though still considered improper by some, split infinitives may provide better clarity and simplicity than the alternatives. As such, avoiding them should not be considered a universal rule.

DOUBLE NEGATIVES

Standard English allows two negatives when a positive meaning is intended. For example, "The team was not displeased with their performance." **Double negatives** that are used to emphasize negation are not part of Standard English.

Negative modifiers (e.g., never, no, and not) should not be paired with other negative modifiers or negative words (e.g., none, nobody, nothing, or neither). The modifiers *hardly, barely*, and *scarcely* are also considered negatives in Standard English. So, they should not be used with other negatives.

PARALLELISM AND SUBORDINATION

PARALLELISM

Parallel structures are used in sentences to highlight similar ideas and to connect sentences that give similar information. **Parallelism** pairs parts of speech, phrases, or clauses together with a matching piece. To write, *I enjoy <u>reading</u> and <u>to study</u>* would be incorrect. An infinitive does not match with a gerund. Instead, you should write *I enjoy <u>reading</u> and <u>studying</u>*.

> **Incorrect**: He stopped at the office, grocery store, and the pharmacy before heading home.
> **Correct**: He stopped at the office, *the* grocery store, and the pharmacy before heading home.

> **Incorrect**: While vacationing in Europe, he went biking, skiing, and climbed mountains.
> **Correct**: While vacationing in Europe, he went biking, skiing, and *mountain climbing*.

SUBORDINATION

When two items are not equal to each other, you can join them by making the more important piece an independent clause. The less important piece can become **subordinate**. To make the less important piece subordinate, you make it a phrase or a dependent clause. The piece of more importance should be the one that readers want or will need to remember.

> **Separated**: The team had a perfect regular season. The team lost the championship.
> **Subordinated**: Despite having a perfect regular season, *the team lost the championship*.

TRANSITIONS

Transitions are bridges between what has been read and what is about to be read. Transitions smooth the reader's path between sentences and inform the reader of major connections to new ideas forthcoming in the text. **Transitional phrases** should be used with care, selecting the appropriate phrase for a transition. **Tone** is another important consideration in using transitional phrases, varying the tone for different audiences. For example, in a scholarly essay, *in summary* would be preferable to the more informal *in short*.

When working with transitional words and phrases, writers usually find a natural **flow** that indicates when a transition is needed. In reading a draft of the text, it should become apparent where the flow is uneven or rough. At this point, the writer can add transitional elements during the revision process. **Revising** can also afford an opportunity to delete transitional devices that seem heavy handed or unnecessary.

Transitional words and phrases are used to transition between paragraphs and also to transition within a single paragraph. Transitions assist the flow of ideas and help to unify an essay. A writer can use certain words to indicate that an example or summary is being presented. The following phrases, among others, can be used as this type of transition: *as a result, as I have said, for example, for instance, in any case, in any event, in brief, in conclusion, in fact, in other words, in short, on the whole,* and *to sum it up.*

> **Review Video: Transitions**
> Visit mometrix.com/academy and enter code: 707563

TRANSITIONAL WORDS

LINK SIMILAR IDEAS

When a writer links ideas that are **similar** in nature, there are a variety of words and phrases he or she can choose, including but not limited to: *also, and, another, besides, equally important, further, furthermore, in addition, likewise, too, similarly, nor, of course,* and *for instance.*

LINK DISSIMILAR OR CONTRADICTORY IDEAS

Writers can link **contradictory** ideas in an essay by using, among others, the following words and phrases: *although, and yet, even if, conversely, but, however, otherwise, still, yet, instead, in spite of, nevertheless, on the contrary,* and *on the other hand.*

INDICATE CAUSE, PURPOSE, OR RESULT

Writers may need to indicate that one thing is the **cause**, **purpose**, or **result** of another thing. To show this relationship, writers can use, among others, the following linking words and phrases: *as, as a result, because, consequently, hence, for, for this reason, since, so, then, thus,* and *therefore.*

INDICATE TIME OR POSITION

Certain words can be used to indicate the **time** and **position** of one thing in relation to another. Writers can use, for example, the following terms to create a timeline of events in an essay: *above, across, afterward, before, beyond, eventually, meanwhile, next, presently, around, at once, at the present time, finally, first, here, second, thereafter,* and *upon.* These words can show the order or placement of items or ideas in an essay.

TONE

Tone may be defined as the writer's **attitude** toward the topic, and to the audience. This attitude is reflected in the language used in the writing. The tone of a work should be **appropriate** to the topic and to the intended audience. Some texts should not contain slang or **jargon**, although these may be fine in a different piece. Tone can range from humorous to serious and all levels in between. It may be more or less formal, depending on the purpose of the writing and its intended audience. All these nuances in tone can flavor the entire writing and should be kept in mind as the work evolves.

WORD USAGE

Word usage, or **diction**, refers to the use of words with meanings and forms that are appropriate for the context and structure of a sentence. A common error in word usage occurs when a word's meaning does not fit the context of the sentence.

> Incorrect: Susie likes chips better then candy.
> Correct: Susie likes chips better than candy.

Incorrect: The cat licked it's coat.
Correct: The cat licked its coat.

Review Video: Word Usage
Visit mometrix.com/academy and enter code: 197863

WORD CONFUSION

Which is used for things only.

Example: John's dog, *which was called Max,* is large and fierce.

That is used for people or things.

Example: Is this the only book *that Louis L'Amour wrote?*
Example: Is Louis L'Amour the author *that wrote Western novels?*

Who is used for people only.

Example: Mozart was the composer *who wrote those operas.*

Improving Paragraphs

LEVEL OF FORMALITY

The relationship between writer and reader is important in choosing a **level of formality** as most writing requires some degree of formality. **Formal writing** is for addressing a superior in a school or work environment. Business letters, textbooks, and newspapers use a moderate to high level of formality. **Informal writing** is appropriate for *private letters, personal e-mails, and business correspondence between close associates.*

For your exam, you will want to be aware of informal and formal writing. One way that this can be accomplished is to watch for shifts in point of view in the essay. For example, unless writers are using a personal example, they will rarely refer to themselves (e.g., "*I* think that *my* point is very clear.") to avoid being informal when they need to be formal.

Also, be mindful of an author who addresses his or her audience **directly** in their writing (e.g., "Readers, *like you*, will understand this argument.") as this can be a sign of informal writing. Good writers understand the need to be consistent with their level of formality. Shifts in levels of formality or point of view can confuse readers and discount the message of an author's writing.

CLICHÉS

Clichés are phrases that have been **overused** to the point that the phrase has no importance or has lost the original meaning. The phrases have no originality and add very little to a passage. Therefore, most writers will avoid the use of clichés. Another option is to make changes to a cliché so that it is not predictable and empty of meaning.

Examples:

> When life gives you lemons, make lemonade.
> Every cloud has a silver lining.

JARGON

Jargon is a **specialized vocabulary** that is used among members of a trade or profession. Since jargon is understood by a small audience, writers tend to leave them to passages where certain readers will understand the vocabulary. Jargon includes exaggerated language that tries to impress rather than inform. Sentences filled with jargon are not precise and difficult to understand.

Examples:

> "He is going to *toenail* these frames for us." (toenailing refers to nailing at an angle)
> "They brought in a *kip* of material today." (a kip is a unit of measure equal to 1000 pounds)

SLANG

Slang is an **informal** and sometimes private language that is understood by some individuals. Slang has some usefulness, but the language can have a small audience. So, most formal writing will not include this kind of language.

Examples:

> "Yes, the event was a *blast*!" (the speaker means that the event was a great experience)
> "That attempt was an *epic fail*." (the speaker means that the attempt was a spectacular failure.)

COLLOQUIALISM

A colloquialism is a word or phrase that is found in informal writing. Unlike slang, **colloquial language** will be familiar to a greater range of people. Colloquial language can include some slang, but these are limited to contractions for the most part.

Examples:

"Can *y'all* come back another time?" (y'all is a contraction of "you all")
"Will you stop him from building this *castle in the air*?" (A "castle in the air" is an improbable or unlikely event.)

POINT OF VIEW

Point of view is the **perspective** from which writing occurs. There are several possibilities:

- **First person** is written so that the *I* of the story is a participant or observer.
- **Second person** is written directly to the reader. is a device to draw the reader in more closely. It is really a variation or refinement of the first-person narrative.
- **Third person**, the most traditional form of point of view, is the omniscient narrator, in which the narrative voice, presumed to be the writer's, is presumed to know everything about the characters, plot, and action. Most writing uses this point of view.

> **Review Video: Point of View**
> Visit mometrix.com/academy and enter code: 383336

PRACTICE MAKES PREPARED WRITERS

Writing is a skill that continues to need development throughout a person's life. For some people, writing seems to be a natural gift. They rarely struggle with writer's block. When you read their papers, they have persuasive ideas. For others, writing is an intimidating task that they endure. As you prepare for the TEAS, believe that you can improve your skills and be better prepared for reviewing several types of writing.

A traditional way to prepare for the English and Language Usage Section is to **read**. When you read newspapers, magazines, and books, you learn about new ideas. You can read newspapers and magazines to become informed about issues that affect many people. As you think about those issues and ideas, you can take a **position** and form **opinions**. Try to develop these ideas and your opinions by sharing them with friends. After you develop your opinions, try **writing** them down as if you were going to spread your ideas beyond your friends.

Remember that you are practicing for more than an exam. Two of the most valuable things in life are the abilities to **read critically** and to **write clearly**. When you work on evaluating the arguments of a passage and explain your thoughts well, you are developing skills that you will use for a lifetime.

BRAINSTORMING

Brainstorming is a technique that is used to find a creative approach to a subject. This can be accomplished by simple **free-association** with a topic. For example, with paper and pen, you write every thought that you have about the topic in a word or phrase. This is done without critical thinking. Everything that comes to your mind about the topic, you should put on your scratch paper. Then, you need to read the list over a few times. Next, you look for *patterns, repetitions, and clusters of ideas*. This allows a variety of fresh ideas to come as you think about the topic.

FREE WRITING

Free writing is a form of brainstorming, but the method occurs in a **structured** way. The method involves a *limited amount of time* (e.g., 2 to 3 minutes) and writing everything that comes to mind about the topic in complete sentences. When time expires, you need to review everything that has been written down. Many of your sentences may make little or no sense, but the insights and observations that can come from free writing make this method a valuable approach. Usually, free writing results in a fuller expression of ideas than brainstorming because thoughts and associations are written in complete sentences. However, both techniques can be used to complement the other.

REVISIONS

A writer's choice of words is a signature of their **style**. Careful thought about the use of words can improve a piece of writing. A passage can be an exciting piece to read when attention is given to the use of specific nouns rather than general ones.

Example:

> **General**: His kindness will never be forgotten.
> **Specific**: His thoughtful gifts and bear hugs will never be forgotten.

Revising sentences is done to make writing more effective. **Editing** sentences is done to correct any errors. Sentences are the building blocks of writing, and they can be changed by paying attention to sentence length, sentence structure, and sentence openings.

You should add **variety** to sentence length, structure, and openings so that the essay does not seem boring or repetitive. A careful analysis of a piece of writing will expose these stylistic problems, and they can be corrected before you finish your essay. Changing up your sentence *structure* and sentence *length* can make your essay more inviting and appealing to readers.

RECURSIVE WRITING PROCESS

However you approach writing, you may find comfort in knowing that the revision process can occur in any order. The **recursive writing process** is not as difficult as the phrase may seem to indicate. Simply put, the recursive writing process means that you may need to revisit steps after completing other steps. Also implied in it is that there is no required order for the steps to take place. Indeed, you may find that **planning**, **drafting**, and **revising** (all a part of the writing process) take place at about the same time. The writing process involves moving back and forth between planning, drafting, and revising, and then more planning, more drafting, and more revising until the writing is satisfactory.

> **Review Video: Recursive Writing Process**
> Visit mometrix.com/academy and enter code: 951611

PARAGRAPHS

After the introduction of a passage, a series of **body paragraphs** will carry a message through to the conclusion. A paragraph should be unified around a **main point**. Normally, a good **topic sentence** summarizes the paragraph's main point. A topic sentence is a general sentence that introduces the paragraph.

The sentences that follow are a **support** to the topic sentence. However, the topic sentence can come as the final sentence to the paragraph if the earlier sentences give a clear explanation of the topic sentence. Overall, the paragraphs need to stay true to the main point. This means that any unnecessary sentences that do not advance the main point should be removed.

The **main point** of a paragraph requires adequate **development** (i.e., a substantial paragraph that covers the main point). A paragraph of only two or three sentences may not adequately cover a main point. An occasional short paragraph is fine as a **transitional device**. However, a well-developed argument will primarily consist of paragraphs with more than a few sentences.

METHODS OF DEVELOPING PARAGRAPHS

A common method of development with paragraphs can be done with **examples**. These examples are the supporting details to the main idea of a paragraph or a passage. When authors write about something that their audience may not understand, they can provide an example to show their point. When authors write about something that is not easily accepted, they can give examples to prove their point.

Illustrations are extended examples that require several sentences. Well-selected illustrations can be a great way for authors to develop a point that may not be familiar to their audience.

Analogies make comparisons between items that appear to have nothing in common. Analogies are employed by writers to provoke fresh thoughts about a subject. These comparisons may be used to explain the unfamiliar, to clarify an abstract point, or to argue a point. Although analogies are effective *literary devices*, they should be used carefully in arguments. Two things may be alike in some respects but completely different in others.

Cause and effect is an excellent device used when the cause and effect are accepted as true. One way that authors can use cause and effect is to state the effect in the topic sentence of a paragraph and add the causes in the body of the paragraph. With this method, an author's paragraphs can have structure which always strengthens writing.

TYPES OF PARAGRAPHS

A **paragraph of narration** tells a story or a part of a story. Normally, the sentences are arranged in chronological order (i.e., the order that the events happened). However, flashbacks (i.e., beginning the story at an earlier time) can be included.

A **descriptive paragraph** makes a verbal portrait of a person, place, or thing. When specific details are used that appeal to one or more of the senses (i.e., sight, sound, smell, taste, and touch), authors give readers a sense of being present in the moment.

A **process paragraph** is related to time order (i.e., First, you open the bottle. Second, you pour the liquid, etc.). Usually, this describes a process or teaches readers how to perform a process.

Comparing two things draws attention to their similarities and indicates a number of differences. When authors **contrast**, they focus only on differences. Both comparisons and contrasts may be used point-by-point or in following paragraphs.

Reasons for starting a new paragraph include:

- To mark off the introduction and concluding paragraphs
- To signal a shift to a new idea or topic
- To indicate an important shift in time or place
- To explain a point in additional detail
- To highlight a comparison, contrast, or cause and effect relationship

Paragraph Length

Most readers find that their comfort level for a paragraph is *between 100 and 200 words*. Shorter paragraphs cause too much starting and stopping, and give a choppy effect. Paragraphs that are too long often test the attention span of readers. Two notable exceptions to this rule exist. In scientific or scholarly papers, longer paragraphs suggest seriousness and depth. In journalistic writing, constraints are placed on paragraph size by the narrow columns in a newspaper format.

The first and last paragraphs of a text will usually be the **introduction** and **conclusion**. These special-purpose paragraphs are likely to be shorter than paragraphs in the body of the work. Paragraphs in the body of the essay follow the subject's **outline**; one paragraph per point in short essays and a group of paragraphs per point in longer works. Some ideas require more development than others, so it is good for a writer to remain flexible. A paragraph of excessive length may be divided, and shorter ones may be combined.

Coherent Paragraphs

A smooth flow of sentences and paragraphs without gaps, shifts, or bumps will lead to paragraph **coherence**. Ties between old and new information can be smoothed by several methods:

- **Linking ideas clearly**, from the topic sentence to the body of the paragraph, is essential for a smooth transition. The topic sentence states the main point, and this should be followed by specific details, examples, and illustrations that support the topic sentence. The support may be direct or indirect. In **indirect support**, the illustrations and examples may support a sentence that in turn supports the topic directly.
- The **repetition of key words** adds coherence to a paragraph. To avoid dull language, variations of the key words may be used.
- **Parallel structures** are often used within sentences to emphasize the similarity of ideas and connect sentences giving similar information.
- Maintaining a **consistent verb tense** throughout the paragraph helps. Shifting tenses affects the smooth flow of words and can disrupt the coherence of the paragraph.

Vocabulary

CONTEXT CLUES

Learning new words is an important part of comprehending and integrating unfamiliar information. When a reader encounters a new word, he can stop and find it in the dictionary or the glossary of terms but sometimes those reference tools aren't readily available or using them at the moment is impractical (e.g., during a test). Furthermore, most readers are usually not willing to take the time.

Another way to determine the meaning of a word is by considering the **context** in which it is being used. These indirect learning hints are called **context clues**. They include definitions, descriptions, examples, and restatements. Because most words are learned by listening to conversations, people use this tool all the time even if they do it unconsciously. But to be effective in written text, context clues must be used judiciously because the unfamiliar word may have several subtle variations, and therefore the context clues could be misinterpreted.

Context refers to *how a word is used in a sentence*. Identifying context can help determine the definition of unknown words. There are different contextual clues such as definition, description, example, comparison, and contrast. The following are examples:

- **Definition**: the unknown word is clearly defined by the previous words. – "When he was painting, his instrument was a ___." (paintbrush)
- **Description**: the unknown word is described by the previous words. – "I was hot, tired, and thirsty; I was ___." (dehydrated)
- **Example**: the unknown word is part of a series of examples. – "Water, soda, and ___ were the offered beverages." (coffee)
- **Comparison**: the unknown word is compared to another word. – "Barney is agreeable and happy like his ___ parents." (positive)
- **Contrast**: the unknown word is contrasted with another word. – "I prefer cold weather to ___ conditions." (hot)

> **Review Video: Context**
> Visit mometrix.com/academy and enter code: 613660

SYNONYMS AND ANTONYMS

When you understand how words relate to each other, you will discover more in a passage. This is explained by understanding **synonyms** (e.g., words that mean the same thing) and **antonyms** (e.g., words that mean the opposite of one another). As an example, *dry* and *arid* are synonyms, and *dry* and *wet* are antonyms.

There are many pairs of words in English that can be considered **synonyms**, despite having slightly different definitions. For instance, the words *friendly* and *collegial* can both be used to describe a warm interpersonal relationship, and one would be correct to call them synonyms. However, *collegial* (kin to *colleague*) is often used in reference to professional or academic relationships, and *friendly* has no such connotation.

If the difference between the two words is too great, then they should not be called synonyms. *Hot* and *warm* are not synonyms because their meanings are too distinct. A good way to determine whether two words are synonyms is to substitute one word for the other word and verify that the meaning of the sentence has not changed. Substituting *warm* for *hot* in a sentence would convey a different meaning. Although warm and hot may seem close in meaning, warm generally means that the temperature is moderate, and hot generally means that the temperature is excessively high.

Antonyms are words with opposite meanings. *Light* and *dark*, *up* and *down*, *right* and *left*, *good* and *bad*: these are all sets of antonyms. Be careful to distinguish between antonyms and pairs of words that are simply different. *Black* and *gray*, for instance, are not antonyms because gray is not the opposite of black. *Black* and *white*, on the other hand, are antonyms.

Not every word has an antonym. For instance, many nouns do not: What would be the antonym of chair? During your exam, the questions related to antonyms are more likely to concern adjectives. You will recall that adjectives are words that describe a noun. Some common adjectives include *purple*, *fast*, *skinny*, and *sweet*. From those four adjectives, *purple* is the item that lacks a group of obvious antonyms.

> **Review Video: Synonyms and Antonyms**
> Visit mometrix.com/academy and enter code: 105612

DESCRIPTION

Occasionally, you will be able to define an unfamiliar word by looking at the **descriptive words** in the context. Consider the following sentence: *Fred dragged the recalcitrant boy kicking and screaming up the stairs.* The words *dragged*, *kicking*, and *screaming* all suggest that the boy does not want to go up the stairs. The reader may assume that *recalcitrant* means something like unwilling or protesting. In this example, an unfamiliar adjective was identified.

Additionally, using description to define an unfamiliar noun is a common practice compared to unfamiliar adjectives, as in this sentence: *Don's wrinkled frown and constantly shaking fist identified him as a curmudgeon of the first order.* Don is described as having a *wrinkled frown and constantly shaking fist* suggesting that a *curmudgeon* must be a grumpy person. **Contrasts** do not always provide detailed information about the unfamiliar word, but they at least give the reader some clues.

When a word has **more than one meaning**, readers can have difficulty with determining how the word is being used in a given sentence. For instance, the verb *cleave*, can mean either *join* or *separate*. When readers come upon this word, they will have to select the definition that makes the most sense. Consider the following sentence: *Hermione's knife cleaved the bread cleanly.* Since, a knife cannot join bread together, the word must indicate separation.

A slightly more difficult example would be the sentence: *The birds cleaved together as they flew from the oak tree.* Immediately, the presence of the word *together* should suggest that in this sentence *cleave* is being used to mean *join*. Discovering the intent of a word with multiple meanings requires the same tricks as defining an unknown word: *look for contextual clues and evaluate the substituted words.*

STRUCTURAL ANALYSIS

An understanding of the basics of language is helpful, and often vital, to understanding what you read. The term **structural analysis** refers to looking at the parts of a word and breaking it down into its different **components** to determine the word's meaning. Parts of a word include prefixes, suffixes, and the root word. By learning the meanings of prefixes, suffixes, and other word fundamentals, you can decipher the meaning of words which may not yet be in your vocabulary.

Prefixes are common letter combinations at the beginning of words, while **suffixes** are common letter combinations at the end. The main part of the word is known as the **root**. Visually, it would look like this: prefix + root word + suffix. Look first at the individual meanings of the root word, prefix and/or suffix. Using knowledge of the meaning(s) of the prefix and/or suffix to see what information it adds to the root.

Even if the meaning of the root is unknown, one can use knowledge of the prefix's and/or suffix's meaning(s) to determine an *approximate meaning* of the word. For example, if one sees the word *uninspired* and does not know what it means, they can use the knowledge that *un-* means 'not' to know that the full word means "not inspired." Understanding the common prefixes and suffixes can illuminate at least part of the meaning of an unfamiliar word.

> **Review Video: Determining Word Meanings**
> Visit mometrix.com/academy and enter code: 894894

AFFIXES

Affixes in the English language are **morphemes** that are added to words to create related but different words. **Derivational affixes** form new words based on and related to the original words. For example, the affix *–ness* added to the end of the adjective *happy* forms the noun *happiness.*

Inflectional affixes form different grammatical versions of words. For example, the plural affix *–s* changes the singular noun *book* to the plural noun *books*, and the past tense affix *–ed* changes the infinitive or present tense verb *look* to the past tense *looked.*

Prefixes are affixes placed in front of words. For example, *heat* means to make hot; *preheat*, using the prefix *pre-*, means to heat in advance. **Suffixes** are affixes placed at the ends of words. The *happiness* example above contains the suffix *–ness.* **Circumfixes** add parts both before and after words, such as how *light* becomes *enlighten* with the prefix *en-* and the suffix *–en.* **Interfixes** compound words via central affixes: *speed* and *meter* become *speedometer* via the interfix *–o–.*

> **Review Video: Prefixes**
> Visit mometrix.com/academy and enter code: 361382
>
> **Review Video: Suffixes**
> Visit mometrix.com/academy and enter code: 212541
>
> **Review Video: Affixes**
> Visit mometrix.com/academy and enter code: 782422

PREFIXES

AMOUNT

Prefix	Definition	Examples
bi-	two	bisect, biennial
mono-	one, single	monogamy, monologue
poly-	many	polymorphous, polygamous
semi-	half, partly	semicircle, semicolon
uni-	one	uniform, unity

NEGATION

Prefix	Definition	Examples
a-	without, lacking	atheist, agnostic
in-	not, opposing	incapable, ineligible
non-	not	nonentity, nonsense
un-	not, reverse of	unhappy, unlock

TIME AND SPACE

Prefix	Definition	Examples
a-	in, on, of, up, to	abed, afoot
ab-	from, away, off	abdicate, abjure
ad-	to, toward	advance, adventure
ante-	before, previous	antecedent, antedate
anti-	against, opposing	antipathy, antidote
cata-	down, away, thoroughly	catastrophe, cataclysm
circum-	around	circumspect, circumference
com-	with, together, very	commotion, complicate
contra-	against, opposing	contradict, contravene
de-	from	depart
dia-	through, across, apart	diameter, diagnose
dis-	away, off, down, not	dissent, disappear
epi-	upon	epilogue
ex-	out	extract, excerpt
hypo-	under, beneath	hypodermic, hypothesis
inter-	among, between	intercede, interrupt
intra-	within	intramural, intrastate
ob-	against, opposing	objection
per-	through	perceive, permit
peri-	around	periscope, perimeter
post-	after, following	postpone, postscript
pre-	before, previous	prevent, preclude
pro-	forward, in place of	propel, pronoun
retro-	back, backward	retrospect, retrograde
sub-	under, beneath	subjugate, substitute
super-	above, extra	supersede, supernumerary
trans-	across, beyond, over	transact, transport
ultra-	beyond, excessively	ultramodern, ultrasonic, ultraviolet

MISCELLANEOUS

Prefix	Definition	Examples
belli-	war, warlike	bellicose
bene-	well, good	benefit, benefactor
equi-	equal	equivalent, equilibrium
for-	away, off, from	forget, forswear
fore-	previous	foretell, forefathers
homo-	same, equal	homogenized, homonym
hyper-	excessive, over	hypercritical, hypertension
in-	in, into	intrude, invade
magn-	large	magnitude, magnify
mal-	bad, poorly, not	malfunction, malpractice
mis-	bad, poorly, not	misspell, misfire
mor-	death	mortality, mortuary
neo-	new	Neolithic, neoconservative
omni-	all, everywhere	omniscient, omnivore
ortho-	right, straight	orthogonal, orthodox
over-	above	overbearing, oversight
pan-	all, entire	panorama, pandemonium
para-	beside, beyond	parallel, paradox
phil-	love, like	philosophy, philanthropic
prim-	first, early	primitive, primary
re-	backward, again	revoke, recur
sym-	with, together	sympathy, symphony
vis-	to see	visage, visible

SUFFIXES

Suffixes are a group of letters, placed behind a root word, that carry a specific meaning. Suffixes can perform one of two possible functions. They can be used to create a new word, or they can shift the tense of a word without changing its original meaning. For example, the suffix -*ability* can be added to the end of the word *account* to form the new word *accountability*. *Account* means a written narrative or description of events, while *accountability* means the state of being liable. The suffix -*ed* can be added to *account* to form the word *accounted*, which simply shifts the word from present tense to past tense.

Sometimes adding a suffix can change the **spelling** of a root word. If the suffix begins with a vowel, the final consonant of the root word must be doubled. This rule applies only if the root word has one syllable or if the accent is on the last syllable. For example, when adding the suffix -*ery* to the root word *rob*, the final word becomes *robbery*. The letter *b* is doubled because *rob* has only one syllable. However, when adding the suffix -*able* to the root word *profit*, the final word becomes *profitable*. The letter *t* is not doubled because the root word *profit* has two syllables.

Spelling is not changed when the suffixes -*less, -ness, -ly*, or -*en* are used. The only exception to this rule occurs when the suffix -*ness* or -*ly* is added to a root word ending in *y*. In this case, the *y* changes to *i*. For example, *happy* becomes *happily*.

Certain suffixes require that the root word be **modified**. If the suffix begins with a vowel, e.g., -*ing*, and the root word ends in the letter *e*, the *e* must be dropped before adding the suffix. For example, the word *write* becomes *writing*. If the suffix begins with a consonant instead of a vowel, the letter *e* at the end of the root word does not need to be dropped. For example, *hope* becomes *hopeless*. The only exceptions to this rule are the words *judgment, acknowledgment,* and *argument.* If a root word ends in the letter *y* and is preceded by a consonant, the *y* is changed to *i* before adding the suffix. This is true for all suffixes except those that begin with *i.* For example, *plenty* becomes *plentiful.*

Here are some common suffixes, their meanings, and some examples of their use:

ADJECTIVE SUFFIXES

Suffix	Definition	Examples
-able (-ible)	capable of being	toler*able*, ed*ible*
-esque	in the style of, like	picturesque, grotesque
-ful	filled with, marked by	thankful, zestful
-ic	make, cause	terrific, beatific
-ish	suggesting, like	churlish, childish
-less	lacking, without	hopeless, countless
-ous	marked by, given to	religious, riotous

NOUN SUFFIXES

Suffix	Definition	Examples
-acy	state, condition	accuracy, privacy
-ance	act, condition, fact	acceptance, vigilance
-ard	one that does excessively	drunkard, sluggard
-ation	action, state, result	occupation, starvation
-dom	state, rank, condition	serfdom, wisdom
-er (-or)	office, action	teach*er*, elevat*or*, hon*or*
-ess	feminine	waitress, duchess
-hood	state, condition	manhood, statehood
-ion	action, result, state	union, fusion
-ism	act, manner, doctrine	barbarism, socialism
-ist	worker, follower	monopolist, socialist
-ity (-ty)	state, quality, condition	acid*ity*, civil*ity*, royal*ty*
-ment	result, action	refreshment, disappointment
-ness	quality, state	greatness, tallness
-ship	position	internship, statesmanship
-sion (-tion)	state, result	revi*sion*, expedi*tion*
-th	act, state, quality	warmth, width
-tude	quality, state, result	magnitude, fortitude

VERB SUFFIXES

Suffix	Definition	Examples
-ate	having, showing	separate, desolate
-en	cause to be, become	deepen, strengthen
-fy	make, cause to have	glorify, fortify
-ize	cause to be, treat with	sterilize, mechanize, criticize

Comprehensive Practice Tests

The table below shows the amount of time and number of questions that are on each practice test. It is recommended that you use a timer when taking the test to properly simulate the test taking conditions.

Reading	Mathematics	Science	English and Language Usage	Total
53 items	36 items	53 items	28 items	170 items
64 minutes	54 minutes	63 minutes	28 minutes	209 minutes

DIRECTIONS: The questions you are about to take are multiple-choice with only one correct answer per question. Read each test item and mark your answer on the appropriate blank on the answer page that precedes each practice test.

When you have completed a practice test, you may check your answers with those on the answer key that follows each test.

Each practice test is followed by detailed answer explanations.

Special feature: In addition to the two full-length practice tests included in this section, you also have access to an **online interactive practice test!** Just follow the link below on your computer or mobile device to get started.

<u>**Online Interactive Practice Test**</u>
Visit mometrix.com/university/teas-bonus-practice-test

TEAS Practice Test #1

	Reading		Mathematics	Science		English and Language Usage

Reading	Number of Questions: **53**
	Time Limit: **64 Minutes**

1. Which of the answer choices gives the best definition for the underlined word in the following sentence?

Adelaide attempted to <u>assuage</u> her guilt over the piece of cheesecake by limiting herself to salads the following day.

    a. increase
    b. support
    c. appease
    d. conceal

2. Which of the following would best support the argument that people cause global climate change?

    a. The average global temperature has increased 1.5 degrees Fahrenheit since 1880.
    b. Common greenhouse gases include carbon dioxide and water vapor.
    c. Most of the greenhouse gases today come from burning things like coal and other fossil fuels for energy.
    d. The average person breathes out about 1.0 kg of carbon dioxide every day, while the average cow produces about 80 kg of methane.

The next three questions are based on the following information.

    <u>The Dewey Decimal Classes</u>

    000 Computer science, information, and general works
    100 Philosophy and psychology
    200 Religion
    300 Social sciences
    400 Languages
    500 Science and mathematics
    600 Technical and applied science
    700 Arts and recreation
    800 Literature
    900 History, geography, and biography

3. Lise is doing a research project on the various psychological theories that Sigmund Freud developed and on the modern response to those theories. She is not sure where to begin, so she consults the chart of Dewey Decimal Classes. To which section of the library should she go to begin looking for research material?

    a. 100
    b. 200
    c. 300
    d. 900

4. During her research, Lise discovers that Freud's theory of the Oedipal complex was based on ancient Greek mythology that was made famous by Sophocles' play *Oedipus Rex*. To which section of the library should she go if she is interested in reading the play?

a. 300
b. 400
c. 800
d. 900

5. Also during her research, Lise learns about Freud's Jewish background, and she decides to compare Freud's theories to traditional Judaism. To which section of the library should she go for more information on this subject?

a. 100
b. 200
c. 800
d. 900

6. Which of the answer choices best describes the appropriateness of Mara's data sample in the following vignette?

Mara is conducting a study that will examine the ideas of middle school teachers, concerning the usage of iPhones in the classroom. She interviews all teachers who teach a computer software course.

a. The sample is biased because it only includes teachers who are immersed in the technology field
b. The sample is biased because the sample size is too small
c. The sample is biased because the sample size is too large
d. The sample is not biased and is appropriate for the study

7. Which of the answer choices gives the best definition for the underlined word in the following sentence?

Although his friends believed him to be enjoying a lavish lifestyle in the large family estate he had inherited, Enzo was in reality <u>impecunious</u>.

a. Penniless
b. Unfortunate
c. Emotional
d. Commanding

8. Follow the instructions below to transform the starting word into a different word.

- **Start with the word ESOTERIC**
- **Remove both instances of the letter E from the word**
- **Remove the letter I from the word**
- **Move the letter T from the middle of the word to the end of the word**
- **Remove the letter C from the word**

What new word has been spelled?

a. SECT
b. SORT
c. SORE
d. TORE

The next two questions are based on the following chart, which reflects the enrollment and the income for a small community college.

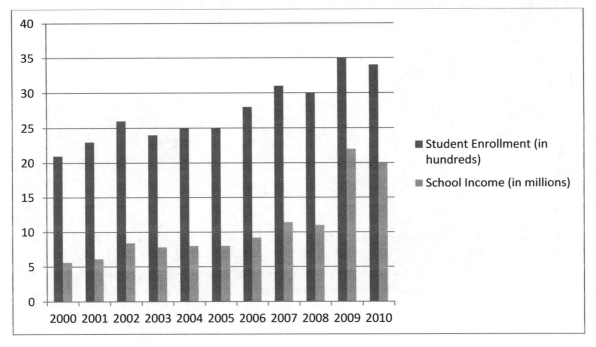

9. Based on the chart, approximately how many students attended the community college in the year 2001?

    a. 2100
    b. 2300
    c. 2500
    d. 2700

10. In order to offset costs, the college administration decided to increase admission fees. Reviewing the chart above, during which year is it most likely that the college raised the price of admission?

    a. 2002
    b. 2007
    c. 2009
    d. 2010

11. If the statements listed below are true, which of the answer choices is a logical conclusion?

Literacy rates are lower today than they were fifteen years ago. Then, most people learned to read through the use of phonics. Today, whole language programs are favored by many educators.

    a. whole language is more effective at teaching people to read than phonics.
    b. phonics is more effective at teaching people to read than whole language.
    c. literacy rates will probably continue to decline over the next 15 years.
    d. the definition of what it means to be literate is much stricter now.

The next four questions are based on the following passage.

The Bermuda Triangle

The area known as the Bermuda Triangle has become such a part of popular culture that it can be difficult to separate fact from fiction. The interest first began when five Navy planes vanished in 1945, officially resulting from "causes or reasons unknown." The explanations about other accidents in the Triangle range from the scientific to the supernatural. Researchers have never been able to find anything truly mysterious about what happens in the Bermuda Triangle, if there even is a Bermuda Triangle. What is more, one of the biggest challenges in considering the phenomenon is deciding how much area actually represents the Bermuda Triangle. Most consider the Triangle to stretch from Miami out to Puerto Rico and to include the island of Bermuda. Others expand the area to include all of the Caribbean islands and to extend eastward as far as the Azores, which are closer to Europe than they are to North America.

The problem with having a larger Bermuda Triangle is that it increases the odds of accidents. There is near-constant travel, by ship and by plane, across the Atlantic, and accidents are expected to occur. In fact, the Bermuda Triangle happens to fall within one of the busiest navigational regions in the world, and the reality of greater activity creates the possibility for more to go wrong. Shipping records suggest that there is not a greater than average loss of vessels within the Bermuda Triangle, and many researchers have argued that the reputation of the Triangle makes any accident seem out of the ordinary. In fact, most accidents fall within the expected margin of error. The increase in ships from East Asia no doubt contributes to an increase in accidents. And as for the story of the Navy planes that disappeared within the Triangle, many researchers now conclude that it was the result of mistakes on the part of the pilots who were flying into storm clouds and simply got lost.

12. Which of the following describes this type of writing?

a. Narrative
b. Persuasive
c. Expository
d. Technical

13. Which of the following sentences is most representative of a summary sentence for this passage?

a. The problem with having a larger Bermuda Triangle is that it increases the odds of accidents.
b. The area that is called the Bermuda Triangle happens to fall within one of the busiest navigational regions in the world, and the reality of greater activity creates the possibility for more to go wrong.
c. One of the biggest challenges in considering the phenomenon is deciding how much area actually represents the Bermuda Triangle.
d. Researchers have never been able to find anything truly mysterious about what happens in the Bermuda Triangle, if there even is a Bermuda Triangle.

14. With which of the following statements would the author most likely agree?

a. There is no real mystery about the Bermuda Triangle because most events have reasonable explanations.
b. Researchers are wrong to expand the focus of the Triangle to the Azores, because this increases the likelihood of accidents.
c. The official statement of "causes or reasons unknown" in the loss of the Navy planes was a deliberate concealment from the Navy.
d. Reducing the legends about the mysteries of the Bermuda Triangle will help to reduce the number of reported accidents or shipping losses in that region.

15. Which of the following represents an opinion statement on the part of the author?

a. The problem with having a larger Bermuda Triangle is that it increases the odds of accidents.
b. The area known as the Bermuda Triangle has become such a part of popular culture that it can be difficult to sort through the myth and locate the truth.
c. The increase in ships from East Asia no doubt contributes to an increase in accidents.
d. Most consider the Triangle to stretch from Miami to Puerto Rico and include the island of Bermuda.

16. Which of the following is a primary source?

a. A report of an original research experiment
b. An academic textbook's citation of research
c. A quotation of a researcher in a news article
d. A website description of another's research

17. The guide words at the top of a dictionary page are *intrauterine* and *invest*. Which of the following words is an entry on this page?

a. Intransigent
b. Introspection
c. Investiture
d. Intone

The next question is based on the following chart.

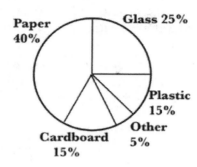

18. A recycling company collects sorted materials from its clients. The materials are weighed and then processed for re-use. The chart shows the weights of various classes of materials that were collected by the company during a representative month. Which of the following statements is NOT supported by the data in the chart?

a. Paper products, including cardboard, make up a majority of the collected materials.
b. One quarter of the materials collected are made of glass.
c. More plastic is collected than cardboard.
d. Plastic and cardboard together represent a larger portion of the collected materials than glass bottles.

19. Ninette has celiac disease, which means that she cannot eat any product containing gluten. Gluten is a protein present in many grains such as wheat, rye, and barley. Because of her health condition, Ninette has to be careful about what she eats to avoid having an allergic reaction. She will be attending an all-day industry event, and she requested the menu in advance. Here is the menu:

- **Breakfast: Fresh coffee or tea, scrambled eggs, bacon or sausage**
- **Lunch: Spinach salad (dressing available on the side), roasted chicken, steamed rice**
- **Cocktail Hour: Various beverages, fruit and cheese plate**
- **Dinner: Spaghetti and sauce, tossed salad, garlic bread**

During which of these meals should Ninette be careful to bring her own food?

a. Breakfast
b. Lunch
c. Cocktail Hour
d. Dinner

20. Which of the following best provides detailed support for the claim that "seatbelts save lives"?

a. A government website containing driving accident information
b. A blog developed by one of the largest car companies in the world
c. An encyclopedia entry on the seatbelt and its development
d. An instant message sent out by a famous race car driver

21. Which of the answer choices presents a valid inference based on the following scenario?

The latest movie by a certain director gets bad reviews before it opens in theatres. Consequently, very few people go to the movie and the director is given much less money to make his next movie, which is also unsuccessful.

   a. This director makes terrible movies
   b. The general public does not pay attention to movie reviews
   c. The movie reviewers were right about the first movie
   d. Movie reviewers exert influence on the movie quality

The next three questions are based on the following table.

NAME	COMPOSITION (PER 100)	WORLD LITERATURE (PER 100)	TECHNICAL WRITING (PER 100)	LINGUISTICS (PER 100)
Textbook-Mania	$4500	$5150	$6000	$6500
Textbook Central	$4350	$5200	$6100	$6550
Bookstore Supply	$4675	$5000	$5950	$6475
University Textbooks	$4600	$5000	$6100	$6650

Note: Shipping is free for all schools that order 100 textbooks or more.

22. A school needs to purchase 500 composition textbooks and 500 world literature textbooks. Which of the textbook suppliers can offer the lowest price?

   a. Textbook Mania
   b. Textbook Central
   c. Bookstore Supply
   d. University Textbooks

23. A school needs to purchase 1000 composition textbooks and 300 linguistics textbooks. Which of the textbook suppliers can offer the lowest price?

   a. Textbook Mania
   b. Textbook Central
   c. Bookstore Supply
   d. University Textbooks

24. A school needs to purchase 400 world literature textbooks and 200 technical writing textbooks. Which of the textbook suppliers can offer the lowest price?

   a. Textbook Mania
   b. Textbook Central
   c. Bookstore Supply
   d. University Textbooks

The next four questions are based on the following graphic.

Table 1. Consumer Price Index for All Urban Consumers (CPI-U): U.S. city average, by expenditure category and commodity and service group

(1982-84=100, unless otherwise noted)

Item and group	Relative importance, December 2008	Unadjusted indexes		Unadjusted percent change to June 2009 from—		Seasonally adjusted percent change from—		
		May 2009	June 2009	June 2008	May 2009	Mar. to Apr.	Apr. to May	May to June
Expenditure category								
All items	100.000	213.856	215.693	-1.4	0.9	0.0	0.1	0.7
All items (1967=100)	-	640.616	646.121	-	-	-	-	-
Food and beverages	15.757	218.076	218.030	2.2	.0	-.2	-.2	.1
Food	14.629	217.826	217.740	2.1	.0	-.2	-.2	.0
Food at home	8.156	215.088	214.824	.8	-.1	-.6	-.5	.0
Cereals and bakery products	1.150	252.714	253.008	3.0	.1	-.7	-.2	.0
Meats, poultry, fish, and eggs	1.898	203.789	204.031	.6	.1	.0	-.9	-.2
Dairy and related products [1]	.910	196.055	194.197	-7.1	-.9	-1.3	-.5	-.9
Fruits and vegetables	1.194	274.006	272.608	-1.9	-.5	.0	-1.0	1.1
Nonalcoholic beverages and beverage materials	.982	162.803	162.571	2.7	-.1	-1.0	-.1	.1
Other food at home	2.022	191.144	191.328	4.1	.1	-.8	-.1	.0
Sugar and sweets	.300	196.403	197.009	6.2	.3	-.5	.0	.2
Fats and oils	.241	200.679	201.127	2.5	.2	-1.4	-.7	.6
Other foods	1.481	205.587	205.654	3.9	.0	-.8	.0	-.2
Other miscellaneous foods [1][2]	.433	122.838	122.224	3.2	-.5	.4	.0	-.5
Food away from home [1]	6.474	223.023	223.163	3.8	.1	.3	.1	.1
Other food away from home [1][2]	.314	155.099	155.841	4.0	.5	.4	.0	.5
Alcoholic beverages	1.127	220.005	220.477	3.1	.2	-.1	.3	.2
Housing	43.421	216.971	218.071	.1	.5	-.1	-.1	.0
Shelter	33.200	249.779	250.243	1.3	.2	.2	.1	.1
Rent of primary residence [3]	5.957	249.069	249.092	2.7	.0	.2	.1	.1
Lodging away from home [2]	2.478	135.680	138.318	-6.9	1.9	.5	.1	.3
Owners' equivalent rent of primary residence [3][4]	24.433	256.875	256.981	1.9	.0	.1	.1	.1
Tenants' and household insurance [1][2]	.333	120.728	121.083	1.7	.3	-.1	.0	.3
Fuels and utilities	5.431	206.358	212.677	-8.1	3.1	-1.7	-1.3	-.8
Household energy	4.460	183.783	190.647	-10.8	3.7	-2.2	-1.8	-1.0
Fuel oil and other fuels	.301	225.164	232.638	-40.3	3.3	-2.1	-3.1	2.0
Gas (piped) and electricity [3]	4.159	189.619	196.754	-7.8	3.8	-2.2	-1.7	-1.2
Water and sewer and trash collection services [2]	.971	159.517	159.831	6.2	.2	.6	.6	.4
Household furnishings and operations	4.790	129.644	129.623	1.6	.0	.0	.0	.0
Household operations [1][2]	.781	149.468	149.995	1.3	.4	-.1	-.9	.4
Apparel	3.691	121.751	118.799	1.5	-2.4	-.2	-.2	.7
Men's and boys' apparel	.923	117.146	112.849	.7	-3.7	-1.7	.4	-.5
Women's and girls' apparel	1.541	109.460	106.455	2.1	-2.7	.2	-.1	1.6
Infants' and toddlers' apparel	.183	114.142	113.915	2.1	-.2	1.3	-1.6	2.2
Footwear	.688	127.519	125.515	1.6	-1.6	.4	.1	.2
Transportation	15.314	175.997	183.735	-13.2	4.4	-.4	.8	4.2
Private transportation	14.189	171.757	179.649	-13.3	4.6	-.3	.9	4.5
New and used motor vehicles [2]	6.931	92.701	93.020	-.6	.3	.4	.5	.4
New vehicles	4.480	135.162	135.719	.9	.4	.4	.5	.7
Used cars and trucks	1.628	122.650	124.323	-8.6	1.4	-.1	1.0	.9
Motor fuel	3.164	193.609	225.021	-35.2	16.2	-2.6	2.7	17.2
Gasoline (all types)	2.964	193.727	225.526	-34.6	16.4	-2.8	3.1	17.3
Motor vehicle parts and equipment [1]	.382	134.347	134.270	5.0	-.1	.1	-.2	-.1
Motor vehicle maintenance and repair [1]	1.188	242.488	242.683	4.1	.1	.2	-.1	.1
Public transportation	1.125	228.878	232.540	-12.1	1.6	-.8	-1.0	-.5

25. Which of the following expense categories decreased in the year prior to June 2009?

a. Rent of primary residence
b. Boys' and men's apparel
c. Transportation
d. Meats, fish, and eggs

26. On a seasonally adjusted basis, which of the following decreased by the greatest percentage between April and May of 2009?

    a. Gasoline
    b. Fuel oil and other fuels
    c. Infants' and toddlers' apparel
    d. Fruits and vegetables

27. According to the organization of the table, which of the following expense categories is not considered to be a component of the "Food at Home" category?

    a. Cereals and bakery products
    b. Fats and oils
    c. Other miscellaneous foods
    d. Alcoholic beverages

28. Which expenditure category was the most important in December of 2008?

    a. Housing
    b. Food and Beverages
    c. Apparel
    d. Transportation

The next question refers to the following image.

Starting Image

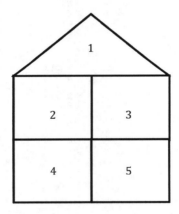

Start with the shape pictured above. Follow the directions to alter its appearance.

- **Rotate section 1 90° clockwise and move it to the right side, against sections 3 and 5.**
- **Remove section 4.**
- **Move section 2 immediately above section 3.**
- **Swap section 2 and section 5.**
- **Remove section 5.**
- **Draw a circle around the shape, enclosing it completely.**

29. Which of the following does the shape now look like?

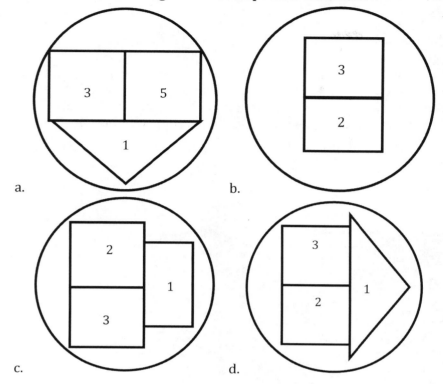

a.

b.

c.

d.

30. Anna is planning a trip to Bretagne, or Brittany, in the northwestern part of France. Since she knows very little about it, she is hoping to find the most up-to-date information with the widest variety of details about hiking trails, beaches, restaurants, and accommodations. Which of the following guides will be the best for her to review?

a. *The Top Ten Places to Visit in Brittany*, published by a non-profit organization in Bretagne looking to draw tourism to the region (2015)

b. *Getting to Know Nantes: Eating, Staying, and Sightseeing in Brittany's Largest City*, published by the French Ministry of Tourism (2014)

c. *Hiking Through Bretagne: The Best Trails for Discovering Northwestern France*, published by a company that specializes in travel for those wanting to experience the outdoors (2013)

d. *The Complete Guide to Brittany*, published by a travel book company that publishes guides for travel throughout Europe (2015)

The next three questions are based on the following passage.

An adult skeleton had 206 bones. The skeleton has two major divisions: the axial skeleton and the appendicular skeleton. Each bone belongs to either the axial skeleton or the appendicular skeleton. The axial skeleton, which consists of 80 bones including the skull, vertebrae, and rib, is located down the center of the body. The axial skeleton protects vital organs such as the brain and heart. The appendicular skeleton consists of 126 bones of the arms, legs, and the bones that attach these bones to the axial skeleton. The appendicular skeleton includes the scapulae (shoulder blades), clavicles (collarbones), and pelvic (hip) bones.

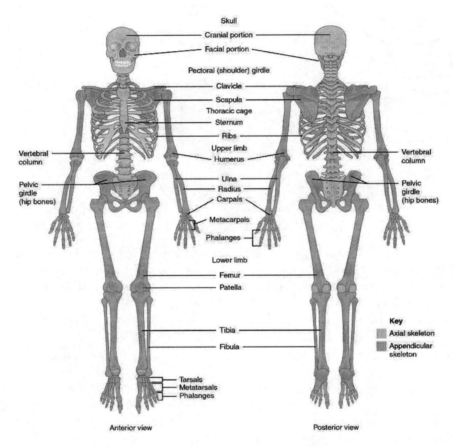

31. Which of the following bones is not associated with the leg?

a. Femur
b. Tibia
c. Patella
d. Radius

32. Which of the following bones is not part of the appendicular skeleton?

a. Skull
b. Clavicle
c. Scapula
d. Pelvic bone

33. Which of the following bones are located in the hand?

a. Fibula

b. Metacarpals

c. Metatarsals

d. Ulna

The next three questions are based on the following passage.

As little as three years before her birth, few would have thought that the child born Princess Alexandrina Victoria would eventually become Britain's longest reigning monarch, Queen Victoria. She was born in 1819, the only child of Edward, Duke of Kent, who was the fourth son of King George III. Ahead of Edward were three brothers, two of whom became king but none of whom produced a legitimate, surviving heir. King George's eldest son, who was eventually crowned King George IV, secretly married a Catholic commoner, Maria Fitzherbert, in 1783. The marriage was never officially recognized, and in 1795, George was persuaded to marry a distant cousin, Caroline of Brunswick. The marriage was bitter, and the two had only one daughter, Princess Charlotte Augusta. She was popular in England where her eventual reign was welcomed, but in a tragic event that shocked the nation, the princess and her stillborn son died in childbirth in 1817.

Realizing the precarious position of the British throne, the remaining sons of King George III were motivated to marry and produce an heir. The first in line was Prince Frederick, the Duke of York. Frederick married Princess Frederica Charlotte of Prussia, but the two had no children. After Prince Frederick was Prince William, the Duke of Clarence. William married Princess Adelaide of Saxe-Meiningen, and they had two sickly daughters, neither of whom survived infancy. Finally, Prince Edward, the Duke of Kent, threw his hat into the ring with his marriage to Princess Victoria of Saxe-Coburg-Saalfeld. The Duke of Kent died less than a year after his daughter's birth, but the surviving Duchess of Kent was not unaware of the future possibilities for her daughter. She took every precaution to ensure that the young Princess Victoria was healthy and safe throughout her childhood.

Princess Victoria's uncle, William, succeeded his brother George IV to become King William IV. The new king recognized his niece as his future heir, but he did not necessarily trust her mother. As a result, he was determined to survive until Victoria's eighteenth birthday to ensure that she could rule in her own right without the regency of the Duchess of Kent. The king's fervent prayers were answered: he died June 20, 1837, less than one month after Victoria turned eighteen. Though young and inexperienced, the young queen recognized the importance of her position and determined to rule fairly and wisely. The improbable princess who became queen ruled for more than sixty-three years, and her reign is considered to be one of the most important in British history.

34. Which of the following is a logical conclusion that can be drawn from the information in the passage above?

a. Victoria's long reign provided the opportunity for her to bring balance to England and right the wrongs that had occurred during the reigns of her uncles.

b. It was the death of Princess Charlotte Augusta that motivated the remaining princes to marry and start families.

c. The Duke of Kent had hoped for a son but was delighted with his good fortune in producing the surviving heir that his brothers had failed to produce.

d. King William IV was unreasonably suspicious of the Duchess of Kent's motivations, as she cared only for her daughter's well-being.

35. What is the author's likely purpose in writing this passage about Queen Victoria?

a. To persuade the reader to appreciate the accomplishments of Queen Victoria, especially when placed against the failures of her forebears.

b. To introduce the historical impact of the Victorian Era by introducing to readers the queen who gave that era its name.

c. To explain how small events in history placed an unlikely princess in line to become the queen of England.

d. To indicate the role that King George III's many sons played in changing the history of England.

36. Based on the context of the passage, the reader can infer that this information is likely to appear in which of the following types of works?

a. A scholarly paper
b. A mystery
c. A fictional story
d. A biography

The next five questions are based on the following passage.

In 1603, Queen Elizabeth I of England died. She had never married and had no heir, so the throne passed to a distant relative: James Stuart, the son of Elizabeth's cousin and one-time rival for the throne, Mary, Queen of Scots. James was crowned King James I of England. At the time, he was also King James VI of Scotland, and the combination of roles would create a spirit of conflict that haunted the two nations for generations to come.

The conflict developed as a result of rising tensions among the people within the nations, as well as between them. Scholars in the 21st century are far too hasty in dismissing the role of religion in political disputes, but religion undoubtedly played a role in the problems that faced England and Scotland. By the time of James Stuart's succession to the English throne, the English people had firmly embraced the teachings of Protestant theology. Similarly, the Scottish Lowlands was decisively Protestant. In the Scottish Highlands, however, the clans retained their Catholic faith. James acknowledged the Church of England and still sanctioned the largely Protestant translation of the Bible that still bears his name.

James's son King Charles I proved himself to be less committed to the Protestant Church of England. Charles married the Catholic Princess Henrietta Maria of France, and there were suspicions among the English and the Lowland Scots that Charles was quietly a Catholic. Charles's own political troubles extended beyond religion in this case, and he was beheaded in 1649. Eventually, his son King Charles II would be crowned, and this Charles is believed to have converted secretly to the Catholic Church. Charles II died without a legitimate heir, and his brother James ascended to the throne as King James II.

James was recognized to be a practicing Catholic, and his commitment to Catholicism would prove to be his downfall. James's wife Mary Beatrice lost a number of children during their infancy, and when she became pregnant again in 1687 the public became concerned. If James had a son, that son would undoubtedly be raised a Catholic, and the English people would not stand for this. Mary gave birth to a son, but the story quickly circulated that the royal child had died and the child named James's heir was a foundling smuggled in. James, his wife, and his infant son were forced to flee; and James's Protestant daughter Mary was crowned the queen.

In spite of a strong resemblance to the king, the young James was generally rejected among the English and the Lowland Scots, who referred to him as "the Pretender." But in the Highlands the Catholic princeling was welcomed. He inspired a group known as *Jacobites*, to reflect the Latin version of his name. His own son Charles, known affectionately as Bonnie Prince Charlie, would eventually raise an army and attempt to recapture what he believed to be his throne. The movement was soundly defeated at the Battle of Culloden in 1746, and England and Scotland have remained ostensibly Protestant ever since.

37. Which of the following sentences contains an opinion on the part of the author?

a. James was recognized to be a practicing Catholic, and his commitment to Catholicism would prove to be his downfall.
b. James' son King Charles I proved himself to be less committed to the Protestant Church of England.
c. The movement was soundly defeated at the Battle of Culloden in 1746, and England and Scotland have remained ostensibly Protestant ever since.
d. Scholars in the 21st century are far too hasty in dismissing the role of religion in political disputes, but religion undoubtedly played a role in the problems that faced England and Scotland.

38. Which of the following is a logical conclusion based on the information that is provided within the passage?

a. Like Elizabeth I, Charles II never married and thus never had children.
b. The English people were relieved each time that James II's wife Mary lost another child, as this prevented the chance of a Catholic monarch.
c. Charles I's beheading had less to do with religion than with other political problems that England was facing.
d. Unlike his son and grandsons, King James I had no Catholic leanings and was a faithful follower of the Protestant Church of England.

39. Based on the information that is provided within the passage, which of the following can be inferred about King James II's son?

a. Considering his resemblance to King James II, the young James was very likely the legitimate child of the king and the queen.

b. Given the queen's previous inability to produce a healthy child, the English and the Lowland Scots were right in suspecting the legitimacy of the prince.

c. James "the Pretender" was not as popular among the Highland clans as his son Bonnie Prince Charlie.

d. James was unable to acquire the resources needed to build the army and plan the invasion that his son succeeded in doing.

40. Which of the following best describes the organization of the information in the passage?

a. Cause-effect

b. Chronological sequence

c. Problem-solution

d. Comparison-contrast

41. Which of the following best describes the author's intent in the passage?

a. To persuade

b. To entertain

c. To express feeling

d. To inform

The next two questions are based on the following statements.

Lisa Grant: "Schools should make students wear uniforms. Everyone would look the same. Students would be able to respect each other based on their ideas and character because they would no longer be judged by their appearance."

Vivian Harris: "Students should not have to wear uniforms. Clothing is an important part of self-expression. Taking away that method of expression is suppressing that student's rights."

42. What is one idea that the students above seem to agree on, based on their statements?

a. Students should be allowed to express themselves through apparel.

b. Schools should give students a certain amount of respect.

c. Students should focus more on school than on appearance.

d. Schools would violate students' basic rights by enforcing a dress code.

43. Which of the following statements could NOT provide support for BOTH arguments?

a. A number of local school districts have recently implemented dress codes.

b. School administrators have been in talks with parents over the issue of uniforms.

c. Students have reported that school uniforms are costly and typically ill-fitting.

d. Several groups of students have been organized to discuss uniform dress codes.

The next three questions are based on the following passage.

NOTE: The instructor of a history class has just finished grading the essay exams from his students, and the results are not good. The essay exam was worth 70% of the final course score. The highest score in the class was a low B, and more than half of the class of 65 students failed the exam. In view of this, the instructor reconsiders his grading plan for the semester and sends out an email message to all students.

Dear Students:

The scores for the essay exam have been posted in the online course grade book. By now, many of you have probably seen your grade and are a little concerned. (And if you're not concerned, you should be—at least a bit!) At the beginning of the semester, I informed the class that I have a strict grading policy and that all scores will stand unquestioned. With each class comes a new challenge, however, and as any good instructor will tell you, sometimes the original plan has to change. As a result,

I propose the following options for students to make up their score:

1. I will present the class with an extra credit project at the next course meeting. The extra credit project will be worth 150% of the point value of the essay exam that has just been completed. While I will not drop the essay exam score, I will give you more than enough of a chance to make up the difference and raise your overall score.
2. I will allow each student to develop his or her own extra credit project. This project may reflect the tenor of option number 1 (above) but will allow the student to create a project more in his or her own line of interest. Bear in mind, however, that this is more of a risk. The scoring for option number 2 will be more subjective, depending on whether or not I feel that the project is a successful alternative to the essay exam. If it is, the student will be awarded up to 150% of the point value of the essay exam.
3. I will provide the class with the option of developing a group project. Students may form groups of 3 to 4 and put together an extra credit project that reflects a stronger response to the questions in the essay exam. This extra credit project will also be worth 150% of the point value of the essay exam. Note that each student will receive an equal score for the project, so there is a risk in this as well. If you are part of a group in which you do most of the work, each member of the group will receive equal credit for it. The purpose of the group project is to allow students to work together and arrive at a stronger response than if each worked individually.

If you are interested in pursuing extra credit to make up for the essay exam, please choose <u>one</u> of the options above. No other extra credit opportunities will be provided for the course.

Good luck!

Dr. Edwards

44. Which of the following describes this type of writing?

a. Technical
b. Narrative
c. Persuasive
d. Expository

45. Which of the following best describes the instructor's purpose in writing this email to his students?

a. To berate students for the poor scores that they made on the recent essay exam.
b. To encourage students to continue working hard in spite of failure.
c. To give students the opportunity to make up the bad score and avoid failing the course.
d. To admit that the essay exam was likely too difficult for most students.

46. Which of the following offers the best summary for the instructor's motive in sending the email to the students?

a. By now, many of you have probably seen your grade and are a little concerned. (And if you're not concerned, you should be—at least a bit!)
b. With each class comes a new challenge, however, and as any good instructor will tell you, sometimes the original plan has to change.
c. The purpose of the group project is to allow students to work together and arrive at a stronger response than if each worked individually.
d. At the beginning of the semester, I informed the class that I have a strict grading policy and that all scores will stand unquestioned.

The next seven questions are based on this passage.

In the United States, where we have more land than people, it is not at all difficult for persons in good health to make money. In this comparatively new field there are so many avenues of success open, so many vocations which are not crowded, that any person of either sex who is willing, at least for the time being, to engage in any respectable occupation that offers, may find lucrative employment.

Those who really desire to attain an independence, have only to set their minds upon it, and adopt the proper means, as they do in regard to any other object which they wish to accomplish, and the thing is easily done. But however easy it may be found to make money, I have no doubt many of my hearers will agree it is the most difficult thing in the world to keep it. The road to wealth is, as Dr. Franklin truly says, "as plain as the road to the mill." It consists simply in expending less than we earn; that seems to be a very simple problem. Mr. Micawber, one of those happy creations of the genial Dickens, puts the case in a strong light when he says that to have annual income of twenty pounds per annum, and spend twenty pounds and sixpence, is to be the most miserable of men; whereas, to have an income of only twenty pounds, and spend but nineteen pounds and sixpence is to be the happiest of mortals.

Many of my readers may say, "we understand this: this is economy, and we know economy is wealth; we know we can't eat our cake and keep it also." Yet I beg to say that perhaps more cases of failure arise from mistakes on this point than almost any other. The fact is, many people think they understand economy when they really do not.

47. Which of the following statements best expresses the main idea of the passage?

a. Getting a job is easier now than it ever has been before.
b. Earning money is much less difficult than managing it properly.
c. Dr. Franklin advocated getting a job in a mill.
d. Spending money is the greatest temptation in the world.

48. What would this author's attitude likely be to a person unable to find employment?

a. descriptive
b. conciliatory
c. ingenuous
d. incredulous

49. According to the author, what is more difficult than making money?

a. managing money
b. traveling to a mill
c. reading Dickens
d. understanding the economy

50. Who is the most likely audience for this passage?

a. economists
b. general readers
c. teachers
d. philanthropists

51. What is the best definition of *economy* as it is used in this passage?

a. exchange of money, goods, and services
b. delegation of household affairs
c. efficient money management
d. less expensive

52. Which word best describes the author's attitude towards those who believe they understand money?

a. supportive
b. incriminating
c. excessive
d. patronizing

53. This passage is most likely taken from a(n) _____.

a. self-help manual
b. autobiography
c. epistle
d. novel

Mathematics	Number of Questions: 36
	Time Limit: 54 Minutes

1. Which of the following is the percentage equivalent of 0.0016?

    a. 16%
    b. 160%
    c. 1.6%
    d. 0.16%

2. Curtis is taking a road trip through Germany, where all distance signs are in metric. He passes a sign that states the city of Dusseldorf is 45 kilometers away. Approximately how far is this in miles?

    a. 42 miles
    b. 37 miles
    c. 28 miles
    d. 16 miles

3. On a floor plan drawn at a scale of 1:100, the area of a rectangular room is 30 cm^2. What is the actual area of the room?

    a. 30,000 cm^2
    b. 300 m^2
    c. 3,000 m^2
    d. 30 m^2

4. Mandy can buy 4 containers of yogurt and 3 boxes of crackers for $9.55. She can buy 2 containers of yogurt and 2 boxes of crackers for $5.90. How much does one box of crackers cost?

    a. $1.75
    b. $2.00
    c. $2.25
    d. $2.50

The next two questions are based on the following information:

    Pernell's scores on her last five chemistry exams were 81, 92, 87, 89, and 94.

5. What is the approximate average of her scores?

    a. 81
    b. 84
    c. 89
    d. 91

6. What is the *median* of Pernell's scores?

    a. 87
    b. 89
    c. 92
    d. 94

7. Gordon purchased a television when his local electronics store had a sale. The television was offered at 30% off its original price of $472. What was the sale price that Gordon paid?

    a. $141.60
    b. $225.70
    c. $305.30
    d. $330.40

8. Simplify the following expression: $\frac{2}{3} \div \frac{4}{15} \times \frac{5}{8}$

    a. $1\frac{9}{16}$
    b. $1\frac{1}{4}$
    c. $2\frac{1}{8}$
    d. 2

9. Simplify the following expression: 0.0178×2.401

    a. 2.0358414
    b. 0.0427378
    c. 0.2341695
    d. 0.3483240

10. Tom needs to buy ink cartridges and printer paper. Each ink cartridge costs $30. Each ream of paper costs $5. He has $100 to spend. Which of the following inequalities may be used to find the combinations of ink cartridges and printer paper that he may purchase?

    a. $30c + 5p \leq 100$
    b. $30c + 5p < 100$
    c. $30c + 5p > 100$
    d. $30c + 5p \geq 100$

11. Solve for x: $4(2x - 6) = 10x - 6$

    a. $x = 5$
    b. $x = -7$
    c. $x = -9$
    d. $x = 10$

12. Erma has her eye on two sweaters at her favorite clothing store, but she has been waiting for the store to offer a sale. This week, the store advertises that all clothing purchases, including sweaters, come with an incentive: 25% off a second item of equal or lesser value. One sweater is $50 and the other is $44. If Erma purchases the sweaters during the sale, what will she spend?

    a. $79
    b. $81
    c. $83
    d. $85

13. Simplify the following expression: $1.034 + 0.275 - 1.294$

    a. 0.015
    b. 0.15
    c. 1.5
    d. −0.15

14. The graph below shows the weekly church attendance among residents in the town of Ellsford, with the town having five different denominations: Episcopal, Methodist, Baptist, Catholic, and Orthodox. Approximately what percentage of church-goers in Ellsford attends Catholic churches?

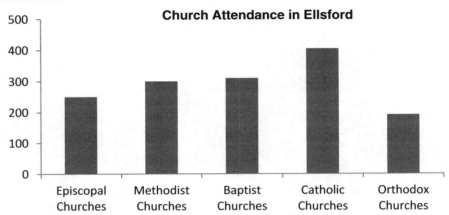

a. 23%
b. 28%
c. 36%
d. 42%

15. Jerry needs to load four pieces of equipment on to a factory elevator that has a weight limit of 800 pounds. Jerry weighs 200 pounds. What would the average weight of each item have to be so that the elevator's weight limit is not exceeded assuming Jerry accompanies the equipment?

a. 128 pounds
b. 150 pounds
c. 175 pounds
d. 180 pounds

16. Simplify the following expression: $4\frac{2}{3} \div 1\frac{1}{6}$

a. 2
b. $3\frac{1}{3}$
c. 4
d. $4\frac{1}{2}$

17. Solve for x: $2x + 4 = x - 6$

a. $x = -12$
b. $x = 10$
c. $x = -16$
d. $x = -10$

18. Solve for x: $2x - 7 = 3$

a. $x = 4$
b. $x = 3$
c. $x = -2$
d. $x = 5$

19. What kind of association does the scatter plot show?

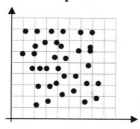

    a. linear, positive
    b. linear, negative
    c. quadratic
    d. no association

20. If Stella's current weight is 56 kilograms, which of the following is her approximate weight in pounds? (Note: 1 kilogram is approximately equal to 2.2 pounds.)

    a. 123 pounds
    b. 110 pounds
    c. 156 pounds
    d. 137 pounds

21. Which of the following is listed in order from *least to greatest*?

    a. $-\frac{3}{4}, -7\frac{4}{5}, -8, 18\%, 0.25, 2.5$
    b. $-8, -7\frac{4}{5}, -\frac{3}{4}, 0.25, 2.5, 18\%$
    c. $18\%, 0.25, -\frac{3}{4}, 2.5, -7\frac{4}{5}, -8$
    d. $-8, -7\frac{4}{5}, -\frac{3}{4}, 18\%, 0.25, 2.5$

22. Between the years 2000 and 2010, the number of births in the town of Daneville increased from 1432 to 2219. Which of the following is the approximate percent of increase in the number of births during those ten years?

    a. 55%
    b. 36%
    c. 64%
    d. 42%

23. Simplify the following expression: $\frac{1}{4} \times \frac{3}{5} \div 1\frac{1}{8}$

    a. $\frac{8}{15}$
    b. $\frac{27}{160}$
    c. $\frac{2}{15}$
    d. $\frac{27}{40}$

24. While at the local ice skating rink, Cora went around the rink 27 times total. She slipped and fell 20 of the 27 times she skated around the rink. What approximate percentage of the times around the rink did Cora *not* slip and fall?

    a. 37%
    b. 74%
    c. 26%
    d. 15%

25. A can has a radius of 1.5 inches and a height of 3 inches. Which of the following best represents the volume of the can?

    a. 17.2 in^3
    b. 19.4 in^3
    c. 21.2 in^3
    d. 23.4 in^3

26. Simplify the following expression: $3\frac{1}{6} - 1\frac{5}{6}$

    a. $2\frac{1}{3}$
    b. $1\frac{1}{3}$
    c. $2\frac{1}{9}$
    d. $\frac{5}{6}$

27. Four more than a number, x, is 2 less than $\frac{1}{3}$ of another number, y. Which of the following algebraic equations correctly represents this sentence?

    a. $x + 4 = \frac{1}{3}y - 2$
    b. $4x = 2 - \frac{1}{3}y$
    c. $4 - x = 2 + \frac{1}{3}y$
    d. $x + 4 = 2 - \frac{1}{3}y$

28. Margery is planning a vacation, and she has added up the cost. Her round-trip airfare will cost $572. Her hotel cost is $89 per night, and she will be staying at the hotel for five nights. She has allotted a total of $150 for sightseeing during her trip, and she expects to spend about $250 on meals. As she books the hotel, she is told that she will receive a discount of 10% per night off the price of $89 after the first night she stays there. Taking this discount into consideration, what is the amount that Margery expects to spend on her vacation?

    a. $1328.35
    b. $1373.50
    c. $1381.40
    d. $1417.60

29. Given the double bar graph shown below, which of the following statements is true?

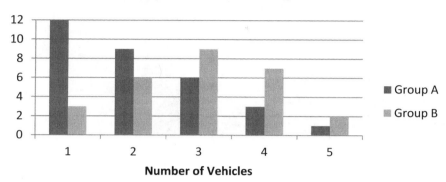

Number of Vehicles Owned

a. Group A is negatively skewed, while Group B is approximately normal.
b. Group A is positively skewed, while Group B is approximately normal.
c. Group A is approximately normal, while Group B is negatively skewed.
d. Group A is approximately normal, while Group B is positively skewed.

30. A gift box has a length of 14 inches, a height of 8 inches, and a width of 6 inches. How many square inches of wrapping paper are needed to wrap the box?

a. 56
b. 244
c. 488
d. 672

31. After a hurricane struck a Pacific island, donations began flooding into a disaster relief organization. The organization provided the opportunity for donors to specify where they wanted the money to be used, and the organization provided four options. When the organization tallied the funds received, they allotted each to the designated need. Reviewing the chart below, what percentage of the funds was donated to support construction costs?

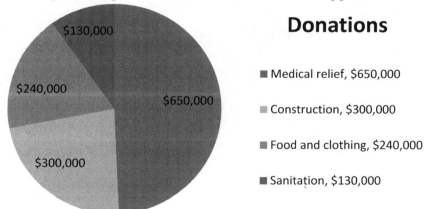

a. 49%
b. 23%
c. 18%
d. 10%

32. Arrange the following numbers above from least to greatest: $\frac{7}{3}, \frac{9}{2}, \frac{10}{9}, \frac{7}{8}$

   a. $\frac{10}{9}, \frac{7}{3}, \frac{9}{2}, \frac{7}{8}$

   b. $\frac{9}{2}, \frac{7}{3}, \frac{10}{9}, \frac{7}{8}$

   c. $\frac{7}{3}, \frac{9}{2}, \frac{10}{9}, \frac{7}{8}$

   d. $\frac{7}{8}, \frac{10}{9}, \frac{7}{3}, \frac{9}{2}$

33. Simplify the following expression: $\frac{2}{7} \div \frac{5}{6}$

   a. $\frac{2}{5}$

   b. $\frac{35}{12}$

   c. $\frac{5}{21}$

   d. $\frac{12}{35}$

34. Simplify the following expression: $7 + 16 - (5 + 6 \times 3) - 10 \times 2$

   a. -42

   b. -20

   c. 23

   d. 20

35. The table below shows the cost of renting a bicycle for 1, 2, or 3 hours. Which answer choice shows the equation that best represents the data? Let C represent the cost of the rental and h stand for the number of hours of rental time.

Hours	1	2	3
Cost	$3.60	$7.20	$10.80

   a. $C = 3.60h$

   b. $C = h + 3.60$

   c. $C = 3.60h + 10.80$

   d. $C = \frac{10.80}{h}$

36. Chan receives a bonus from his job. He pays 30% in taxes, gives 30% to charity, and uses another 25% to pay off an old debt. He has $600 remaining from his bonus. What was the total amount of Chan's bonus?

   a. $3000

   b. $3200

   c. $3600

   d. $4000

Science	Number of Questions: **53**
	Time Limit: **63 Minutes**

1. The first four steps of the scientific method are as follows:

I. Identify the problem.
II. Ask questions.
III. Develop a hypothesis.
IV. Collect data and experiment on that data.

Which of the following is the fifth step in the scientific method?

    a. Observe the data.
    b. Analyze the results.
    c. Measure the data.
    d. Develop a conclusion.

2. Which of the following is FALSE regarding the use of qualitative and quantitative data in scientific research?

    a. Quantitative data is collected through numerical measurements.
    b. Quantitative data is more accurate than qualitative data.
    c. Qualitative data is focused on perspectives and behavior.
    d. Qualitative data is collected through observation and interviews.

The next question refers to the following graphic.

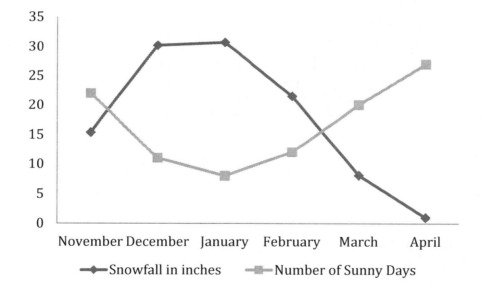

3. The chart above shows the average snowfall in inches for a town on Michigan's Upper Peninsula, during the months November through April. Which of the following can be concluded based on the information that is provided in the chart?

    a. April is not a good month to go skiing in the Upper Peninsula.
    b. Snowfall blocks the sunshine and reduces the number of sunny days.
    c. The fewest sunny days occur in the months with the heaviest snowfall.
    d. There is no connection between the amount of snowfall and the number of sunny days.

4. Which of the following statements correctly describes the function of the corresponding physiologic structure?

a. The trachea connects the throat and the stomach, encouraging food to follow this path through contractions.
b. The esophagus is the cylindrical portion of the respiratory tract that joins the larynx with the lungs.
c. The diaphragm is a muscle that controls the height of the thoracic cavity, decreasing the height on contraction, and increasing the height on relaxation causing expiration.
d. The epiglottis covers the trachea during swallowing, preventing food from entering the airway.

5. Which of the following is an example of the location and function of cartilage in the body?

a. The dense connective tissue that comprises the better part of the structural skeleton.
b. The supportive pads that provide cushion at joints, such as between the vertebrae of the spinal cord.
c. The connective structure made of fibrous collagen that connects muscles and bones, such as the connection of the patella to the quadricep.
d. The layer beneath the skin and on the outside of internal organs that provides cushioning and protection.

6. Two criteria for classifying epithelial tissue are:

a. cell type and cell function.
b. cell shape and cell type.
c. cell layers and cell shape.
d. cell function and cell layers.

7. Where is the parathyroid gland located?

a. On the lateral lobes of the thyroid gland, on the posterior aspect.
b. On the pyramidal lobe of the thyroid gland, on the posterior aspect.
c. On the lateral lobes of the thyroid gland, on the anterior aspect.
d. On the left lateral lobe of the thyroid gland, on the anterior aspect.

8. How many organ systems are in the human body?

a. 12
b. 15
c. 9
d. 11

9. Which element or structure within the respiratory system is responsible for removing foreign matter from the lungs?

a. Bronchial tubes
b. Cilia
c. Trachea
d. Alveoli

10. Organized from highest to lowest, what is the hierarchy of the human body's structures is as follows: organism, organ systems, organs, tissues. Which of the following comes next?

    a. Organs, cells, tissues, molecules, atoms.

    b. Organ system, organism, organ, cells, tissues, atoms, molecules.

    c. Organism, organ systems, organs, tissues, cells, molecules, atoms.

    d. Organism, organ, cells, tissues, molecules, atoms.

The next two questions are based on the periodic table.

Note: The row labeled with * is the <u>Lanthanide Series</u>, and the row labeled with ^ is the <u>Actinide Series</u>.

11. On average, how many neutrons does one atom of bromine (Br) have?

    a. 35

    b. 44.90

    c. 45

    d. 79.90

12. On average, how many protons does one atom of zinc (Zn) have?

    a. 30

    b. 35

    c. 35.39

    d. 65.39

13. Which statement below correctly describes the movement of molecules in the body and/or in relation to the external environment?

a. Osmosis is the movement of a solution from and area of low solute concentration to an area of high solute concentration.

b. Diffusion is the process in the lungs by which oxygen is transported from the air to the blood.

c. Dissipation is the transport of molecules across a semipermeable membrane from an area of low concentration to high concentration, requiring energy.

d. Reverse osmosis is the movement of molecules in a solution from an area of high concentration to an area of lower concentration.

14. Which gland is responsible for the regulation of calcium levels?

a. The parathyroid glands

b. The pituitary gland

c. The adrenal glands

d. The pancreas

15. Which statement matches the function to the organ of the digestive system?

a. The large intestine reabsorbs water into the body to form solid waste.

b. The duodenum is the middle section of the small intestine in which acids, fat, and sugar are absorbed.

c. The jejunum is the first part of the small intestine that receives chyme from the stomach and further digests it prior to entering the large intestine.

d. The gallbladder produces insulin to assist in the transport of sugars from the blood to the organs.

16. In your garden, you noticed that the tomato plants did better on the north side of your house than the west side and you decided to figure out why. They are both planted with the same soil that provides adequate nutrients to the plant, and they are watered at the same time during the week. Over the course of a week, you begin to measure the amount of sunlight that hits each side of the house and determine that the north side gets more light because the sunlight is blocked by the house's shadow on the west side. What is the name of the factor in your observations that affected the tomato plants growth?

a. The control

b. The independent variable

c. The dependent variable

d. The conclusion

17. Which of the following describes one responsibility of the integumentary system?

a. Distributing vital substances (such as nutrients) throughout the body

b. Blocking pathogens that cause disease

c. Sending leaked fluids from cardiovascular system back to the blood vessels

d. Storing bodily hormones that influence gender traits

18. When are the parasympathetic nerves active within the nervous system?

a. When an individual experiences a strong emotion, such as fear or excitement.

b. When an individual feels pain or heat.

c. When an individual is either talking or walking.

d. When an individual is either resting or eating.

19. Which of the following best describes the relationship between the circulatory system and the integumentary system?

a. Removal of excess heat from body.
b. Hormonal influence on blood pressure.
c. Regulation of blood's pressure and volume.
d. Development of blood cells within marrow.

20. Which of the following statements describes the path of blood entering into the heart?

a. Blood enters the heart through the pulmonary vein, into the right atrium, through the tricuspid valve to the right ventricle.
b. Once the right ventricle is full, blood exits into the pulmonary artery and then empties into the left ventricle.
c. After traveling through the lungs, oxygenated blood enters into the left atrium, then through the mitral valve to the left ventricle.
d. Once the left ventricle is full, the left tricuspid valve shuts, the ventricle contracts, and blood exits through the aorta.

21. The part of the human excretory system most responsible for maintaining normal body temperature is the:

a. kidney.
b. bladder.
c. liver.
d. sweat glands.

22. A part of which body system controls fluid loss, protects deep tissues, and synthesizes vitamin D?

a. The skeletal system.
b. The muscular system.
c. The lymphatic system.
d. The integumentary system.

23. There are three insects that are being compared under a microscope. As a scientist, you decide that measuring them would be an important part of recording their data. Which unit of measurement would best for this situation?

a. Centimeters.
b. Meters.
c. Micrometers.
d. Kilometers.

24. The respiratory system _____ oxygen for and _____ carbon dioxide from the circulatory system.

a. creates; filters
b. provides; removes
c. ionizes; absorbs
d. eliminates; destroys

25. Which statement below accurately describes the function of its element?

a. Collagen is a spongy fatty compound that creates a padding between bones and other structures.
b. Hemoglobin is the amount of red blood cells that are present in blood, which can reflect disease states, hydration, and blood loss.
c. Lymph is tissue that forms into nodes through which blood is filtered and cleaned.
d. An antigen stimulates the production of antibodies.

26. Which group of major parts and organs make up the immune system?

a. Lymphatic system, spleen, tonsils, thymus, and bone marrow.
b. Brain, spinal cord, and nerve cells.
c. Heart, veins, arteries, and capillaries.
d. Nose, trachea, bronchial tubes, lungs, alveolus, and diaphragm.

The next two questions are based on the following information.

A student is conducting an experiment using a ball that is attached to the end of a string on a pendulum. The student pulls the ball back so that it is at an angle to its resting position. As the student releases the ball, it swings forward and backward. The student measures the time it takes the ball to make one complete period. A period is defined as the time it takes the ball to swing forward and back again to its starting position. This is repeated using different string lengths.

27. The student formed the following hypothesis:

Lengthening the string of the pendulum increases the time it takes the ball to make one complete period.

What correction would you have the student make to the hypothesis?

a. Turn it into an "if/then" statement.
b. Add the word "will" in the middle after the word "pendulum."
c. Switch the order of the sentence so that the phrase about the period comes first, and the phrase about the string's length is last.
d. No corrections are needed.

28. What would be an appropriate control variable for this experiment?

a. The period
b. The length of the string
c. The mass of the ball
d. The color of the ball

29. Which of the following does not exist in RNA?

a. Uracil
b. Thymine
c. Cytosine
d. Guanine

30. In which of the following muscle types are the filaments arranged in a disorderly manner?

a. Cardiac.
b. Smooth.
c. Skeletal.
d. Rough.

31. Which of the following hormones is correctly matched with the gland/organ it is produced by?

a. Insulin; kidney.
b. Testosterone; thyroid.
c. Melatonin; pineal.
d. Epinephrine; gall bladder.

32. Which of the following best describes a section that divides the body into equal right and left parts?

a. Midsagittal plane.
b. Coronal plane.
c. Oblique plane.
d. Frontal plane.

33. In the development of genetic traits, one gene must match to one _____ for the traits to develop correctly.

a. Codon
b. Protein
c. Amino acid
d. Chromosome

34. Which of the following is not composed of striated muscle?

a. Quadriceps.
b. Uterus.
c. Triceps.
d. Gastrocnemius.

35. Which of the following is NOT found in the dorsal cavity of the body?

a. Cerebellum
b. Heart
c. Brainstem
d. Spine

36. Which of the following best describes the careful ordering of molecules within solids that have a fixed shape?

a. Physical bonding
b. Polar molecules
c. Metalloid structure
d. Crystalline order

37. Which of the following statement properly describes how the structure moves during inspiration?

    a. The lungs contract on inspiration.
    b. The diaphragm moves downward on inspiration.
    c. The ribs remain fixed during inspiration.
    d. The heart moves inward on inspiration.

38. Which of the following describes the transport network that is responsible for the transference of proteins throughout a cell?

    a. Golgi apparatus
    b. Endoplasmic reticulum
    c. Mitochondria
    d. Nucleolus

39. What occurs during the *anaphase* of mitosis?

    a. Chromosomes, originally in pairs, separate from their daughters and move to the opposite ends (or poles) of the cell.
    b. The mitotic spindle fibers begin to form.
    c. The chromosomes align in the middle of the cell.
    d. Two nuclei form, surrounded each by a nuclear membrane.

40. Using the table below, what conclusions can be made about the students' scores?

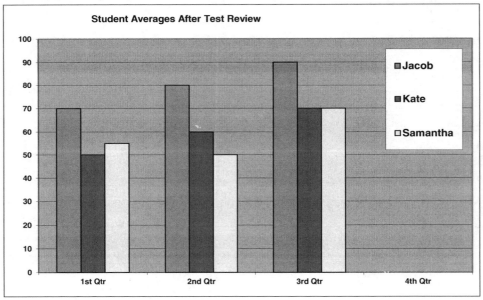

    a. The scores increased as the year progressed.
    b. The girls did better than the boys on the test each quarter.
    c. The test was about math.
    d. The scores were heavily impacted by the test reviews that were provided.

41. Which of the following statements is correct about normal human lung anatomy?

a. The right lung has three lobes; the left lung has two lobes.
b. The right lung has two lobes; the left lung has three lobes.
c. Both lungs have two lobes.
d. Both lungs have three lobes.

42. All of the following are parts of the cardiac system EXCEPT the:

a. ventricle.
b. alveoli.
c. atrium.
d. septum.

43. If a biologist is describing the physical and visible expression of a genetic trait, which of the following is he referring to?

a. Phenotype.
b. Allele.
c. Gamete.
d. Genotype.

44. Which of the following does NOT produce hormones?

a. Pituitary gland.
b. The Pons.
c. Pancreas.
d. Ovaries.

45. Which organ is correctly matched with the cavity in which it is found?

a. Spleen; pelvic cavity.
b. Brain; vertebral canal.
c. Bladder; abdominal cavity.
d. Heart; thoracic cavity.

46. A substance is considered *acidic* if it has a pH of less than which of the following?

a. 12
b. 9
c. 7
d. 4

47. Which of the following choices best describes the location of the trachea in relation to the esophagus?

a. Lateral
b. Anterior
c. Posterior
d. Dorsal

48. A triple beam balance would show the units of measurement in which form?

a. Liters
b. Grams
c. Meters
d. Gallons

49. Which of the following best describes a section that divides the body into equal upper and lower portions?

    a. Coronal
    b. Transverse
    c. Oblique
    d. Median

50. Which of the following best describes one of the roles of RNA?

    a. Manufacturing the proteins needed for DNA
    b. Creating the bonds between the elements that compose DNA
    c. Sending messages about the correct sequence of proteins in DNA
    d. Forming the identifiable "*double helix*" shape of DNA

51. Which of the following do *catalysts* alter to control the rate of a chemical reaction?

    a. Substrate energy
    b. Activation energy
    c. Inhibitor energy
    d. Promoter energy

52. Which of the following components of the human integumentary system is the deepest?

    a. Stratum basale.
    b. Epidermis.
    c. Hypodermis.
    d. Dermis.

53. The Punnett square shown here indicates a cross between two parents, one with alleles BB and the other with alleles Bb. Select the correct entry for the upper right box in the Punnett square, which is indicated with the letter, *x*:

	B	B
B		*x*
b		

    a. Bb
    b. bB
    c. BB
    d. bb

English and Language Usage	Number of Questions: **28**
	Time Limit: **28 Minutes**

1. Which of the following nouns represents the correct plural form of the word *syllabus*?

    a. Syllabus
    b. Syllaba
    c. Syllabi
    d. Syllabis

2. Which of the following words functions as an adjective in the sentence below?

The Welsh kingdom of Gwynedd existed as an independent state from the early 5th century, when the Romans left Britain, until the late 13th century, when the king of England took control of Wales.

    a. Independent
    b. Century
    c. King
    d. Control

3. *Bi, re,* and *un* are:

    a. Suffixes, appearing at the beginning of base words to change their meaning
    b. Suffixes, appearing at the end of base words to enhance their meaning
    c. Prefixes, appearing at the beginning of base words to emphasize their meaning
    d. Prefixes, appearing at the beginning of base words to change their meanings

4. Which of the following sentences shows the correct use of quotation marks?

    a. Grady asked Abe, 'Did you know that an earthquake and a tsunami hit Messina, Italy, in 1908?'
    b. Grady asked Abe, "Did you know that an earthquake and a tsunami hit Messina, Italy, in 1908"?
    c. Grady asked Abe, "Did you know that an earthquake and a tsunami hit Messina, Italy, in 1908?"
    d. Grady asked Abe, " 'Did you know that an earthquake and a tsunami hit Messina, Italy, in 1908'?"

5. *Since, whether,* and *accordingly* are examples of which type of signal words?

    a. Common, or basic, signal words
    b. Compare/contrast words
    c. Cause–effect words
    d. Temporal sequencing words

6. Which of the answer choices identifies the misspelled word in the sentence below?

Donald considered the job offer carefully, but he ultimately decided that the low salary was not acceptable given his previous experience.

    a. carefully
    b. decided
    c. salary
    d. acceptable

7. Which of the answer choices best combines the following four sentences into two sentences?

I'm usually good about keeping track of my keys. I lost them. I spent hours looking for them. I found them in the freezer.

a. I lost my keys, even though I'm usually good about keeping track of them. I found them in the freezer and spent hours looking for them.

b. I spent hours looking for my keys and found them in the freezer. I had lost them, even though I'm usually good about keeping track of them.

c. I'm usually good about keeping track of my keys, but I lost them. After spending hours looking for them, I found them in the freezer.

d. I'm usually good about keeping track of my keys, but I lost them in the freezer. I had to spend hours looking for them.

8. Which of the answer choices gives the best definition of the underlined word in the following sentence?

The warning against smoking may have been <u>tacit</u>, but Beryl instinctively knew that her mother wanted her to avoid picking up the habit.

a. complicated

b. empty

c. wordy

d. unstated

9.Which of the answer choices shows the correct punctuation of the city and the state in the following sentence?

After living in Oak Ridge Missouri all her life, Cornelia was excited about her trip to Prague.

a. After living in Oak Ridge, Missouri, all her life, Cornelia was excited about her trip to Prague.

b. After living in Oak Ridge, Missouri all her life, Cornelia was excited about her trip to Prague.

c. After living in Oak, Ridge, Missouri all her life, Cornelia was excited about her trip to Prague.

d. After living in Oak Ridge Missouri all her life, Cornelia was excited about her trip to Prague.

10. What transition should be added to the beginning of sentence 2 below?

(1) I zoned out in class, turned work in late, talked out in class, and handed in assignments after the due date. (2) Mr. Shanbourne just nodded.

a. Surprisingly

b. Actually

c. Furthermore

d. Instead

11. The following words all end in the same suffix, *-ism*: polytheism, communism, nationalism. Considering the meaning of these three words, how does the suffix *-ism* apply to all of them?

a. Doctrine

b. Condition

c. Characteristic

d. State of being

12. What is the most effective way to rewrite the following sentence?

She is saying that some of the students are wearing to school is being distracting and inappropriate.

    a. Some of the outfits students wear to school, she is saying, are distracting and not appropriate.
    b. The outfits are distracting and inappropriate, she says, that students wear to school.
    c. She says that some of the outfits that students wear to school are distracting and inappropriate.
    d. She says that it is distracting and inappropriate that students wear outfits to school.

13. Which of the following is an example of a correctly punctuated sentence?

    a. Beatrice is very intelligent, she just does not apply herself well enough in her classes to make good grades.
    b. Beatrice is very intelligent: she just does not apply herself well enough in her classes to make good grades.
    c. Beatrice is very intelligent she just does not apply herself well enough in her classes to make good grades
    d. Beatrice is very intelligent; she just does not apply herself well enough in her classes to make good grades.

14. What is the most effective way to combine the two sentences below?

Some members of the Sons of Liberty constructed a paper obelisk. An obelisk is the same shape as the Washington Monument.

    a. Some members of the Sons of Liberty constructed a paper obelisk, which is the same shape as the Washington Monument.
    b. Some members of the Sons of Liberty constructed a paper obelisk which is the same shape as the Washington Monument.
    c. Some members of the Sons of Liberty constructed a paper obelisk, that is the same shape as the Washington Monument.
    d. Some members of the Sons of Liberty constructed a paper obelisk; which is the same shape as the Washington Monument.

15. Which of the following is a compound sentence?

    a. Tabitha and Simon started the day at the zoo and then went to the art museum for the rest of the afternoon.
    b. Tabitha and Simon started the day at the zoo, and then they went to the art museum for the rest of the afternoon.
    c. After starting the day at the zoo, Tabitha and Simon then went to the art museum for the rest of the afternoon.
    d. Tabitha and Simon had a busy day, because they started at the zoo, and then they went to the art museum for the rest of the afternoon.

16. Which of the following follows the rules of capitalization?

    a. Dashiell visited his Cousin Elaine on Tuesday.
    b. Juniper sent a card to Uncle Archibald who has been unwell.
    c. Flicka and her Mother spent the day setting up the rummage sale.
    d. Lowell and his twin Sister look alike but have very different personalities.

17. What is the most likely meaning of the underlined phrase in the sentence below?

The Western perspective expects moral actions to be <u>quid pro quo</u>; to put it another way, a Westerner assumes that if he or she does something considered "good," then he or she should and will be rewarded.

    a. "something for nothing."
    b. "good merits money."
    c. "to each his own."
    d. "this for that."

18. Which of the following sets of words correctly fill in the blanks in the sentence below?

We cannot allow the budget cuts to _____ the plans to improve education; the futures of _____ children are at stake.

    a. effect; your
    b. affect; you're
    c. effect; you're
    d. affect; your

19. Which of the answer choices gives the best definition of the underlined word in the following sentence?

The experience of being the survivor of a plane crash left an <u>indelible</u> impression on Johanna, and she suffered from nightmares for years afterwards.

    a. candid
    b. permanent
    c. inexpressible
    d. indirect

20. Which of the following sentences contains an incorrect use of capitalization?

    a. For Christmas, we are driving to the South to visit my grandmother in Mississippi.
    b. Last year, we went to East Texas to go camping in Piney Woods.
    c. Next month, we will visit my Aunt Darla who lives just East of us.
    d. When my sister-in-law Susan has her baby, I will take the train north to see her.

21. Which of the following sentences is grammatically correct?

    a. Krista was not sure who to hold responsible for the broken window.
    b. Krista was not sure whom was responsible for the broken window.
    c. Krista was not sure whom to hold responsible for the broken window.
    d. Krista was not sure on who she should place responsibility for the broken window.

22. The word *capacity* functions as which part of speech in the following sentence?

    Irish politician Constance Markiewicz was the first woman elected to the British House of Commons, but she never served in that capacity due to her activity in forming the Irish Republic.

    a. Verb
    b. Noun
    c. Adverb
    d. Pronoun

23. Which of the following sentences represents the best style and clarity of expression?

    a. Without adequate preparation, the test was likely to be a failure for Zara.
    b. The test was likely to be a failure for Zara without adequate preparation.
    c. Without adequate preparation, Zara expected to fail the test.
    d. Zara expected to fail the test without adequate preparation.

24. Which of the following sentences contains a correct example of subject-verb agreement?

    a. All of the board members are in agreement on the issue.
    b. Each of the students were concerned about the test scores for the final exam.
    c. Neither of the children are at home right now.
    d. Any of the brownie recipes are perfect for the bake sale.

25. Which of the answer choices gives the best definition of the underlined word in the following sentence?

Despite the important achievement of the election of our first African American president, the need for knowledge and education about African American history is still unmet to a <u>substantial</u> degree.

    a. base
    b. considerable
    c. minor
    d. trivial

26. Which of the following is a simple sentence?

    a. Phillippa walked the dog, and Primula gave the dog a bath.
    b. Phillippa walked and bathed the dog, and Primula helped.
    c. Phillippa walked the dog, while Primula gave the dog a bath.
    d. Phillippa and Primula walked the dog and gave the dog a bath.

27. Which of the following sentences is most correct in terms of style, clarity, and punctuation?

    a. The possible side effects of the medication that the doctor had prescribed for her was a concern for Lucinda, and she continued to take the medication.
    b. The medication that the doctor prescribed had side effects concerning Lucinda who continued to take it.
    c. Lucinda was concerned about side effects from the medication that her doctor had prescribed, so she continued to take it.
    d. Although Lucinda was concerned about the possible side effects, she continued to take the medication that her doctor had prescribed for her.

28. What does the prefix _poly-_ mean in the word _polygon?_

    a. few
    b. several
    c. none
    d. many

Answer Key and Explanations for Test #1

Reading

1. C: To *assuage* is to lessen the effects of something, in this case Adelaide's guilt over eating the piece of cheesecake. The context of the sentence also suggests that she feels sorry for eating it and wants to compensate the following day.

2. C: This choice shows how greenhouse gases are released from burning coal and other fuels, which people need for power. The first, second, and third choices are facts, but don't show a relationship to the main idea.

3. A: To find information on Freud's psychological theories, Lise should go to class 100.

4. C: In this case, Lise needs to find a work of literature instead of a work of psychology, so she should consult the 800s.

5. B: To study Jewish traditions further, Lise should consult the 200s, which is devoted to books on religion.

6. A: The sample is biased because the study wishes to examine all middle school teachers' ideas, regarding usage of iPhones in the classroom, while the sample only represents ideas of those teachers teaching technology courses.

7. A: The sentence indicates a contrast between the appearance and the reality. Enzo's friends believe him to be wealthy, due to the large home that he inherited, but he is actually penniless.

8. B: The word SORT results from following all of the directions that are provided.

9. B: The enrollment in 2001 falls directly between 2000 and 2500, so 2300 is accurate. Note that the enrollment for 2000 falls much closer to 2000, so 2100 is a best estimate for that year.

10. C: The tuition appears to rise alongside the enrollment, until the year 2009 when it jumps significantly. Since the enrollment between 2008 and 2009 does not justify the immediate jump in income for the school, an increase in tuition costs makes sense.

11. B: It can be concluded that phonics is a more effective way to learn to read for two reasons. First, the passage states that literacy rates are lower now than they were 15 years ago, meaning that more people knew how to read 15 years ago. Then, the passage states that phonics was the main way people learned how to read then. Therefore, based on these two facts, it can be concluded that phonics is more effective.

12. C: The passage is *expository* in the sense that it looks more closely into the mysteries of the Bermuda Triangle and *exposes* information about what researchers have studied and now believe.

13. D: This sentence is the best summary statement for the entire passage, because it wraps up clearly what the author is saying about the results of studies on the Bermuda Triangle.

14. A: Of all the sentences provided, this is the one with which the author would most likely agree. The passage suggests that most of the "mysteries" of the Bermuda Triangle can be explained in a reasonable way. The passage mentions that some expand the Triangle to the Azores, but this is a point of fact, and the author makes no mention of whether or not this is in error. The author quotes the Navy's response to the disappearance of the planes, but there is no reason to believe the author questions this response. The author raises questions about the many myths surrounding the Triangle, but at no point does the author connect these myths with what are described as accidents that fall "within the expected margin of error."

15. C: The inclusion of the statement about the ships from East Asia is an opinion statement, as the author provides no support or explanation. The other statements within the answer choices offer supporting evidence and explanatory material, making them acceptable for an expository composition.

16. A: When a researcher has conducted an original experiment and reports the results, findings, and associated conclusions in a research report, that report is considered a primary source. Academic textbooks, journal articles, articles in other periodicals, and authoritative databases may all be primary sources. When an academic textbook cites research (B) by others, that citation is considered a secondary source as it refers to information originally presented by others. When a news article quotes a researcher's writing (C), that is also a secondary source. So is a description given on a website of another person's research (D).

17. B: Only the word *introspection* can fall between *intrauterine* and *invest*. The words *intransigent* and *intone* come before, and the word *investiture* follows.

18. C: The chart shows that plastic and cardboard materials both comprise 15% of the collected materials, and therefore it is incorrect to say that there is more plastic than cardboard. They are present in equal quantities.

19. D: The spaghetti and the garlic bread are definitely concerns for Ninette if she is unable to consume products with wheat in them. With all other meals, there appear to be gluten-free options that she can eat.

20. A: The government website would publish the most recent data on seatbelt information, like how many people wore seatbelts in the accident and how many survived. Choices B and C are more likely to be opinion-based. Choice D is tempting, but it would not give someone the most up-to-date information.

21. D: The negative reviews led to the poor quality of the second movie.

22. B: This question and the two that follow require simple multiplication and addition. Since the quantities needed are the same for both texts, one need only find the supplier with the lowest combined price (per 100) for the two texts. Textbook Central's combined price for 100 each of the two texts is $9,550. The closest competitor is University Textbook with a combined price of $9,600. The other two suppliers come in at $9,650 and $9,675. The total for the transaction with Textbook Central is $47,750.

23. B: Once again, Textbook Central prevails. In this case, it is not even necessary to do the calculations. The cost for composition textbooks is $4350 (per 100) and for linguistics textbooks is $6550 (per 100). The lower cost for the composition textbooks–$150 less per 100 than the closest company in cost–outweighs the slight difference in cost for the linguistics textbooks.

24. C: Bookstore Supply has the lowest cost of the four for the technical writing textbooks, and it has a comparable cost to University Textbook for the world literature textbooks. The slight difference for the technical writing textbooks will make the overall cost lower than University Textbook's and give Bookstore Supply the competitive edge in cost.

25. C: This should be read from the column labeled "Unadjusted percent change to June 2009 from June 2008", a period of one year. For transportation, the index is down 13.2%. This is the only negative change among the choices given.

26. B: Read this answer in the second column from the right. Fuel oil and other fuels decreased by 3.1% during this period. Gasoline increased by 3.1%. The other commodities decreased, but by lesser amounts.

27. D: In the table, components of each category are shown by indentation under the name of the category itself. There may be sub-categories within each category that are further indented. All of the Choices are indented under "Food at Home" except for "Alcoholic Beverages", which is a separate category.

28. A: Read this from the second column in the table, "Relative Importance December 2008". These numbers represent the average percentage of household budgets that are spent on the expenditure category. The greatest number, 43.421%, is on the row corresponding to housing.

29. D: Answer choice D is the only option that correctly follows the instructions in the question. Sections 4 and 5 are removed; section 1 is placed on the right sides along sections 3 and 2; and there is a circle drawn around the entire shape. Answer choice A places section 1 in the wrong location and fails to switch sections 2 and 5. Answer choice B incorrectly removes section 1 altogether. Answer choice C changes the shape of section 1 to a rectangle and reverses sections 2 and 3.

30. D: Anna is ultimately looking for a good all-around guidebook for the region. *The Top Ten Places to Visit in Brittany* might have some useful information, but it will not provide enough details about hiking trails, beaches, restaurants, and accommodations. *Getting to Know Nantes* limits the information to one city, and Anna's destination in Brittany is not identified. *Hiking Through Bretagne* limits the information to one activity. These three guidebooks might offer great supplemental information, but *The Complete Guide to Brittany* is the most likely to offer *all* of the information that Anna needs for her trip.

31. D: According to Figure 1, the radius is a bone in the lower arm. The femur, tibia, and patella are located in the leg. Therefore, choice D is correct.

32. A: According to the passage, the skull is part of the axial skeleton. Therefore, choice A is correct.

33. B: According to Figure 1, the metacarpals are located in the hand. The metatarsals are located in the foot. The fibula is in the leg, and the ulna is in the arm. Therefore, choice B is correct.

34. B: The passage does not state this outright, but the author indicates that the younger sons of King George III began considering the option of marrying and producing heirs *after* Princess Charlotte Augusta died. Since she was the heir-apparent, her death left the succession undetermined. The author mentions very little about any "wrongs" that Victoria's uncles committed, so this cannot be a logical conclusion. The passage says nothing about the Duke of Kent's preference for a male heir over a female. (In fact, it was likely that he was delighted to have any heir.) And the author does not provide enough detail about the relationship between the Duchess of Kent and King William IV to infer logically that his suspicions were "unreasonable" or that the duchess cared only for her daughter's well-being.

35. C: The author actually notes in the last paragraph that Victoria was an "improbable princess who became queen" and the rest of the passage demonstrates how it was a series of small events that changed the course of British succession. The passage is largely factual, so it makes little sense as a persuasive argument. The author mentions the Victorian Era, but the passage is more about Queen Victoria's family background than it is about the era to which she gave her name. And the passage is more about how the events affected Victoria (and through her, England) than it is about the direct effect that George III's sons had on English history.

36. D: This passage is most likely to belong in some kind of biographical reference about Queen Victoria. A scholarly paper would include more analysis instead of just fact. The information in the passage does not fit the genre of mystery at all. And since the passage recounts history, it is not an obvious candidate for a fictional story.

37. D: All other sentences in the passage offer some support or explanation. Only the sentence in answer choice D indicates an unsupported opinion on the part of the author.

38. C: The author actually says, "Charles's own political troubles extended beyond religion in this case, and he was beheaded in 1649." This would indicate that religion was less involved in this situation than in other situations. There is not enough information to infer that Charles II never married; the passage only notes that he had no legitimate children. (In fact, he had more than ten illegitimate children by his mistresses.) And while the chance of a Catholic king frightened many in England, it is reaching beyond logical inference to assume that people were relieved when the royal children died. Finally, the author does not provide enough detail for the reader to assume that James I had *no* Catholic leanings. The author only says that James recognized the importance of committing to the Church of England.

39. A: The author notes, "In spite of a strong resemblance to the king, the young James was generally rejected among the English and the Lowland Scots, who referred to him as "the Pretender." This indicates that there *was* a resemblance, and this increases the likelihood that the child was, in fact, that of James and Mary Beatrice. Answer choice B is too much of an opinion statement that does not have enough support in the passage. The passage essentially refutes answer choice C by pointing out that James "the Pretender" was welcomed in the Highlands. And there is little in the passage to suggest that James was unable to raise an army and mount an attack.

40. B: The passage is composed in a chronological sequence with each king introduced in order of reign.

41. D: The passage is largely informative in focus, and the author provides extensive detail about this period in English and Scottish history. There is little in the passage to suggest persuasion, and the tone of the passage has no indication of a desire to entertain. Additionally, the passage is historical, so the author avoids expressing feelings and instead focuses on factual information (with the exception of the one opinion statement).

42. B: Both of the speakers are arguing over the respect due to an individual, but they are going about it in different ways.

43. C: This detail would only really support the argument against wearing school uniforms, while the other three choices could all appear as details in support of either side of the argument.

44. A: Technical passages focus on presenting specific information and have a tone of formality. Narrative writing focuses on telling a story, and the passage offers no indication of this. Persuasive writing attempts to persuade the reader to agree with a certain position; the instructor offers the students information but leaves the decision up to each student. Expository passages reveal analytical information to the reader. The instructor is more focused on providing the students with information than with offering the students analytical details. (The analysis, it appears, will be up to the students if they choose to complete an extra credit project.)

45. C: Answer choice C fits the tone of the passage best. The instructor is simply offering students the chance to make up the exam score (which is worth 70% of their grade) and thus avoid failing the course. The instructor does not berate students at any point, nor does the instructor admit that the exam was too difficult. Additionally, the instructor offers encouragement to the students should they choose to complete an extra credit project, but that is not the primary purpose of this email.

46. B: This question asks for the best summary of the instructor's motive. In the opening paragraph, the instructor notes that his original grading plan has to change to reflect the exam scores. Because they were low, he now wants to give students a chance to make up for their low scores. Answer choice B thus summarizes his motive effectively. The instructor introduces his email with the notes about the scores being posted, but, given the information that is provided in the message, this is not the sole motive for his writing. Answer choice A limits the motive to the details about the group project, and the instructor provides three options. Answer choice D overlooks the instructor's further note about how the grading policy sometimes has to bend to reflect circumstances.

47. B: The author asserts both that earning money is increasingly easy and that managing money is difficult.

48. D: The author seems to believe that there are plenty of lucrative jobs for everyone.

49. A: The author insists that many people who have no trouble earning money waste it through lavish spending.

50. B: This passage is clearly intended for a non-expert adult readership.

51. C: Here, the author is speaking of money management on a personal or household level.

52. D: The author suggests that many people who believe they understand economy in fact do not.

53. A: It seems clear that the author is about to describe the correct means of personal economy for a self-help manual.

Mathematics

1. D: To derive a percentage from a decimal, multiply by 100: $0.0016(100) = 0.16\%$.

2. C: One kilometer is about 0.62 miles, so $45(0.62)$ is 27.9, or approximately 28 miles.

3. D: Since there are 100 cm in a meter, on a 1:100 scale drawing, each centimeter represents one meter. Therefore, an area of one square centimeter on the drawing represents one square meter in actuality. Since the area of the room in the scale drawing is 30 cm^2, the room's actual area is 30 m^2.

Another way to determine the area of the room is to write and solve an equation, such as this one: $l/100 \times w/100 = 30$ cm^2, where l and w are the dimensions of the actual room

$$lw/1000 = 30 \text{ cm}^2$$

$$\text{Area} = 300,000 \text{ cm}^2$$

Since this is not one of the answer choices, convert cm² to m²:

$$300{,}000 \text{ cm}^2 \times \frac{1 \text{ m}}{100 \text{ cm}} \times \frac{1 \text{ m}}{100 \text{ cm}} = 30 \text{ m}^2.$$

4. C: The situation may be modeled by the system:

$$4x + 3y = 9.55$$
$$2x + 2y = 5.90$$

Multiplying the bottom equation by −2 gives:

$$4x + 3y = 9.55$$
$$-4x - 4y = -11.80$$

Addition of the two equations gives $-y = -2.25$ or $y = 2.25$. Thus, one box of crackers costs $2.25.

5. C: To find the average of Pernell's scores, add them up and then divide by the number of scores (5 in this case). In other words,

$$81 + 92 + 87 + 89 + 94 = 443$$

$$443/5 = 88.6, \text{ or approximately } 89$$

6. B: To find the median, list the series of numbers from least to greatest. The middle number represents the median—in this case 81, 87, 89, 92, 94. The number 89 is in the middle, so it is the median.

7. D: The television is 30% off its original price of $472. 30% of 472 is 141.60, and 141.60 subtracted from 472 is 330.40. Thus, Gordon paid $330.40 for the television.

8. A: To simplify, proceed in the order of the operations: $\frac{2}{3} \div \frac{4}{15}$ is $\frac{2}{3} \times \frac{15}{4}$, or $\frac{30}{12}$, which simplifies to $\frac{5}{2}$. Next, multiply $\frac{5}{2}$ by $\frac{5}{8}$. The result is $\frac{25}{16}$, or $1\frac{9}{16}$.

9. B: This is a simple matter of multiplication. The product is 0.0427378.

10. A: The inequality will be less than or equal to, since he may spend $100 or less on his purchase.

11. C: Multiplying the equation results in the following:

$$8x - 24 = 10x - 6$$
$$-18 = 2x$$
$$-\frac{18}{2} = x = -9$$

12. C: Erma's sale discount will be applied to the less expensive sweater, so she will receive the $44 sweater for 25% off. This amounts to a discount of $11, so the cost of the sweater will be $33. Added to the cost of the $50 sweater, which is not discounted, Erma's total is $83.

13. A: Start by adding the first two expressions, and then subtract 1.294 from the sum:

$$1.034 + 0.275 - 1.294 = 1.309 - 1.294 = 0.015$$

14. B: Adding up the number of church-goers in Ellsford results in about 1450 residents who attend a church in the town each week. There are approximately 400 people in Ellsford who attend a Catholic church each week. This number represents about 28% of the 1450 church-goers in the town.

15. B: To solve, first subtract Jerry's weight from the total permitted: $800 - 200 = 600$. Divide 600 by 4 (the four pieces of equipment) to get 150, the average weight.

16. C: Turn both expressions into fractions, and then multiply the first by the reverse of the second:

$$= \frac{14}{3} \div \frac{7}{6}$$
$$= \frac{14}{3} \times \frac{6}{7}$$

The result is the whole number 4.

17. D: Begin by subtracting 4 from both sides, then subtract x from both sides:

$$2x + 4 - 4 = x - 6 - 4$$
$$2x = x - 10$$
$$2x - x = x - 10 - x$$
$$x = -10$$

18. D: To solve the equation for x, you can follow the steps below:

$$2x - 7 = 3$$
$$2x - 7 + 7 = 3 + 7$$
$$2x = 10$$
$$\frac{2x}{2} = \frac{10}{2}$$
$$x = 5$$

19. D: The points do not show any trend line or trend curve at all. So, there is no association in the scatter plot.

20. A: To find the correct answer, simply multiply 56 by 2.2. The result is 123.2, or approximately 123. This is Stella's weight in pounds.

21. D: The smallest negative integers are those that have the largest absolute value. Therefore, the negative integers, written in order from least to greatest, are $-8, -7\frac{4}{5}, -\frac{3}{4}$. The percentage, 18%, can be written as the decimal, 0.18; 0.18 is less than 0.25. The decimal, 2.5, is the greatest rational number given. Thus, the values, $-8, -7\frac{4}{5}, -\frac{3}{4}, 18\%, 0.25, 2.5$, are written in order from least to greatest.

22. A: Begin by subtracting 1432 from 2219. The result is 787. Then, divide 787 by 1432 to find the percent of increase: 0.549, or 54.9%. Rounded up, this is approximately a 55% increase in births between 2000 and 2010.

23. C: Solve the equation in the order of operations: $\frac{1}{4} \times \frac{3}{5}$, or $\frac{3}{20}$. Follow this up with division, which requires a reversal of the fraction: $\frac{3}{20} \div \frac{9}{8}$, or $\frac{3}{20} \times \frac{8}{9}$, which equals $\frac{24}{180}$. The result simplifies to $\frac{2}{15}$.

24. C: Cora did *not* fall 7 out of 27 times. To find the solution, simply divide 7 by 27 to arrive at 0.259, or 25.9%. Rounded up, this is approximately 26%.

25. C: The volume of a cylinder may be calculated using the formula $V = \pi r^2 h$, where r represents the radius and h represents the height. Substituting 1.5 for r and 3 for h gives $V = \pi (1.5)^2 (3)$, which simplifies to $V \approx 21.2$.

26. B: Since the denominator is the same for both fractions, this is simple subtraction. Start by turning each expression into a fraction: $\frac{19}{6} - \frac{11}{6}$. The result is $\frac{8}{6}$, or $1\frac{2}{6} = 1\frac{1}{3}$.

27. A: The expression "Four more than a number, x" can be interpreted as $x + 4$. This is equal to "2 less than $\frac{1}{3}$ of another number, y," or $\frac{1}{3}y - 2$. Thus, the equation is $x + 4 = \frac{1}{3}y - 2$.

28. C: Start by adding up the costs of the trip, excluding the hotel cost: $572 + $150 + $250 = $972. Then, calculate what Margery will spend on the hotel. The first of her five nights at the hotel will cost her $89. For each of the other four nights, she will get a discount of 10% per night, or $8.90. This discount of $8.90 multiplied by the four nights is $35.60. The total she would have spent on the five nights without the discount is $445. With the discount, the amount goes down to $409.40. Add this amount to the $972 for a grand total of $1381.40.

29. B: Data is said to be positively skewed when there are a higher number of lower values, indicating data that is skewed right. An approximately normal distribution shows an increase in frequency, followed by a decrease in frequency, of approximately the same rate.

30. C: The surface area of a rectangular prism may be calculated using the formula

$$SA = 2lw + 2wh + 2hl$$

Substituting the dimensions of 14 inches, 6 inches, and 8 inches gives:

$$SA = 2(14)(6) + 2(6)(8) + 2(8)(14)$$

Thus, the surface area is 488 square inches.

31. B: Start by locating the section of the pie chart that represents construction. It looks close to a quarter of the pie chart, which means that it is probably 23%, but you can verify by adding up the numbers. The total amount of all donations is about $1.3 million and the amount given for construction is $0.3 million. $\frac{0.3}{1.3} = 0.227 \approx 23\%$.

32. D: Turn the fractions into mixed numbers to see the amounts more clearly. The result is that $\frac{7}{8}$ is smaller than $\frac{10}{9}$, or $1\frac{1}{9}$, which is smaller than $\frac{7}{3}$, or $2\frac{1}{3}$, which is smaller than $\frac{9}{2}$, or $4\frac{1}{2}$.

33. D: In order to divide the terms, they must first be rearranged as a multiplication by keeping the first fraction as is, changing the division sign to multiplication, and taking the reciprocal of the second fraction: $\frac{2}{7} \times \frac{6}{5}$. Then, multiply the new terms: $\frac{2}{7} \times \frac{6}{5} = \frac{12}{35}$. In Answer A, a common denominator was found, but the numerators were not also adjusted. Therefore, $\frac{2}{7}$ became $\frac{2}{42}$ and $\frac{5}{6}$ became $\frac{5}{42}$. Then, the fraction division process resulted in $\frac{2}{42} \div \frac{5}{42} = \frac{2}{42} \times \frac{42}{5} = \frac{2}{5}$. In Answer B, the reciprocal was taken of the first fraction instead of the second fraction before multiplying the terms. In Answer C, the fractions were incorrectly just multiplied as is.

34. B: Start by calculating the amount in parentheses, completing the multiplication first: $5 + 6 \times 3$, which is $5 + 18$ or 23. Then calculate the product at the end: 10×2 which is 20 and complete the equation:

$$= 7 + 16 - 23 - 20$$
$$= 23 - 23 - 20$$
$$= 0 - 20$$
$$= -20$$

35. A: This equation is a linear relationship that has a slope of 3.60 and passes through the origin. The table shows that for each hour of rental, the cost increases by $3.60. This matches with the slope of the equation. Of course, if the bicycle is not rented at all (0 hours), there will be no charge ($0). If plotted on the Cartesian plane, the line would have a y intercept of 0. Choice A is the only one that follows these requirements.

36. D: The correct answer is $4000. Chan has paid out a total of $30\% + 30\% + 25\% = 85\%$ of his bonus for the items in the question. So, the $600 is the remaining 15%. To find out his total bonus, solve $\frac{100}{15} \times 600 = \$4000$.

Science

1. B: There are six steps in the scientific process, the fifth of which is "Analyze the results" (the results of the experiments that were conducted in step four). The results of step four must be analyzed before reaching the final step, "Develop a conclusion."

2. B: The two types of measurement important in science are quantitative (when a numerical result is used) and qualitative (when descriptions or qualities are reported). Qualitative data is collected through observation and interviews, and focuses on the informant's behavior and perspectives. Both qualitative and quantitative data are equally important in scientific research, and when combined and analyzed together provide a full picture of the focus of the question at hand. Additionally, both qualitative and quantitative data can be accurate, or may be skewed by bias, therefore both should be thoroughly analyzed.

3. C: The chart shows two specific changes: snowfall levels from November to April and sunny days from November to April. Based on the chart alone, the only information that can be determined is that the fewest sunny days coincide with the months that have the heaviest snowfall. Anything further reaches beyond the immediate facts of the chart and moves into the territory of requiring other facts. As for answer choice D, it uses the word "relationship," which is not required in the question. The question only asks for what can be concluded.

4. D: The epiglottis covers the trachea during swallowing, thus preventing food from entering the airway. The trachea, also known as the windpipe, is a cylindrical portion of the respiratory tract that joins the larynx with the lungs. The esophagus connects the throat and the stomach. When a person swallows, the esophagus contracts to force the food down into the stomach. Like other structures in the respiratory system, the esophagus secretes mucus for lubrication. The diaphragm is a muscle that controls the height of the thoracic cavity, increasing the height on contraction (inspiration), and decreasing the height on relaxation (expiration).

5. B: The pads that support the vertebrae are made up of cartilage. Cartilage, a strong form of connective tissue, cushions and supports the joints. Cartilage also makes up the larynx and the outer ear. Bone is a form of connective tissue that comprises the better part of the skeleton. It includes both organic and inorganic substances. Tendons connect the muscles to other structures of the body, typically bones. Tendons can increase and decrease in length as the bones move. Fat is a combination of lipids; in humans, fat forms a layer beneath the skin and on the outside of the internal organs.

6. C: Cell layers and cell shape are the criteria for classifying epithelial tissue. Cell layers refers to the amount of cells that separate the basement membrane from the surface, such as a simple single layer, a stratified layer (2 or more), or a pseudostratified layer. Cell shapes refer to the shape of the outer cells and can be squamous, columnar or cuboidal.

7. A: The parathyroid gland is located on the lateral lobes of the thyroid gland in the neck, on the posterior aspect. It is part of the endocrine system. When the supply of calcium in blood diminishes to unhealthy levels, the parathyroid gland motivates the secretion of a hormone that encourages the bones to release calcium into the bloodstream. The parathyroid gland also regulates the amount of phosphate in the blood by stimulating the excretion of phosphates in the urine.

8. D: There are 11 organ systems in the human body: circulatory, digestive, endocrine, integumentary, lymphatic, muscular, nervous, reproductive, respiratory, skeletal, and urinary.

9. B: The cilia are the tiny hairs in the respiratory system that are responsible for removing foreign matter from the lungs. The cilia are located within the bronchial tubes, but it is the cilia that have the responsibility for removing inappropriate materials before they enter the lungs.

10. C: The order of hierarchy of human body structures is as follows: Organism, organ systems, organs, tissues, cells, molecules, and atoms. Muscles are types of tissues, so muscles do not have a separate place in the hierarchy but instead fall within the types of tissues.

11. B: To determine the average number of neutrons in one atom of an element, subtract the atomic number from the average atomic mass. For Bromine (Br), subtract its atomic number (35) from its average atomic mass (79.9) to acquire the average number of neutrons, 44.9.

12. A: The number of protons is the same for every atom of a given element and is the element's atomic number: in this case, 30 for Zinc (Zn).

13. B: In the lungs, oxygen is transported from the air to the blood through the process of *diffusion*, in which molecules passively move from an area of high concentration to low concentration. Specifically, the alveolar membranes withdraw the oxygen from the air in the lungs into the bloodstream. *Osmosis* is the passive movement of a water from an area of low solute concentration to an area of higher solute concentration through a permeable membrane. *Reverse osmosis* is the active transport of water opposite the concentration gradient from an area of low solute concentration to high solute concentration. *Dissipation* is a more general reference of the spread or loss of energy.

14. A: The parathyroid glands are four small glands that sit on top of the thyroid gland and regulate calcium levels by secreting parathyroid hormone. The hormone regulates the amount of calcium and magnesium that is excreted by the kidneys into the urine.

15. A: The large intestine's main function is the reabsorption of water into the body to form solid waste. It also allows for the absorption of vitamin K produced by microbes living inside the large intestine. The duodenum is the first section of the small intestine that receives partially digested food from the stomach, also called chyme, further digesting it with the help of enzymes released by the gall bladder, before it enters into the small intestine. The pancreas (not the gall bladder) releases insulin to assist in the removal and transport of sugar in the body. The jejunum is the second portion of the small intestine in which amino acids, fatty acids, and sugars are absorbed.

16. B: The conclusion was that the amount of sunlight received by the plants was affecting their growth. The independent variable was the amount of light that was given to the plants and could have been manipulated by the experimenter by moving the plants or adding equal parts of light. No control was used in this experiment.

17. B: The integumentary system includes skin, hair, and mucous membranes, all of which are responsible–in part, at least–for blocking disease-causing pathogens from entering the blood stream. The circulatory system distributes vital substances through the body. The lymphatic system sends leaked fluids from the cardiovascular system back to the blood vessels. The reproductive system stores bodily hormones that influence gender traits.

18. D: The parasympathetic nerves are active when an individual is either resting or eating. The sympathetic nerves are active when an individual experiences a strong emotion, such as fear or excitement. Feeling pain and heat fall under the responsibility of the sensory neurons. Talking and walking fall under the responsibility of the ganglia within the sensory-somatic nervous system.

19. A: The integumentary system (i.e., the skin, hair, mucous membranes, etc.) coordinates with the circulatory system to remove excess heat from the body. The superficial blood vessels (those nearest the surface of the skin) dilate to allow the heat to exit the body. The hormonal influence on blood pressure is the result of the relationship between the circulatory system and the endocrine system. The urinary system is responsible for assisting in the regulation of blood's pressure and volume. The skeletal system is responsible for assisting in the development of blood vessels within the marrow.

20. C: Blood returns to the heart from both the inferior and superior vena cava, entering into the right atrium, through the tricuspid valve, and into the right ventricle. Once the right ventricle is full, the tricuspid valve closes, and upon heart contraction, the blood is pumped through the pulmonary artery, becoming oxygenated in the lungs. The blood returns to the heart from the lungs through the pulmonary vein, into the left atrium, through the mitral valve, and into the left ventricle. When the left ventricle is full, the mitral valve closes, and the heart contracts and distributes the newly oxygenated blood throughout the body through the aortic valve and into the aorta.

21. D: Blood is cooled as it passes through capillaries surrounding the sweat glands. Heat is absorbed along with excess salt and water and transferred to the glands as sweat. Droplets of sweat then evaporate from the skin surface to dissipate heat and cool the body. The kidney, bladder, and liver are not involved in regulating body temperature.

22. D: The skin is a part of the integumentary system, along with the hair, nails, nerves, and glands. The skin controls fluid loss, protects deep tissues, and synthesizes vitamin D. The skeletal system gives the body its bony supporting structure, protects vital organs, collaborates with muscles in body movement, stores calcium, and produces red blood cells. The muscular system maintains posture, collaborates with the bones in body movement, uses energy, and generates heat. The lymphatic system retrieves fluids leaked from capillaries and contains white blood cells, and parts of it support parts of the immune system.

23. C: The best use of the International System of Units (SI) for this situation would be the use of the micrometer as it is the smallest unit of measurement provided and the scientist is using a microscope to view the insects.

24. B: The respiratory system inhales air, of which oxygen is one component. From that inhaled air, the respiratory system delivers oxygen to the circulatory system through gas exchange. It then removes carbon dioxide (CO_2) from the circulatory system as we exhale. The respiratory system does not create or destroy anything (A, D). It also does not ionize the oxygen (C).

25. D: The name for a substance that stimulates the production of antibodies is an *antigen*. An antigen is any substance perceived by the immune system as dangerous. When the body senses an antigen, it produces an antibody. *Collagen* is one of the components of bone, tendon, and cartilage. It is a spongy protein that can be turned into gelatin by boiling. *Hemoglobin* is the part of red blood cells that carries oxygen. In order for the blood to carry enough oxygen to the cells of the body, there has to be a sufficient amount of hemoglobin. *Lymph* is a near-transparent fluid that performs a number of functions in the body: It removes bacteria from tissues, replaces lymphocytes in the blood, and moves fat away from the small intestine. Lymph contains white blood cells. The lymph *node* is the tissue through which lymph travels in this filtering process.

26. A: The immune system consists of the lymphatic system, spleen, tonsils, thymus, and bone marrow. The nervous system consists of the brain, spinal cord, and nerve cells. The circulatory system consists of the heart, veins, arteries, and capillaries. The respiratory system consists of the nose, trachea, bronchial tubes, lungs, alveolus, and diaphragm.

27. A: Turn it into an "if/then" statement. A formalized hypothesis written in the form of an if/then statement can then be tested. A statement may make a prediction or imply a cause/effect relationship, but that does not necessarily make it a good hypothesis. In this example, the student could rewrite the statement in the form of an if/then statement such as, "If the length of the string of the pendulum is varied, then the time it takes the ball to make one complete period changes." This hypothesis is testable, and doesn't simply make a prediction or a conclusion. The validity of the hypothesis can then be supported or disproved by experimentation and observation.

28. C: The mass of the ball. The mass of the ball is appropriately called a control variable for the experiment. A control or controlled variable is a factor that could be varied, but for testing purposes should remain the same throughout all experiments, otherwise, it could affect the results. In this case, if the mass of the ball was changed, it could also affect the length of the period. The length of the string is meant to be an independent variable, one that is changed during experiments to observe the results upon the dependent variable, which is the variable (or variables) that are affected. In this case, the period would be the dependent variable.

29. B: The substance thymine does not exist in RNA. The bases of RNA include uracil, cytosine, guanine, and adenine.

30. B: Smooth muscle tissue is said to be arranged in a disorderly fashion because it is not striated like the other two types of muscle: cardiac and skeletal. Striations are lines that can only be seen with a microscope. *Smooth* muscle is typically found in the supporting tissues of hollow organs and blood vessels. *Cardiac* muscle is found exclusively in the heart; it is responsible for the contractions that pump blood throughout the body. *Skeletal* muscle, by far the most preponderant in the body, controls the movements of the skeleton. The contractions of skeletal muscle are responsible for all voluntary motion. There is no such thing as *rough* muscle.

31. C: *Melatonin* is produced by the pineal gland. One of the primary functions of melatonin is regulation of the circadian cycle, which is the rhythm of sleep and wakefulness. *Insulin* helps regulate the amount of glucose in the blood. Without insulin, the body is unable to convert blood sugar into energy. *Testosterone* is the main hormone produced by the testes; it is responsible for the development of adult male sex characteristics. *Epinephrine*, also known as adrenaline, performs a number of functions: It quickens and strengthens the heartbeat and dilates the bronchioles. Epinephrine is one of the hormones secreted when the body senses danger.

32. A: The midsagittal plane refers to a lengthwise cut that divides the body into equal right and left portions; it is also called the medial plane. The frontal or coronal plane refers to a cut that divides the body into anterior and posterior sections. The oblique plane is when a cylindrical organ is sectioned with an angular cut across the organ.

33. B: In the development of genetic traits, one gene must match to a protein for a genetic trait to develop correctly.

34. B: Skeletal or striated muscles are voluntary muscles that help support the skeletal structures. Examples of striated muscles are the biceps, triceps, quadriceps, gluteus, and gastrocnemius muscles to name a few. Smooth or involuntary muscles are muscles primarily found in the visceral organs such as the intestines, prostate, reproductive organs, bladder and trachea.

35. B: The vertebral cavity (containing the spine) can be found in the dorsal cavity along with the cranial cavity (containing the brain). The ventral body cavity is divided into several subsections: the thoracic and abdominopelvic cavities. The heart is in the thoracic cavity, the stomach is in the abdominal cavity, and the testes are in the pelvic cavity.

36. D: Solids with a fixed shape have a crystalline order that defines and maintains that shape.

37. B: The diaphragm moves downward or contracts to increase the space in the thoracic cavity. This downward motion inflates the lungs and contracts the ribs. The heart's position does not change during inspiration or expiration.

38. B: The endoplasmic reticulum is the cell's transport network that moves proteins from one part of the cell to another. The Golgi apparatus assists in the transport but is not the actual transport network. Mitochondria are organelles ("tiny organs") that help in the production of ATP, which the cells need to operate properly. The nucleolus participates in the production of ribosomes that are needed to generate proteins for the cell.

39. A: There are four phases of mitosis: the prophase, metaphase, anaphase, and telophase. During the prophase of mitosis, the mitotic spindle fibers begin to form. Next, during the metaphase, the chromosomes line up in the middle of the cell. Next, in the anaphase of mitosis, the chromosomes, originally in pairs, separate and move to the opposite ends of the cells. Then, during the telophase, two nuclei form around the separated chromosomes, each surrounded by a nuclear membrane.

40. A: The table reflects student scores for each quarter. The trend that can be seen in the graph is an increase in scores as the year progressed. The graph label mentions a test review, but there is not enough information about that to know if that is the reason for the scores changing.

41. A: The right lung has three segments: upper, medial and lower. The left lung has two lobes: upper and lower. The lobes are further divided into segments. The right lung comprises ten segments: three in the right upper, two in the right medial lobe, and five in the right lower lobe. The left lung comprises eight segments: four in the left upper lobe and four in the left lower lobe.

42. B: Alveoli are air sacs found within the lung parenchyma and are not part of the cardiac system. The septum is dividing wall between the right and left sides of the heart. The heart has four chambers: the upper two chambers are the right and left atrium and the lower two chambers are the right and left ventricles.

43. A: The physical expression—such as hair color—is the result of the phenotype. The genotype is the basic genetic code. Allele are two or more alternative gene forms that generally arises via mutation, and are located in the same part of a chromosome. A gamete is a germ cell (female or male) that can unite with the opposite sex germ cell in the process of zygote formation of sexual reproduction.

44. B: The endocrine system is made up of the pituitary gland, thyroid gland, parathyroid glands, adrenal glands, pancreas, ovaries, and testicles. They secrete hormones which help regulate mood, growth and development, tissue function, metabolism, and sexual function and reproductive processes. The Pons is located in the brain stem and relays nerve signals that coordinate messages between the brain and the body.

45. D: The heart is located in the thoracic cavity. The thoracic cavity extends from the neck to the diaphragm, which divides the abdominal cavity from the thoracic cavity. Some of the major structures contained in the thoracic cavity are the ribs, heart, lungs, mediastinum, trachea, and the esophagus. The spleen is located in the abdominal cavity. The brain is located in the cranial cavity. The bladder is located in the pelvic cavity.

46. C: The number of 7 is the "breaking point" between basic and acidic. Above 7 solutions are considered basic; below 7 solutions are considered acidic. For instance, milk, with a pH of 6.5, is actually considered acidic. Bleach, with a pH of 12.5, is considered basic.

47. B: The trachea is anterior or ventral to the esophagus. The trachea is separated from the esophagus by the epiglottis, which is a flap of cartilage that covers one while the other is in use. The trachea's proximal portion is connected to the larynx and the distal portion splits off into the right and left bronchi.

48. B: All of the answers use the System of International Units (SI) of measurement with the exception of gallons. A liter is the measurement of a liquid. Grams are a unit of measurement for the weight of an object, which would be measured on the triple beam balance. Meters measure length.

49. B: The transverse plane separates the body into equal upper and lower portions. The oblique plane is when a cylindrical organ is sectioned with an angular cut across the organ. The midsagittal or medial plane refers to a lengthwise cut that divides the body into equal right and left portions. The frontal or coronal plane refers to a cut that divides the body into anterior and posterior sections.

50. C: RNA has several roles, one of which is to act as the messenger and deliver information about the correct sequence of proteins in DNA. The ribosomes do the actual manufacturing of the proteins. Hydrogen, oxygen, and nitrogen work to create the bonds within DNA. And far from having a double helix shape, RNA has what would be considered a more two-dimensional shape.

51. B: Catalysts alter the activation energy during a chemical reaction and therefore control the rate of the reaction. The substrate is the actual surface that enzymes use during a chemical reaction (and there is no such term as *substrate energy*). Inhibitors and promoters participate in the chemical reaction, but it is the activation energy that catalysts alter to control the overall rate as the reaction occurs.

52. C: The stratum basale is the lowest level of the epidermis, which is the surface level. The dermis is a layer of connective tissue immediately beneath the epidermis. The hypodermis, while not a layer of skin, is part of the integumentary system and it is just below the dermis.

53. C: Crossing the corresponding alleles from each parent will yield a result of BB in the upper right box of this Punnett square.

English and Language Usage

1. C: The word *syllabi* is the correct plural form of *syllabus*. The other answer choices reflect incorrect plural forms. Specifically, *syllabus* does not change the form at all, and the Latin root of *syllabus* would require some change. At the same time, *syllaba*—while an accurate plural for some words with Latin roots—is incorrect in this case. And *syllabis* is a double form of the plural, so it cannot be correct.

2. A: The word *independent* is an adjective that modifies the word *state*, describing what kind of state the kingdom of Gwynedd was. The words *century*, *king*, and *control* are all nouns in this context.

3. D: Prefixes, appearing at the beginning of base words to change their meanings. Suffixes appear at the end of words. Prefixes are attached to the beginning of words to change their meanings. *Un+happy, bi+monthly,* and *re+examine* are prefixes that, by definition, change the meanings of the words to which they are attached.

4. C: Answer choice C is correct, because the quotation is a standard quotation (requiring double quotes) as well as a question. Additionally, the question mark belongs inside the quotation marks. Answer choice A correctly places the question mark inside the quotation marks, but the use of single quotes is incorrect for standard quotations. Answer choice B is incorrect, because it places the question mark outside the quotation marks. Answer choice D uses the layered quotes, which are unnecessary in this case, since the sentence presents only one quotation instead of more than one.

5. C: Cause–effect words. Signal words give the reader hints about the purpose of a particular passage. Some signal words are concerned with comparing/contrasting, some with cause and effect, some with temporal sequencing, some with physical location, and some with a problem and its solution. The words *since, whether,* and *accordingly* are words used when describing an outcome. Outcomes have causes.

6. D: *Acceptable* is the correct spelling of the word.

7. C: Answer choice C offers the most effective combination of the sentences with the use of the conjunction *but* and the dependent clause starting with *after*. All other answer choices result in choppy or unclear combinations of the four sentences.

8. D: If Beryl knew something instinctively, it is safe to say that her mother's warning was not stated outright. Therefore, answer choice D is the best option. Answer choice A makes little sense. Answer choice B makes sense only if Beryl suspects her mother does not care whether or not she smokes. Answer choice C has a meaning that is the opposite of the one implied in the sentence.

9. A: Correct punctuation requires a comma after both city and state when both fall within the sentence, even when the city and state fall within an opening dependent clause that has a comma after it. All answer choices that do not have a comma after the state as well as the city are incorrect.

Answer choice C is incorrect because it adds a comma after *Oak* for no clear reason as the name of the city in full is clearly *Oak Ridge*.

10. A: The transition "surprisingly" indicates that the reaction was unexpected, or even contradictory to the circumstance of the speaker not turning his work in on time and talking-out in class. The other answer choices do not make as much sense to coordinate these two sentences.

11. A: The suffix *-ism* here suggests a doctrine that is followed, whether that be the doctrine of polytheism (a religious doctrine), communism (a social doctrine), or nationalism (a political doctrine).

12. C: This version begins with a subject and verb and is followed by a clause. Choice A is incorrect because the words are out of order and don't logically follow the previous sentence. The sentence should begin with 'She says' because it is the school principal's opinion being expressed. This choice is also incorrect because it uses the words *not appropriate* instead of *inappropriate*. Choice B is incorrect because the clause "that students wear to schools" should come after the word *outfits*. Choice D is incorrect because the word order changes the meaning of the sentence by stating that any outfits are distracting and inappropriate.

13. D: The semicolon correctly joins the two sentences. Answer choice A is incorrect, because it uses a comma splice to join two independent clauses. (To join two independent clauses, a comma needs to be accompanied by a coordinating conjunction.) The colon in answer choice B is incorrect because the information in the second clause does not clearly define or explain the previous clause. Answer choice C is incorrect because it offers no punctuation to separate the two independent clauses and thus creates more confusion than clarity.

14. A: A comma should be used to separate the independent clause beginning with *some members* from the non-essential phrase beginning with *which is*. Choice B is incorrect because it is missing the comma. Choice C is incorrect because it incorrectly uses *that* instead of *which*. Choice D is incorrect because it uses a semicolon instead of a comma.

15. B: Answer choice B contains two independent clauses that are joined with a comma and the coordinating conjunction *and*. Answer choice A, though it contains a compound subject and a compound verb, is still a simple sentence. Answer choice C opens with a dependent clause, so it is a complex sentence. Answer choice D is a compound-complex sentence because it includes a dependent clause as well as two independent clauses.

16. B: Answer choice B correctly capitalizes *Uncle Archibald*, where *Uncle Archibald* is used as one whole to a specific name, which makes it a proper noun. If the sentence said "her uncle Archibald," then *uncle* would remain lower case. In answer choice A, the word *cousin* needs no capitalization, because it is used to describe Elaine but is not used as part of her name. (The only distinctions are when the word is used within a direct address or opens a sentence.) Similarly, *mother* and *sister* do not need to be capitalized unless they are the first word of the sentence or are used to directly address someone.

17. D: Within the context of the sentence, it seems as if "*quid pro quo*" means something like "if I do something, then I will be rewarded with something good." Choice A is not a good choice because it says "if I don't do anything, I will get something good." Choice B is inappropriate because money is not mentioned. While choice C might seem like a good choice, the phrase is not put in another way to talk about what people deserve as much as it talks about what people should do or how they should behave. Choice D is the best choice because "something for something" implies the sort of exchange described in the passage.

18. D: The word *affect* is a verb in this context and is the correct usage within the sentence. The possessive pronoun *your* also correctly modifies *children*, so answer choice D is correct. All other answer choices incorrectly apply the words to the sentence.

19. B: The context of the sentence suggests that the trauma of surviving the plane crash left long-term memories that haunted Johanna for many years. As a result, *permanent* is the best meaning of *indelible*. The other meanings make little sense in the context of the sentence. The only possible option is *indirect*, but there is nothing about the sentence to suggest that the nightmares are indirect impressions of a traumatic experience.

20. C: The word *east* in answer choice C is simply a directional indication and does not need to be capitalized in the context of the sentence. All other uses of capitalization are correct in the context of the sentences. The word *South* should be capitalized when it refers to a region of the United States (as indicated by the mention of Mississippi). The word *East* should be capitalized when it refers to the region of Texas. And the word *north* does not need to be capitalized when it is simply a directional indication (as in answer choice D).

21. C: The word *whom* correctly indicates the objective case—as in "to hold him/her responsible"—so answer choice C is correct. The word *who* in answer choice A incorrectly indicates the subjective case. Similarly, answer choice B is incorrect because it incorrectly applies the objective *whom* instead of the subjective *who*. Answer choice D is incorrect because the word *who* is the subjective case (instead of the objective case) here.

22. B: The word *capacity* is a noun in this context, so answer choice B is correct. Because the word functions as the object of the preposition, the options of verb and adverb cannot be correct. Answer choice D is incorrect because the word *capacity* is not a pronoun in any context.

23. C: Answer choice C summarizes the ideas within the sentence simply and clearly. Answer choice A moves the ideas around to make them awkward instead of effective. Answer choice B creates a dangling modifier with the phrase *without adequate preparation*, so it cannot be correct. Similarly, answer choice D makes this phrase a dangling modifier that makes the flow of thought awkward instead of clear.

24. A: The pronoun *all* is plural, so it requires the plural verb *are*. The pronouns *each* and *neither* are singular and require singular verbs (not provided in answer choices B and C). The pronoun *any* can be either singular or plural depending on the context of the sentence. In this case, *any* suggests a singular usage, so answer choice D is incorrect with the plural verb.

25. B: The use of *substantial* in this sentence has a meaning that is closest to "considerable." The other choices are antonyms of *substantial*.

26. D: While answer choice D is arguably the longest of the four sentences, it is actually a simple sentence. It contains a compound subject and a compound verb, but because it represents only one independent clause it still functions as a simple sentence. Answer choices A and B contain two independent clauses and are thus compound sentences. Answer choice C contains a dependent clause, so it is a complex sentence.

27. D: Answer choice D correctly arranges the ideas to reflect the most effective meaning of the sentence. All other answer choices place the ideas in such a way as to create confusion or incorrect punctuation instead of clarity.

28. D: The prefix poly- means "many." A is incorrect because the prefix *poly-* does not mean "few." B is incorrect because the prefix poly- does not mean "several." C is incorrect because the prefix poly- does not mean "none."

TEAS Practice Test #2

Reading		*Mathematics*	*Science*		*English and Language Usage*

Reading

1. _____   46. _____
2. _____   47. _____
3. _____   48. _____
4. _____   49. _____
5. _____   50. _____
6. _____   51. _____
7. _____   52. _____
8. _____   53. _____
9. _____
10. _____
11. _____
12. _____
13. _____
14. _____
15. _____
16. _____
17. _____
18. _____
19. _____
20. _____
21. _____
22. _____
23. _____
24. _____
25. _____
26. _____
27. _____
28. _____
29. _____
30. _____
31. _____
32. _____
33. _____
34. _____
35. _____
36. _____
37. _____
38. _____
39. _____
40. _____
41. _____
42. _____
43. _____
44. _____
45. _____

Mathematics

1. _____
2. _____
3. _____
4. _____
5. _____
6. _____
7. _____
8. _____
9. _____
10. _____
11. _____
12. _____
13. _____
14. _____
15. _____
16. _____
17. _____
18. _____
19. _____
20. _____
21. _____
22. _____
23. _____
24. _____
25. _____
26. _____
27. _____
28. _____
29. _____
30. _____
31. _____
32. _____
33. _____
34. _____
35. _____
36. _____

Science

1. _____   46. _____
2. _____   47. _____
3. _____   48. _____
4. _____   49. _____
5. _____   50. _____
6. _____   51. _____
7. _____   52. _____
8. _____   53. _____
9. _____
10. _____
11. _____
12. _____
13. _____
14. _____
15. _____
16. _____
17. _____
18. _____
19. _____
20. _____
21. _____
22. _____
23. _____
24. _____
25. _____
26. _____
27. _____
28. _____
29. _____
30. _____
31. _____
32. _____
33. _____
34. _____
35. _____
36. _____
37. _____
38. _____
39. _____
40. _____
41. _____
42. _____
43. _____
44. _____
45. _____

English and Language Usage

1. _____
2. _____
3. _____
4. _____
5. _____
6. _____
7. _____
8. _____
9. _____
10. _____
11. _____
12. _____
13. _____
14. _____
15. _____
16. _____
17. _____
18. _____
19. _____
20. _____
21. _____
22. _____
23. _____
24. _____
25. _____
26. _____
27. _____
28. _____

| Reading | Number of Questions: **53** |
| | Time Limit: **64 Minutes** |

At first, the woman's contractions were only <u>intermittent</u>, so the nurse had trouble determining how far her labor had progressed.

1. Which of the following is the definition for the underlined word?

    a. frequent
    b. irregular
    c. painful
    d. dependable

2. Which of the following would be the best source to begin developing a position about civil rights for an oral debate?

    a. A blog created by a proponent of civil rights.
    b. An interview with someone who took part in a civil rights march.
    c. A history textbook detailing civil rights.
    d. A speech by a famous civil rights leader.

The heavy spring rain resulted in a <u>plethora</u> of zucchini in Kit's garden, and left her desperately giving the vegetables to anyone who was interested.

3. Which of the following is the definition for the underlined word in the sentence?

    a. irritation
    b. quantity
    c. abundance
    d. waste

4. The guide words at the top of a dictionary page are *needs* and *negotiate*. Which of the following words is an entry on this page?

    a. needle
    b. neigh
    c. neglect
    d. nectar

The next question is based on the following information.

    <u>Chapter 4: The Fictional Writings of Dorothy L. Sayers</u>

    Plays
    Novels
    Short Stories
    Letters
    Mysteries

5. Analyze the headings above. Which of the following does not belong?

    a. Novels
    b. Plays
    c. Mysteries
    d. Letters

The next three questions are based on the following passage.

Among the first females awarded a degree from Oxford University, Dorothy L. Sayers proved to be one of the most versatile writers in post-war England. Sayers was born in 1893, the only child of an Anglican chaplain, and she received an unexpectedly good education at home. For instance, her study of Latin commenced when she was only six years old. She entered Oxford in 1912, at a time when the university was not granting degrees to women. By 1920, this policy had changed, and Sayers received her degree in medieval literature and modern languages after finishing university. That same year, she also received a master of arts degree.

Sayers's first foray into published writing was a collection of poetry released in 1916. Within a few years, she began work on the detective novels and short stories that would make her famous, due to the creation of the foppish, mystery-solving aristocrat Lord Peter Wimsey. Sayers is also credited with the short story mysteries about the character Montague Egg. In spite of her success as a mystery writer, Sayers continued to balance popular fiction with academic work; her translation of Dante's *Inferno* gained her respect for her ability to convey the poetry in English while still remaining true to the Italian *terza rima*. She also composed a series of twelve plays about the life of Christ, and wrote several essays about education and feminism. In her middle age, Dorothy L. Sayers published several works of Christian apologetics, one of which was so well-received that the archbishop of Canterbury attempted to present her with a doctorate of divinity. Sayers, for reasons known only to her, declined.

6. Which of the following describes the type of writing used to create the passage?

    a. narrative
    b. persuasive
    c. expository
    d. technical

7. Which of the following sentences is the best summary of the passage?

    a. Among the first females awarded a degree from Oxford University, Dorothy L. Sayers proved to be one of the most versatile writers in post-war England.
    b. Sayers was born in 1893, the only child of an Anglican chaplain, and she received an unexpectedly good education at home.
    c. Within a few years, she began work on the detective novels and short stories that would make her famous, due to the creation of the foppish, mystery-solving aristocrat Lord Peter Wimsey.
    d. In her middle age, Dorothy L. Sayers published several works of Christian apologetics, one of which was so well-received that the archbishop of Canterbury attempted to present her with a doctorate of divinity.

8. Which of the following sentences contains an opinion statement by the author?

    a. Among the first females awarded a degree from Oxford University, Dorothy L. Sayers proved to be one of the most versatile writers in post-war England.
    b. Sayers was born in 1893, the only child of an Anglican chaplain, and she received an unexpectedly good education at home.
    c. Her translation of Dante's Inferno gained her respect for her ability to convey the poetry in English while still remaining true to the Italian terza rima.
    d. Sayers, for reasons known only to her, declined.

The next four questions are based on the following information.

The Dewey Decimal Classes

> 000 Computer science, information, and general works
> 100 Philosophy and psychology
> 200 Religion
> 300 Social sciences
> 400 Languages
> 500 Science and mathematics
> 600 Technical and applied science
> 700 Arts and recreation
> 800 Literature
> 900 History, geography, and biography

9. Jorgen is doing a project on the ancient Greek mathematician and poet Eratosthenes. In his initial review, Jorgen learns that Eratosthenes is considered the first person to calculate the circumference of the earth, and that he is considered the first to describe geography as it is studied today. To which section of the library should Jorgen go to find one of the early maps created by Eratosthenes?

> a. 100
> b. 300
> c. 600
> d. 900

10. Due to his many interests and pursuits, Eratosthenes dabbled in a variety of fields, and he is credited with a theory known as the sieve of Eratosthenes. This is an early algorithm used to determine prime numbers. To which section of the library should Jorgen go to find out more about the current applications of the sieve of Eratosthenes?

> a. 000
> b. 100
> c. 400
> d. 500

11. One ancient work claims that Eratosthenes received the nickname "beta" from those who knew him. This is a word that represents the second letter of the Greek alphabet, and it represented Eratosthenes's accomplishments in every area that he studied. To which section of the library should Jorgen go to learn more about the letters of the Greek alphabet and the meaning of the word "beta"?

> a. 200
> b. 400
> c. 700
> d. 900

12. Finally, Jorgen learns that Eratosthenes was fascinated by the story of the Trojan War, and that he attempted to determine the exact dates when this event occurred. Jorgen is unfamiliar with the story of the Fall of Troy, so he decides to look into writings such as *The Iliad* and *The Odyssey*, by Homer. To which section of the library should Jorgen go to locate these works?

    a. 100
    b. 200
    c. 700
    d. 800

13. Which of the answer choices gives the best definition for the underlined word in the following sentence?

With all of the planning that preceded her daughter's wedding, Marci decided that picking out a new paint color for her own living room was largely <u>peripheral</u>.

    a. meaningless
    b. contrived
    c. unimportant
    d. disappointing

The next two questions are based on the following chart.

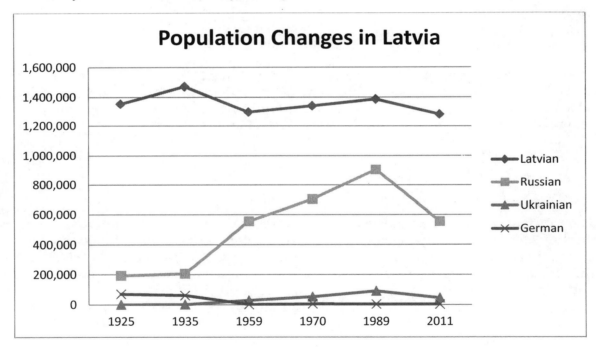

14. Between 1925 and 1991, Latvia was part of the Soviet Union. Since 1991, the population of which ethnic group in Latvia appears to have decreased the most?

    a. Latvian
    b. Russian
    c. Ukrainian
    d. German

15. After World War II ended in 1945, large numbers of non-Latvian workers entered the country, primarily to work at construction jobs. Among these non-Latvian ethnic groups, the increase in workers represented a population percentage shift of less than one percent before 1945 to more than three percent by the time of the Soviet Union's collapse. Which ethnic group shown on the chart best represents this shift?

    a. Latvian
    b. Russian
    c. Ukrainian
    d. German

16. Which answer choice represents the most useful resource for Hilaire in the following vignette?

Hilaire's professor instructed him to improve the word choice in his papers. As the professor noted, Hilaire's ideas are good, but he relies too heavily on simple expressions when a more complex word would be appropriate.

    a. Roget's Thesaurus
    b. Webster's Dictionary
    c. Encyclopedia Britannica
    d. University of Oxford Style Guide

17. Follow the instructions below to transform the starting word into a different word.

- **Start with the word CORPOREAL.**
- **Remove the C from the beginning of the word.**
- **Remove the O from the beginning of the word.**
- **Remove the O from the middle of the word.**
- **Move the E to follow the first R.**
- **Move the L to follow the P.**
- **Remove the second R.**
- **Add the letter Y to the end of the word.**

What is the new word?

    a. REALLY
    b. PRETTY
    c. REPLAY
    d. POWER

18. Which answer choice gives the best definition for the underlined word in the following sentence?

Although not considered the smartest student in her class, Klara was willing to work hard for her grades, and her <u>sedulous</u> commitment to her studies earned her top scores at graduation.

    a. diligent
    b. silent
    c. moderate
    d. complicated

19. Flemming is on a new diet that requires him to avoid all dairy products, as well as dairy byproducts. This will be a big change for him, so his doctor gives him information about foods that he might not realize often contain dairy products. These include bread, granola, deli meat, dry breakfast cereal, and energy bars. Which of the following items from Flemming's standard diet will still be safe to eat?

  a. puffed rice cereal
  b. breaded chicken parmesan
  c. sliced turkey sandwich
  d. yogurt made from coconut milk

The next two questions are based on the following information.

  Car Owner's Manual: Table of Contents:

  Chapter I: Vehicle Instruments
  Chapter II: Safety Options
  Chapter III: Audio, Climate, and Voice Controls
  Chapter IV: Pre-Driving and Driving
  Chapter V: Routine Maintenance
  Chapter VI: Emergencies
  Chapter VII: Consumer Resources

20. To which chapter should Regina turn if she needs to locate information about adjusting the air conditioning in the vehicle?

  a. I
  b. II
  c. III
  d. IV

21. To which chapter should Regina turn if she needs to find out what to do if the car begins overheating?

  a. II
  b. III
  c. IV
  d. VI

22. Of the resource options listed in the answer choices, which would not be considered a reliable, scholarly source for Nora in the following vignette?

Nora is preparing a large research project for the end of the term, and the instructor has required that all students make sure they are using reliable, scholarly resources in their papers.

  a. Encyclopedia Britannica
  b. Wikipedia
  c. Science.gov
  d. LexisNexis

The next five questions are based on the following passage.

In the United States, the foreign language requirement for high school graduation is decided at the state level. This means the requirement varies, with some states deciding to forego a foreign language requirement altogether (www.ncssfl.org). It is necessary that these states reconsider their position and amend their requirements to reflect compulsory completion of a course of one or more foreign languages. Studying a foreign language has become increasingly important for the global economy. As technology continues to make international business relations increasingly easy, people need to keep up by increasing their communication capabilities. High school graduates with foreign language credits have been shown to have an increased college acceptance rate. In addition, students who have mastered more than one language typically find themselves in greater demand when they reach the job market. Students who did not study a foreign language often find themselves unable to obtain a job at all.

23. What is the main idea of this passage?

a. Studying a foreign language will help graduating students find jobs after high school.
b. Studying a foreign language should be a mandatory requirement for high school graduation.
c. Studying a foreign language helps students gain an understanding of other cultures.
d. Studying a foreign language is essential if a student hopes to get into college.

24. Which of the following statements represents the best summary of the claims made in this passage?

a. Studying a foreign language is important if you want to graduate from high school and get a job.
b. Studying a foreign language is important for the global economy because of the technological advances that have been made in international communications.
c. Studying a foreign language is important for the global economy, college acceptance rates, and becoming a sought-after candidate in the job market.
d. Studying a foreign language is important for college acceptance rates and obtaining a job after college.

25. Which of the following statements represents an EXAGGERATED claim in support of the argument presented in this passage?

a. In the United States, the foreign language requirement for high school graduation is decided at the state level.
b. Studying a foreign language has become increasingly important for the global economy.
c. High school graduates with foreign language credits have been shown to have an increased college acceptance rate.
d. Students who did not study a foreign language often find themselves unable to obtain a job at all.

26. Which of the following would be a useful source of information to determine the validity of the argument presented in this passage?

a. A survey of high school students' preferences with regard to foreign language requirements.

b. A comparison of the correlation between a second language introduced at home and subsequent college acceptance rates.

c. A survey that asks parents to select the foreign language they would like their children to study in high school.

d. A comparison of the correlation between high school students' study of a foreign language and subsequent college acceptance rates.

27. Which of the following would be the best concluding statement for this passage?

a. States should consider how important foreign languages are for the global economy when making their policies regarding foreign language requirements for graduation from high school.

b. Policies regarding a foreign language requirement for graduation from high school should take into account the importance of foreign languages for the global economy and the correlation between foreign languages and increased college acceptance rates and employment opportunities.

c. High school graduation requirements should include a foreign language class because of the influence knowledge of a second language has on college acceptance rates.

d. Policies regarding a foreign language requirement for graduation from high school should take into account how difficult it is to obtain a job in today's economy for those who do not have knowledge of more than one language.

The next four questions are based on the following information.

The Big Book of Herbs and Herbal Medicine

Part I: How to Grow Herbs
Chapter 1: Choosing Your Herbs
Chapter 2: Planting Your Herbs
Chapter 3: Caring for Your Herbs

Part II: How to Cook with Herbs
Chapter 4: Herbs in Food
Chapter 5: Herbs in Beverages
Chapter 6: Herbs in Oils and Vinegars

Part III: How to Heal with Herbs
Chapter 7: Herbs for Children's Needs
Chapter 8: Herbs for Adult Needs
     Section 8–A: Women's Needs
     Section 8–B: Men's Needs
Chapter 9: Herbs for Immunity
Chapter 10: Herbs for Respiratory Conditions
Chapter 11: Herbs for Digestive Conditions
Chapter 12: Herbs for Detox
     Section 12–A: Circulatory Conditions
     Section 12–B: Musculoskeletal Conditions
     Section 12–C: Endocrine Conditions
     Section 12–D: Topical Conditions

Part IV: Alphabetical Herb Listing
Chapter 13: Herbs, A–I
Chapter 14: Herbs, J–O
Chapter 15: Herbs, P–Z

28. Clothilde is looking for an herbal remedy to combat a recent outbreak of eczema. In which chapter should she look for more information?

    a. Chapter 8
    b. Chapter 10
    c. Chapter 11
    d. Chapter 12

29. Clothilde's sister has asked her to recommend an herbal therapy for her five-year-old daughter's chronic cough. In which chapter should Clothilde look for more information?

    a. Chapter 7
    b. Chapter 9
    c. Chapter 10
    d. Chapter 12

30. Clothilde's elderberry plant is nearly overgrown, and she is hoping to trim it back and use the elderflower to prepare a blend of tea, as well as a homemade wine. In which chapter should she look for more information about how to do this?

 a. Chapter 3
 b. Chapter 4
 c. Chapter 5
 d. Chapter 13

31. Clothilde realizes that she failed to maintain her elderberry plant as she should have, and she needs tips about how to keep the plant in good condition to avoid another overgrowth. In which chapter should she look for more information?

 a. Chapter 2
 b. Chapter 3
 c. Chapter 13
 d. Chapter 14

The next question is based on the following information.

> LOOKING FOR ROOMMATE – CLEAN HOUSE / QUIET AREA / CLOSE TO UNIVERSITY
> Need one more female roommate for 3-bd house w/in walking distance of univ. Current occupants quiet, house clean/smoke-free. No pets. Long-term applicants preferred. Rent: $800/mo. Utilities/Internet included. Avail: Aug 15. Call Florence at 985-5687, or send an email to f.carpenter@email.com.

32. Florence receives a number of calls about the roommate advertisement. Of the individuals described below, who seems like the best applicant?

 a. Frances is a research assistant in the science department; she has a Yorkshire terrier.
 b. Adelaide works in the humanities department; she is looking for a three-month rental.
 c. Cosette is allergic to cigarette smoke; she needs a quiet place to study.
 d. Felix is a graduate student in the history department; he doesn't have a car.

33. Which answer choice gives the best definition for the underlined word in the following sentence?

Based on the student's <u>florid</u> complexion, Vivienne knew that his nerves were getting the better of him before the debate.

 a. rambling
 b. flushed
 c. unclear
 d. weak

The next two questions are based on the following table.

COMPANY	ENGLISH BREAKFAST	EARL GREY	DARJEELING	OOLONG	GREEN
Tea Heaven	$25	$27	$26	$32	$30
Wholesale Tea	$24	$24	$24	$26	$27
Tea by the Pound	$22	$25	$30	$28	$29
Tea Express	$25	$28	$26	$29	$30

Note: Prices per 16 oz. (1 pound)

34. Noella runs a small tea shop and needs to restock. She is running very low on English Breakfast and Darjeeling tea, and she needs two pounds of each. Which company can offer her the best price on the two blends?

    a. Tea Heaven
    b. Wholesale Tea
    c. Tea by the Pound
    d. Tea Express

35. After reviewing her inventory, Noella realizes that she also needs one pound of Earl Grey and two pounds of green tea. Which company can offer her the best price on these two blends?

    a. Tea Heaven
    b. Wholesale Tea
    c. Tea by the Pound
    d. Tea Express

The next question is based on the following passage.

When people are conducting research, particularly historical research, they usually rely on primary and secondary sources. Primary sources are the more direct type of information. They are accounts of an event that are produced by individuals who were actually present. Some examples of primary sources include a person's diary entry about an event, an interview with an eyewitness, a newspaper article, or a transcribed conversation. Secondary sources are pieces of information that are constructed through the use of other, primary sources. Often, the person who creates the secondary source was not actually present at the event. Secondary sources could include books, research papers, and magazine articles.

36. From the passage it can be assumed that

    a. primary sources are easier to find than secondary sources.
    b. primary sources provide more accurate information than secondary sources.
    c. secondary sources give more accurate information than primary sources.
    d. secondary sources are always used when books or articles are being written.

The next question refers to the following graphic.

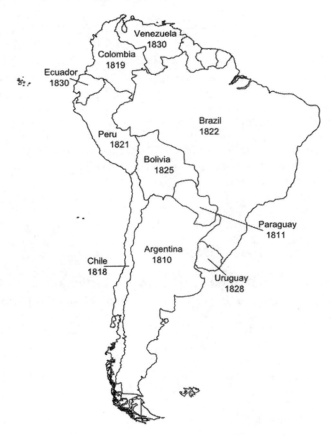

37. The year listed with each country is when the nation gained independence. Which of the following conclusions is true?

a. The nations of North America were also fighting for independence at the same time as nations in South America.

b. France lost most of its control in the New World because of these revolutions.

c. Nations on the west coast gained independence first.

d. South America had many revolutions in the first three decades of the 19th century.

The next two questions are based on the following information.

Dear library patrons:

    To ensure that all visitors have the opportunity to use our limited number of computers, we ask that each person restrict himself or herself to 30 minutes on a computer. For those needing to use a computer beyond this time frame, there will be a $3 charge for each 15-minute period.

We thank you in advance for your cooperation.

Pineville Library

38. Which of the following is a logical conclusion that can be derived from the announcement above?

    a. The library is planning to purchase more computers, but cannot afford them yet.

    b. The library is facing budget cuts, and is using the Internet fee to compensate for them.

    c. The library has added the fee to discourage patrons from spending too long on the computers.

    d. The library is offsetting its own Internet service costs by passing on the fee to patrons.

39. Raoul has an upcoming school project, and his own computer is not working. He needs to use the library computer, and he has estimated that he will need to be on the computer for approximately an hour and a half. How much of a fee can Raoul expect to pay for his computer use at the library?

    a. $6

    b. $9

    c. $12

    d. $15

The next question is based on the following passage.

    Victims of Marah's disease, a virtually unknown neurological condition, appear pain-free and content. Often, they also have a desire to engage in vigorous physical activities such as contact sports. Beneath it all, they are in great physical pain but have an inability to express it or act to reduce it, making diagnosis difficult. As a result, they are inaccurately diagnosed as very low on the pain scale, their discomfort level much lower than victims of severe sprains, despite the fact that sprains, although more painful, are temporary and comparatively easy to manage nature.

40. This passage makes the argument that

    a. the pain scale is not an accurate or adequate way to measure the physical discomfort of certain people, such as those suffering from Marah's disease

    b. sprain victims have more intense pain than Marah's sufferers, but they can manage their pain more easily

    c. the pain scale seems to put more emphasis on intensity of pain than duration

    d. victims of Marah's syndrome are often unable to deal effectively with their discomfort

The next question is based on the following passage.

    There is a clear formula that many students are taught when it comes to writing essays. The first is to develop an introduction, which outlines what will be discussed in the work. It also includes the thesis statement. Next come the supporting paragraphs. Each paragraph contains a topic sentence, supporting evidence, and finally a type of mini-conclusion that restates the point of the paragraph. Finally, the conclusion sums up the purpose of the paper and emphasizes that the thesis statement was proven.

41. After the topic sentence,

    a. a thesis statement is included.

    b. supporting evidence is presented.

    c. the conclusion is stated.

    d. the author outlines what will be discussed.

The next question is based on the following passage.

At one time, the use of leeches to treat medical problems was quite common. If a person suffered from a snake bite or a bee sting, leeches were believed to be capable of removing the poison from the body if they were placed on top of the wound. They have also been used for bloodletting and to stop hemorrhages, although neither of these leech treatments would be considered acceptable by present-day physicians. Today, leeches are still used on a limited basis. Most often, leeches are used to drain blood from clogged veins. This results in little pain for the patient and also ensures the patient's blood will not clot while it is being drained.

42. The main purpose of the passage is

a. to discuss the benefits of using leeches to treat blocked veins.
b. to give an overview of how leeches have been used throughout history.
c. to compare which uses of leeches are effective and which are not.
d. to explain how leeches can be used to remove poison from the body.

The next two questions are based on the following passage.

For lunch, she likes ham and cheese (torn into bites), yogurt, raisins, applesauce, peanut butter sandwiches in the fridge drawer, or any combo of these. She's not a huge eater. Help yourself too. Bread is on counter if you want to make a sandwich.

It's fine if you want to go somewhere, leave us a note of where you are. Make sure she's buckled and drive carefully! Certain fast food places are fun if they have playgrounds and are indoors. It's probably too hot for playground, but whatever you want to do is fine. Take a sippy cup of water and a diaper wherever you go. There's some money here for you in case you decide to go out for lunch with her.

As for nap, try after lunch. She may not sleep, but try anyway. Read her a couple of books first, put cream on her mosquito bites (it's in the den on the buffet), then maybe rock in her chair. Give her a bottle of milk, and refill as needed, but don't let her drink more than $2\frac{1}{2}$ bottles of milk or she'll throw up. Turn on music in her room, leave her in crib with a dry diaper and bottle to try to sleep. She likes a stuffed animal too. Try for 30–45 minutes. You may have to start the tape again. If she won't sleep, that's fine. We just call it "rest time" on those days that naps won't happen.

43. To whom is this passage probably being written?

a. a mother
b. a father
c. a babysitter
d. a nurse

44. You can assume the writer of the passage is:

a. a mom
b. a dad
c. a teacher
d. a parent

The next two questions are based on the following passage.

Volleyball is easy to learn and fun to play in a physical education class. With just one net and one ball, an entire class can participate. The object of the game is to get the ball over the net and onto the ground on the other side. At the same time, all players should be in the ready position to keep the ball from hitting the ground on their own side. After the ball has been served, the opposing team may have three hits to get the ball over the net to the other side. Only the serving team may score. If the receiving team wins the volley, the referee calls, "side out" and the receiving team wins the serve. Players should rotate positions so that everyone gets a chance to serve. A game is played to 15 points, but the winning team must win by two points. That means if the score is 14 to 15, the play continues until one team wins by two. A volleyball match consists of three games. The winner of the match is the team that wins two of the three games.

45. Who can score in a volleyball game?

a. the receiving team
b. the serving team
c. either team
d. there is no score

46. How many people can participate in a volleyball game?

a. 14
b. 15
c. half of a class
d. an entire class

The next five questions are based on the following passage.

Global warming and the depletion of natural resources are constant threats to the future of our planet. All people have a responsibility to be proactive participants in the fight to save Earth by working now to conserve resources for later. Participation begins with our everyday choices. From what you buy to what you do to how much you use, your decisions affect the planet and everyone around you. Now is the time to take action.

When choosing what to buy, look for sustainable products made from renewable or recycled resources. The packaging of the products you buy is just as important as the products themselves. Is the item minimally packaged in a recycled container? How did the product reach the store? Locally grown food and other products manufactured within your community are the best choices. The fewer miles a product traveled to reach you, the fewer resources it required.

You can continue to make a difference for the planet in how you use what you bought and the resources you have available. Remember the locally grown food you purchased? Don't pile it on your plate at dinner. Food that remains on your plate is a wasted resource, and you can always go back for seconds. You should try to be aware of your consumption of water and energy. Turn off the water when you brush your teeth, and limit your showers to five minutes. Turn off the lights, and don't leave appliances or chargers plugged in when not in use.

Together, we can use less, waste less, recycle more, and make the right choices. It may be the only chance we have.

47. What is the author's tone?

a. The author's tone is optimistic.
b. The author's tone is pessimistic.
c. The author's tone is matter-of-fact.
d. The author's tone is angry.

48. Why does the author say it is important to buy locally grown food?

a. Buying locally grown food supports people in your community.
b. Locally grown food travels the least distance to reach you, and therefore uses fewer resources.
c. Locally grown food uses less packaging.
d. Locally grown food is healthier for you because it has been exposed to fewer pesticides.

49. What does the author imply will happen if people do not follow his suggestions?

a. The author implies we will run out of resources in the next 10 years.
b. The author implies water and energy prices will rise sharply in the near future.
c. The author implies global warming and the depletion of natural resources will continue.
d. The author implies local farmers will lose their farms.

50. "You should try to be aware of your consumption of water and energy."

What does the word "consumption" mean in the context of this selection?

a. Using the greatest amount
b. Illness of the lungs
c. Using the least amount
d. Depletion of goods

51. The author makes a general suggestion to the reader: "You should try to be aware of your consumption of water and energy." Which of the following is one way the author specifies that this suggestion be carried out?

a. Food that remains on your plate is a wasted resource, and you can always go back for a second helping.
b. Locally grown food and other products manufactured within your community are the best choices.
c. Turn off the lights, and don't leave appliances or chargers plugged in when not in use.
d. Participation begins with our everyday choices.

The next question is based on the following passage.

The butterfly effect is a somewhat poorly understood mathematical concept, primarily because it is interpreted and presented incorrectly by the popular media. It refers to systems, and how initial conditions can influence the ultimate outcome of an event. The best way to understand the concept is through an example. You have two rubber balls. There are two inches between them, and you release them. Where will they end up? Well, that depends. If they're in a sloped, sealed container, they will end up two inches away from each other at the end of the slope. If it's the top of a mountain, however, they may end up miles away from each other. They could bounce off rocks; one could get stuck in a snow bank while the other continues down the slope; one could enter a river and get swept away. The fact that even a tiny initial difference can have a significant overall impact is known as the butterfly effect.

52. The purpose of this passage is:
   a. To discuss what could happen to two rubber balls released on top of a mountain.
   b. To show why you can predict what will happen to two objects in a sloped, sealed container.
   c. To discuss the primary reason why the butterfly effect is a poorly understood concept.
   d. To give an example of how small changes at the beginning of an event can have large effects.

The next question refers to the following graphic.

THE ROYAL FAMILY

QUEEN VICTORIA *m.* PRINCE ALBERT of Saxe-Coburg and Gotha
1840

Victoria, Princess Royal (Empress Frederick of Germany) born 1840

Prince Alfred, Duke of Edinburgh (Duke of Saxe-Coburg and Gotha) born 1844

Princess Louise (Duchess of Argyll) born 1848

Princess Beatrice (Princess Henry of Battenberg) born 1857

Prince Arthur (Duke of Connaught) born 1850

Princess Alice (Grand Duchess of Hesse) born 1843

Princess Helena (Princess Christian of Schleswig-Holstein) born 1846

Prince Leopold (Duke of Albany) born 1853

Albert Edward, Prince of Wales, *m.* Princess Alexandra born 1841   1863   of Denmark (King Edward VII)

Albert Victor (Duke of Clarence) born 1864

George Frederick, Prince of Wales, born 1865 (King George V), *m.*, 1893, Princess Victoria Mary of Teck

Princess Louise (Duchess of Fife) born 1867

Princess Victoria born 1868

Princess Maud (Queen of Norway) born 1869

Prince Alexander born 1870

53. In what way is the family tree organized?
   a. The oldest generation at the bottom, and the youngest generation at the top.
   b. The youngest children on right and the oldest children on the left.
   c. The youngest children on the left and the oldest children on the right.
   d. The grandparents (Queen Victoria and Prince Albert) are on the top, followed by their children, grandchildren, and great-grandchildren on the bottom layers.

| **Mathematics** | Number of Questions: **36** |
| | Time Limit: **54 Minutes** |

1. Within a certain nursing program, 25% of the class wanted to work with infants, 60% of the class wanted to work with the elderly, 10% of the class wanted to assist general practitioners in private practices, and the rest were undecided. What fraction of the class wanted to work with the elderly?

    a. $\frac{1}{4}$

    b. $\frac{1}{10}$

    c. $\frac{3}{5}$

    d. $\frac{1}{20}$

2. Veronica has to create the holiday schedule for the neonatal unit at her hospital. She knows that 35% of the staff members will not be available because they are taking vacation days during the holiday. Of the remaining staff members who will be available, only 20% are certified to work in the neonatal unit. What percentage of the TOTAL staff is certified and available to work in the neonatal unit during the holiday?

    a. 7%
    b. 13%
    c. 65%
    d. 80%

3. A patient requires a 30% decrease in the dosage of his medication. His current dosage is 340 mg. What will his dosage be after the decrease?

    a. 70 mg
    b. 238 mg
    c. 270 mg
    d. 340 mg

4. A study about anorexia was conducted on 100 patients. Within that patient population 70% were women, and 10% of the men were overweight as children. How many male patients in the study were NOT overweight as children?

    a. 3
    b. 10
    c. 27
    d. 30

5. University Q has an extremely competitive nursing program. Historically, $\frac{3}{4}$ of the students in each incoming class major in nursing but only $\frac{1}{5}$ of those who major in nursing actually complete the program. If this year's incoming class has 100 students, how many students will complete the nursing program?

    a. 75
    b. 20
    c. 15
    d. 5

The next two questions are based on the following information.

> Four nurse midwives open a joint practice together. They use a portion of the income to pay for various expenses for the practice. Each nurse midwife contributes $2000 per month.

6. The first midwife uses $\frac{2}{5}$ of her monthly contribution to pay the rent and utilities for the office space. She saves half of the remainder for incidental expenditures, and uses the rest of the money to purchase medical supplies. How much money does she spend on medical supplies each month?

    a. $600
    b. $800
    c. $1000
    d. $1200

7. The second midwife allocates $\frac{1}{2}$ of her funds to pay an office administrator, plus another $\frac{1}{10}$ for office supplies. What is the total fraction of the second midwife's budget that is spent on the office administrator and office supplies?

    a. $\frac{3}{5}$
    b. $\frac{2}{12}$
    c. $\frac{2}{20}$
    d. $\frac{1}{20}$

8. A mathematics test has a 4:2 ratio of data analysis problems to algebra problems. If the test has 18 algebra problems, how many data analysis problems are on the test?

    a. 24
    b. 28
    c. 36
    d. 38

9. Jonathan pays a $65 monthly flat rate for his cell phone. He is charged $0.12 per minute for each minute used, in a roaming area. Which of the following expressions represents his monthly cell phone bill for x roaming minutes?

    a. $65 + 0.12x$
    b. $65x + 0.12$
    c. $65.12x$
    d. $65.12 + 0.12x$

10. Robert is planning to drive 1,800 miles on a cross-country trip. If his car gets 30 miles to the gallon, and his tank holds 12 gallons of gas, how many tanks of gas will he need to complete the trip?

    a. 3 tanks of gas
    b. 5 tanks of gas
    c. 30 tanks of gas
    d. 60 tanks of gas

11. A patient was taking 310 mg of antidepressant each day. However, the doctor determined that this dosage was too high and reduced the dosage by a fifth. Further observation revealed the dose was still too high, so he reduced it again by 20 mg. What is the final dosage of the patient's antidepressant?

    a. 20 mg
    b. 42 mg
    c. 228 mg
    d. 248 mg

12. A lab technician took 100 hairs from a patient to conduct several tests. The technician used $\frac{1}{7}$ of the hairs for a drug test. How many hairs were used for the drug test? Round your answer to the nearest hundredth.

    a. 14.00
    b. 14.20
    c. 14.29
    d. 14.30

13. What kind of association does the scatter plot show?

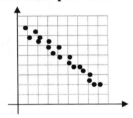

    a. Positive, Linear Association
    b. Negative, Linear Association
    c. Non-linear Association
    d. No association can be determined

14. Joshua has to earn more than 92 points on the state test in order to qualify for an academic scholarship. Each question is worth 4 points, and the test has a total of 30 questions. Let x represent the number of test questions. Which of the following inequalities can be solved to determine the number of questions Joshua must answer correctly?

    a. $4x < 30$
    b. $4x < 92$
    c. $4x > 30$
    d. $4x > 92$

15. Susan decided to celebrate getting her first nursing job by purchasing a new outfit. She bought a dress for $69.99 and a pair of shoes for $39.99. She also bought accessories for $34.67. What was the total cost of Susan's outfit, including accessories?

    a. $69.99
    b. $75.31
    c. $109.98
    d. $144.65

16. Given the histograms shown below, which of the following statements is true?

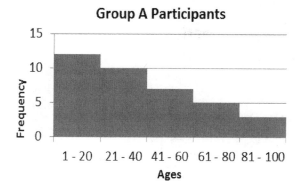

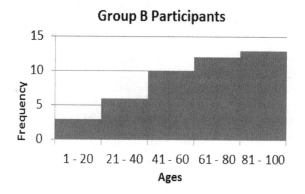

a. Group A is negatively skewed and has a mean that is less than the mean of Group B.
b. Group A is positively skewed and has a mean that is more than the mean of Group B.
c. Group B is negatively skewed and has a mean that is more than the mean of Group A.
d. Group B is positively skewed and has a mean that is less than the mean of Group A.

17. Complete the following equation:

$$2 + (2)(2) - 2 \div 2 = ?$$

a. 5
b. 3
c. 2
d. 1

18. Which of the following is listed in order from *least to greatest*?

a. $-2, -\frac{3}{4}, -0.45, 3\%, 0.36$
b. $-\frac{3}{4}, -0.45, -2, 0.36, 3\%$
c. $-0.45, -2, -\frac{3}{4}, 3\%, 0.36$
d. $-2, -\frac{3}{4}, -0.45, 0.36, 3\%$

19. As part of a study, a set of patients will be divided into three groups: $\frac{4}{15}$ of the patients will be in Group Alpha, $\frac{2}{5}$ of the patients will be in Group Beta, and $\frac{1}{3}$ of the patients will be in Group Gamma. Order the groups from smallest to largest, according to the number of patients in each group.

a. Group Alpha, Group Beta, Group Gamma
b. Group Alpha, Group Gamma, Group Beta
c. Group Gamma, Group Alpha, Group Beta
d. Group Gamma, Group Beta, Group Alpha

20. Solve for *x*:

$$2x + 6 = 14$$

    a. $x = 4$
    b. $x = 8$
    c. $x = 10$
    d. $x = 13$

21. In the 2008 Olympic Games, the semifinal heat for the Women's 200m event had the following results:

Time (in seconds)
22.33
22.50
22.50
22.61
22.71
22.72
22.83
23.22

What was the mean time for the women who ran this 200m event?

    a. 22.50 sec
    b. 22.66 sec
    c. 22.68 sec
    d. 22.77 sec

22. During week 1, Nurse Cameron worked 5 shifts. During week 2, she worked twice as many shifts as she did during week 1. During week 3, she added 4 shifts to the number of shifts she worked during week 2. Which equation below describes the number of shifts Nurse Cameron worked during week 3?

    a. shifts $= (2)(5) + 4$
    b. shifts $= (4)(5) + 2$
    c. shifts $= 5 + 2 + 4$
    d. shifts $= (5)(2)(4)$

23. Simplify the following expression:

$$(3)(-4) + (3)(4) - 1$$

    a. −1
    b. 1
    c. 23
    d. 24

24. How many cubic inches of water could this aquarium hold if it were filled completely?

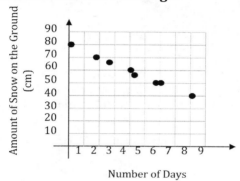

12 *in*

10 *in*

30 *in*

    a. 3600 cubic inches
    b. 52 cubic inches
    c. 312 cubic inches
    d. 1144 cubic inches

25. What statement best describes the rate of change?

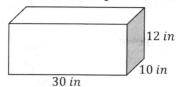

Number of Days

    a. Every day, the snow melts 10 centimeters.
    b. Every day, the snow melts 5 centimeters.
    c. Every day, the snow increases by 10 centimeters.
    d. Every day, the snow increases by 5 centimeters.

26. What are the dependent and independent variables in the graph below?

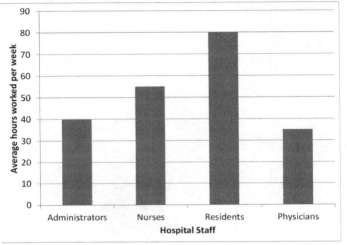

a. The dependent variable is Nurses. The independent variable is Physicians.
b. The dependent variable is Physicians. The independent variable is Nurses.
c. The dependent variable is Hospital Staff. The independent variable is Average hours worked per week.
d. The dependent variable is Average hours worked per week. The independent variable is Hospital Staff.

27. How many milligrams are in 5 grams?

a. 0.005 mg
b. 50 mg
c. 500 mg
d. 5000 mg

28. 9.5% of the people in a town voted for a certain proposition in a municipal election. If the town's population is 51,623, about how many people in the town voted for the proposition?

a. 3,000
b. 5,000
c. 7,000
d. 10,000

29. A charter bus driver drove at an average speed of 65 mph for 305 miles. If he stops at a gas station for 15 minutes, then drives another 162 miles at an average speed of 80 mph, how long, will it have been since he began the trip?

a. 0.96 hours
b. 6.44 hours
c. 6.69 hours
d. 6.97 hours

30. A box in the form of a rectangular solid has a square base of 5 feet in length, a width of 5 feet, and a height of h feet. If the volume of the rectangular solid is 200 cubic feet, which of the following equations may be used to find h?

    a. $5h = 200$
    b. $5h^2 = 200$
    c. $25h = 200$
    d. $h = 200 \div 5$

31. Two even integers and one odd integer are multiplied together. Which of the following could be their product?

    a. 3.75
    b. 9
    c. 16.2
    d. 24

32. There are $\frac{80\ mg}{0.8\ ml}$ in Acetaminophen Concentrated Infant Drops. If the proper dosage for a four-year-old child is 240 mg, how many milliliters should the child receive?

    a. 0.8 mL
    b. 1.6 mL
    c. 2.4 mL
    d. 3.2 mL

33. Using the chart below, which equation describes the relationship between x and y?

x	y
2	6
3	9
4	12
5	15

    a. $x = 3y$
    b. $y = 3x$
    c. $y = \frac{1}{3}x$
    d. $\frac{x}{y} = 3$

34. On a highway map, the scale indicates that 1 inch represents 45 miles. If the distance on the map is 3.2 inches, how far is the actual distance?

    a. 45 miles
    b. 54 miles
    c. 112 miles
    d. 144 miles

35. Andy has already saved $15. He plans to save $28 per month. Which of the following equations represents the amount of money he will have saved?

    a. $y = 15 + 28x$
    b. $y = 43x + 15$
    c. $y = 43x$
    d. $y = 28 + 15x$

36. Given the double bar graph shown below, which of the following statements is true?

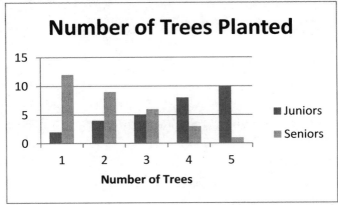

a. The number of trees planted by the Juniors is positively skewed, while the number of trees planted by the Seniors is approximately normal.

b. The number of trees planted by the Juniors is negatively skewed, while the number of trees planted by the Seniors is positively skewed.

c. The number of trees planted by the Juniors is positively skewed, while the number of trees planted by the Seniors is negatively skewed.

d. The number of trees planted by the Juniors is approximately normal, while the number of trees planted by the Juniors is positively skewed.

Science	Number of Questions: **53**
	Time Limit: **63 Minutes**

1. Which of the following is NOT a function of the circulatory system?

a. Pumping blood throughout the body to provide tissues and organs with nutrients and oxygen.
b. Removing toxins and waste from the blood
c. Transmitting nerve impulses between the brain and the rest of the body.
d. Transporting important hormones released from glands to their sites of action.

2. Which item below is NOT a disease of the digestive system?

a. Crohn's disease.
b. Diabetes.
c. Ulcerative colitis.
d. Diverticulosis.

3. Which item below best describes the primary function of the nervous system?

a. The nervous system is the center of communication in the body.
b. The nervous system is primarily responsible for helping the body breathe.
c. The nervous system transports blood throughout the body.
d. The nervous system helps the body break down food.

4. Which of the following is NOT an element of the respiratory system?

a. Ribs.
b. Trachea.
c. Diaphragm.
d. Alveoli.

5. Which of the following cells is NOT part of the immune system?

a. Neurons.
b. Dendritic cells.
c. Macrophages.
d. Mast cells.

6. Which of the following is NOT one of the major types of bones in the human body?

a. Dense bone.
b. Long bone.
c. Short bone.
d. Irregular bone.

7. Which of the following bone types is embedded in tendons?

a. Long bones.
b. Sesamoid bones.
c. Flat bones.
d. Vertical bones.

8. Two nursing students will be completing a scientific experiment measuring the mass of chewed gum after one-minute chewing increments. Which lab equipment will the students most likely use?

    a. Triple beam balance.
    b. Anemometer.
    c. Hot plate.
    d. Microscope.

9. Which of the following is not a product of respiration?

    a. Carbon dioxide.
    b. Water.
    c. Oxygen.
    d. ATP.

10. Of the following, the blood vessel containing the least-oxygenated blood is:

    a. the aorta.
    b. the vena cava.
    c. the pulmonary artery.
    d. the capillaries.

11. Which layer of the heart contains striated muscle fibers for contraction of the heart?

    a. Pericardium.
    b. Epicardium.
    c. Endocardium.
    d. Myocardium.

12. Which blood vessel carries oxygenated blood back to the heart?

    a. Pulmonary vein.
    b. Pulmonary artery.
    c. Aorta.
    d. Superior vena cava.

13. Mrs. Jones's class conducted an experiment on the effects of sugar and artificial sweetener on the cookie recipe's overall color when baked. What would be the independent variable in the cookie experiment?

    a. The students should use the same ingredients in both recipes, but bake the cookies with sugar at 450 degrees and those with artificial sweetener at 475 degrees. They should increase the baking time on the artificial sweetener cookies, since the package instructs them to do so.
    b. The students should use the same ingredients in both recipes, but increase the baking time on the artificial sweetener cookies, since the package instructs them to do so.
    c. The students should use the same ingredients, same baking temperatures, and same baking times for both recipes.
    d. The students should use the same ingredients and baking times in both recipes, but bake the cookies with sugar at 450 degrees and the artificial sweetener cookies at 475 degrees.

14. Which part of the cell is often called the cell "power house" because it provides energy for cellular functions?

a. Nucleus.
b. Cell membrane.
c. Mitochondria.
d. Cytoplasm.

15. What function do ribosomes serve within the cell?

a. Ribosomes are responsible for cell movement.
b. Ribosomes aid in protein synthesis.
c. Ribosomes help protect the cell from its environment.
d. Ribosomes have enzymes that help with digestion.

16. What is the most likely reason that cells differentiate?

a. Cells differentiate to avoid looking like all the cells around them.
b. Cells differentiate so that simple, non-specialized cells can become highly specialized cells.
c. Cells differentiate so that multicellular organisms will remain the same size.
d. Cells differentiate for no apparent reason.

17. How is meiosis similar to mitosis?

a. Both produce daughter cells that are genetically identical.
b. Both produce daughter cells that are genetically different.
c. Both occur in humans, animals, and plants.
d. Both occur asexually.

18. In the suburban neighborhood of Northwoods, there have been large populations of deer, and residents have complained about them eating flowers and garden plants. What would be a logical explanation, based on observations, for the large increase in the deer population over the last two seasons?

a. Increased quantity of food sources in surrounding areas.
b. Decreased population of a natural predator in Northwoods.
c. Deer migration from surrounding areas.
d. Increase in hunting licenses sold.

19. How do DNA and RNA function together as part of the human genome?

a. DNA carries genetic information from RNA to the cell cytoplasm.
b. RNA carries genetic information from DNA to the cell cytoplasm.
c. DNA and RNA carry genetic information from the cell nucleus to the cytoplasm.
d. DNA and RNA do not interact within the cell.

20. The majority of nutrient absorption occurs in the:

a. mouth.
b. stomach.
c. small intestine.
d. large intestine.

21. What process should the DNA within a cell undergo before cell replication?

a. The DNA should quadruple so that daughter cells have more than enough DNA material after cell division.

b. The DNA should triple so that daughter cells have three times the amount of DNA material after cell division.

c. The DNA should replicate so that daughter cells have the same amount of DNA material after cell division.

d. The DNA should split so that daughter cells have half the amount of DNA material after cell division.

22. What basic molecular unit enables hereditary information to be transmitted from parent to offspring?

a. Genes.

b. Blood.

c. Traits.

d. Cell.

23. Which statement most accurately compares and contrasts the structures of DNA and RNA?

a. Both DNA and RNA have 4 nucleotide bases. Three of the bases are the same but the fourth base is thymine in DNA and uracil in RNA.

b. Both DNA and RNA have the same 4 nucleotide bases. However, the nucleotides bond differently in the DNA when compared to RNA.

c. Both DNA and RNA have 6 nucleotide bases. However, the shape of DNA is a triple helix and the shape of RNA is a double helix.

d. Both DNA and RNA have a double helix structure. However, DNA contains 6 nucleotide bases and RNA contains 4 nucleotide bases.

24. Which of the following characteristics is part of a person's genotype?

a. Brown eyes that appear hazel in the sunlight.

b. CFTR genes that causes cystic fibrosis.

c. Black hair that grows rapidly.

d. Being a fast runner.

The next two questions are based on the following information.

Let *B* represent the dominant gene for a full head of hair, and let *b* represent the recessive gene for male pattern baldness. The following Punnett square represents the offspring of two people with recessive genes for baldness.

	B	**b**
B	Possibility 1	Possibility 2
b	Possibility 3	Possibility 4

25. According to the Punnett square, which selection includes all outcomes that would produce an offspring with male pattern baldness?

a. Possibility 1.

b. Possibility 4.

c. Possibilities 1, 2, and 3.

d. Possibilities 2, 3, and 4.

26. According to the Punnett square, which selection includes all outcomes that would produce an offspring with a full head of hair?

    a. Possibility 1.
    b. Possibility 4.
    c. Possibilities 1, 2, and 3.
    d. Possibilities 2, 3, and 4.

27. Where is the interstitial fluid found?

    a. In the blood and lymphatic vessels.
    b. In the tissues around cells.
    c. In the cells.
    d. In the ventricles of the brain.

28. Which type of cell secretes antibodies?

    a. Bacterial cell.
    b. Viral cell.
    c. Lymph cell.
    d. Plasma cells.

29. Chemical C is a catalyst in the reaction between chemical A and chemical B. What is the effect of chemical C?

    a. Chemical C increases the rate of the reaction between A and B.
    b. Chemical C decreases the rate of the reaction between A and B.
    c. Chemical C initiates the reaction between A and B.
    d. Chemical C converts A from a base to an acid.

30. What type of molecules are enzymes?

    a. Water molecules.
    b. Protein molecules.
    c. Tripolar molecules.
    d. Inorganic molecules.

31. Which structure controls the hormones secreted by the pituitary gland?

    a. Hypothalamus.
    b. Adrenal gland.
    c. Testes.
    d. Pancreas.

32. Where does gas exchange occur in the human body?

    a. Alveoli.
    b. Bronchi.
    c. Larynx.
    d. Pharynx.

33. All of the following are parts of the respiratory system EXCEPT the:

    a. trachea.
    b. bronchi.
    c. esophagus.
    d. larynx.

34. What lab equipment would most likely be used to measure a liquid solution?

a. Flask.
b. Triple beam balance.
c. Graduated cylinder.
d. Test tube.

35. An atom has 5 protons, 5 neutrons, and 6 electrons. What is the electric charge of this atom?

a. Neutral.
b. Positive.
c. Negative.
d. Undetermined.

36. All of the following are components of the genitourinary system EXCEPT:

a. the kidneys.
b. the urethra.
c. the rectum.
d. the bladder.

37. Which of the following best describes the structures found underneath each rib in descending order?

a. Vein, nerve, artery.
b. Artery, vein, nerve.
c. Vein, artery, nerve.
d. Nerve, vein, artery.

The table below contains information from the periodic table of elements.

Element	Atomic number	Approximate atomic weight
H	1	1
He	2	4
Li	3	7
Be	4	9

38. Which pattern below best describes the elements listed in the table?

a. The elements are arranged in order by weight with H being the heaviest atom and Be being the lightest atom.
b. The elements are arranged in order by electron charge with H having the most electrons and Be having the fewest electrons.
c. The elements are arranged in order by protons with H having the most protons and Be having the fewest protons.
d. The elements are arranged in order by protons with H having the fewest protons and Be having the most protons.

39. Which of the following is true regarding the primary function of the spleen?

a. It produces bile to emulsify fats.
b. It filters microorganisms and other foreign substances from the blood.
c. It helps control blood glucose levels and regulates blood pressure.
d. It regulates blood clotting factors.

40. The process of changing from a liquid to a gas is called _____.

a. freezing
b. condensation
c. vaporization
d. sublimation

41. A nurse wants to investigate how different environmental factors affect her patients' body temperatures. Which tool would be the most helpful when the nurse conducts her investigation?

a. Scale.
b. Yard stick.
c. Thermometer.
d. Blood pressure monitor.

42. A scientific study has over 2000 data points. Which of the following methods is most likely to help the researcher gain usable information from the data?

a. Use statistical analysis to understand trends in the data.
b. Look at each individual data point, and try to create a trend.
c. Eliminate 90% of the data so that the sample size is more manageable.
d. Stare at the data until a pattern pops out.

The next question is based on the following information.

Many years ago, people believed that flies were created from spoiled food because spoiled food that was left out in the open often contained fly larvae. So a scientist placed fresh food in a sealed container for an extended period of time. The food spoiled, but no fly larvae were found in the food that was sealed.

43. Based on this evidence, what is the most likely reason that spoiled food left out in the open often contained fly larvae?

a. The spoiled food evolved into fly larvae.
b. Since the food was left out in the open, flies would lay eggs in the food.
c. Fly larvae were spontaneously generated by the spoiled food.
d. People only imagined they saw fly larvae in the spoiled food.

44. The average life expectancy in the 21st century is about 75 years. The average life expectancy in the 19th century was about 40 years. What is a possible explanation for the longer life expectancy in the present age?

a. Advances in medical technology enable people to live longer.
b. Knowledge about how basic cleanliness can help avoid illness has enabled people to live longer.
c. The creation of various vaccines has enabled people to live longer.
d. All of the statements above offer reasonable explanations for longer life expectancy.

45. A doctor needs to convince his boss to approve a test for a patient. Which statement below best communicates a scientific argument that justifies the need for the test?

a. The patient looks like he needs this test.
b. The doctor feels that the patient needs this test.
c. The patient's symptoms and health history suggest that this test will enable the correct diagnosis to help the patient.
d. The patient has excellent insurance that will pay for several tests, and the doctor would like to run as many tests as possible.

46. Which of the following is a protein that interferes with virus production?

a. Lysozyme.
b. Prion.
c. Interferon.
d. Keratin.

47. Which of the following does not contain blood vessels?

a. Hyperdermis.
b. Hypodermis.
c. Dermis.
d. Epidermis.

48. What structure is responsible for the release of hormones that stimulate the gonads during puberty?

a. Hypothalamus.
b. Midbrain.
c. Basal ganglia.
d. Hippocampus.

49. Which of the following structures has the lowest blood pressure?

a. Arteries.
b. Arteriole.
c. Venule.
d. Vein.

50. Which of the heart chambers is the most muscular?

a. Left atrium.
b. Right atrium.
c. Left ventricle.
d. Right ventricle.

51. Which part of the brain interprets sensory information?

a. Cerebrum.
b. Hindbrain.
c. Cerebellum.
d. Medulla oblongata.

52. A vaccination is a way of acquiring which type of immunity?

  a. Passive natural immunity.
  b. Active natural immunity.
  c. Active artificial immunity.
  d. Passive artificial immunity.

53. Which component of the nervous system is responsible for lowering the heart rate?

  a. Central nervous system.
  b. Sympathetic nervous system.
  c. Parasympathetic nervous system.
  d. Distal nervous system.

English and Language Usage	Number of Questions: 28
	Time Limit: 28 Minutes

1. Which of the following sentences shows the correct way to separate the items in the series?

    a. These are actual cities in the United States: Unalaska, Alaska; Yreka, California; Two Egg, Florida; and Boring, Maryland.
    b. These are actual cities in the United States: Unalaska; Alaska, Yreka; California, Two Egg; Florid, and Boring; Maryland.
    c. These are actual cities in the United States: Unalaska, Alaska, Yreka, California, Two Egg, Florida, and Boring, Maryland.
    d. These are actual cities in the United States: Unalaska Alaska, Yreka California, Two Egg Florida, and Boring Maryland.

2. Choose the sentence that most effectively follows the conventions of Standard Written English:

    a. Wilbur and Orville Wright were two brothers, and they tested their prototype airplane on a beach in Kitty Hawk, North Carolina.
    b. The two brothers, Wilbur and Orville Wright, tested their prototype airplane on a beach in Kitty Hawk, North Carolina.
    c. Testing their prototype airplane on a beach in Kitty Hawk, North Carolina, were the two brothers, Wilbur and Orville Wright.
    d. The beach in Kitty Hawk, North Carolina was where the two brothers, Wilbur and Orville Wright, came and tested their prototype airplane.

3. Which of the following types of language are not appropriate in a research paper?

    a. colloquialisms
    b. contractions
    c. relative pronouns
    d. both A and B

4. Which of the following sentences demonstrates the correct use of an apostrophe?

    a. Lyle works for the courthouse, and among his responsibilities is getting the jurors meal's.
    b. Lyle works for the courthouse, and among his responsibilities is getting the juror's meals.
    c. Lyle works for the courthouse, and among his responsibilities is getting the jurors' meals.
    d. Lyle works for the courthouse, and among his responsibilities is getting the jurors meals'.

5. Which of the following is a complex sentence?

    a. Milton's favorite meal is spaghetti and meatballs, along with a side salad and garlic toast.
    b. Before Ernestine purchases a book, she always checks to see if the library has it.
    c. Desiree prefers warm, sunny weather, but her twin sister Destiny likes a crisp, cold day.
    d. Ethel, Ben, and Alice are working together on a school project about deteriorating dams.

6. Which of the answer choices gives the best definition of the underlined word in the following sentence?

Finlay flatly refused to take part in the piano recital, so his parents had to <u>cajole</u> him with the promise of a trip to his favorite toy store.

    a. prevent
    b. threaten
    c. insist
    d. coax

7. Which of the following nouns is the correct plural form of the word *tempo*?

    a. tempo
    b. tempae
    c. tempi
    d. tempos

8. Which of the following sentences follows the rules of capitalization?

    a. Kristia knows that her aunt Jo will be visiting, but she is not sure if her uncle will be there as well.
    b. During a visit to the monastery, Jess interviewed brother Mark about the daily prayer schedule.
    c. Leah spoke to her Cousin Martha about her summer plans to drive from Colorado to Arizona.
    d. Justinia will be staying with family in Chicago during the early Fall.

9. Which of the answer choices gives the best definition of the underlined word in the following sentence?

The discussion over the new park had begun well, but it soon descended into an <u>acrimonious</u> debate over misuse of tax revenues.

    a. shocking
    b. childish
    c. rancorous
    d. revealing

10. Which of the following sentences does NOT use correct punctuation to separate independent clauses?

    a. Anne likes to add salsa to her scrambled eggs; Gordon unaccountably likes his with peanut butter.
    b. Anne likes to add salsa to her scrambled eggs, however Gordon unaccountably likes his with peanut butter.
    c. Anne likes to add salsa to her scrambled eggs. Gordon unaccountably likes his with peanut butter.
    d. Anne likes to add salsa to her scrambled eggs, but Gordon unaccountably likes his with peanut butter.

11. Considering both style and clarity, which of the answer choices best combines the following sentences?

Fenella wanted to attend the concert. She also wanted to attend the reception at the art gallery. She tried to find a way to do both in one evening. She failed.

a. Although Fenella wanted to attend the concert, she also wanted to attend the reception at the art gallery, so she tried to find a way to do both in one evening. She failed.
b. Fenella wanted to attend both the concert and the reception at the art gallery, but she failed to find a way to do both in one evening.
c. Fenella failed to find a way to attend both the concert and the reception at the art gallery.
d. Because Fenella wanted to attend both the concert and the reception at the art gallery, she tried to find a way to do both in one evening. Unfortunately, she failed.

12. Which of the answer choices gives the best definition of the underlined word in the following sentence?

Mara enjoyed great <u>felicity</u> when her missing dog found his way home.

a. Discomfort
b. Anxiety
c. Disbelief
d. Happiness

13. Based on the definition of the word *permeate* "to penetrate or pervade," which of the following is the most likely meaning of the prefix *per-*?

a. across
b. by
c. with
d. through

14. The following words share a common Greek-based suffix: *anthropology*, *cosmetology*, *etymology*, and *genealogy*. What is the most likely meaning of the suffix *-logy*?

a. record
b. study
c. affinity
d. fear

15. Which of the following words functions as an adverb in the sentence below?

Jacob had been worried about the speech, but in the end he did well.

a. worried
b. about
c. but
d. well

16. Which of the following would belong in a formal speech?

a. We all need to work together to make this school better. First, we need to organize a list of our issues. Then we need to form small groups to discuss them and find solutions. Finally, we need to implement those solutions.

b. Our purpose is to work together to improve the quality of education at this school. Ideally, we need to organize a list of our issues. Secondly, we need to form small groups to discuss them and find solutions. Then, we need to implement some solutions.

c. We all got to work together to make this school much better than before. First, we need to say what is on our mind. We got to form small groups to discuss them and find solutions. And, we need to talk about those solutions.

d. It is possible for us to talk about the problems in school and solve them. Of course, we need to organize a list of our issues. For example, we should form small groups to discuss them and find solutions. Finally, we need to implement those solutions.

17. Which of the following sentences contains a correct example of subject-verb agreement?

a. Neither Jeanne nor Pauline like the dinner options on the menu.

b. All of the council likes the compromise that they have reached about property taxes.

c. The faculty of the math department were unable to agree on the curriculum changes.

d. Both Clara and Don feels that they need to be more proactive in checking on the contractors.

18. Which of the answer choices gives the best definition of the underlined word in the following sentence?

The guest speaker was undoubtedly an <u>erudite</u> scholar, but his comments on nomological determinism seemed to go over the heads of the students in the audience.

a. authentic

b. arrogant

c. faulty

d. knowledgeable

19. What is the correct spelling of the word that completes the following sentence?

Wearing white to a funeral is considered by many to be ____.

a. sacrelegious

b. sacriligious

c. sacrilegious

d. sacreligious

20. What is the most effective way to combine the two sentences below?

German cuisine is known for its hearty, meat and potato dishes. Families often enjoy a rich Sunday dinner of roast meat, potatoes, and cabbage.

a. German cuisine is known for its hearty, meat and potato dishes but families often enjoy a rich Sunday dinner of roast meat, potatoes, and cabbage.

b. German cuisine is known for its hearty, meat and potato dishes, but families often enjoy a rich Sunday dinner of roast meat, potatoes, and cabbage.

c. German cuisine is known for its hearty, meat and potato dishes, and families often enjoy a rich Sunday dinner of roast meat, potatoes and cabbage.

d. German cuisine is known for its hearty, meat and potato dishes, and families often enjoy a rich Sunday dinner of roast meat, potatoes, and cabbage.

21. Which of the following is a simple sentence?

a. Ben likes baseball, but Joseph likes basketball.
b. It looks like rain; be sure to bring an umbrella.
c. Although he was tired, Edgar still attended the recital.
d. Marjorie and Thomas planned an exciting trip to Maui.

22. Which of the following words functions as a pronoun in the sentence below?

Anne-Charlotte and I will be driving together to the picnic this weekend.

a. be
b. this
c. together
d. I

23. Which of the following sentences is the best in terms of style, clarity, and conciseness?

a. Ava has a leap year birthday; she is really twenty, and her friends like to joke that she is only five years old.
b. Because Ava has a leap year birthday, her friends like to joke that she is only five years old when she is really twenty.
c. Ava is twenty years old, her friends like to joke that she is five because she has a leap year birthday.
d. Although Ava has a leap year birthday, she is twenty years old, but her friends like to joke that she is five.

24. Which of the answer choices gives the best definition of the underlined word in the following sentence?

The housekeeper Mrs. Vanderbroek had a fixed daily routine for running the manor and was not particularly <u>amenable</u> to any suggested changes.

a. capable
b. agreeable
c. obstinate
d. critical

25. Which of the following words does not function as an adjective in the sentence below?

A quick review of all available housing options indicated that Casper had little choice but to rent for now and wait for a better time to buy.

a. quick
b. available
c. little
d. rent

26. What is the most effective way to combine the two sentences below?

A lot of teens express themselves through fashion. Since many teens start earning their own money, they can buy their own clothes and choose the fashions that they want.

a. A lot of teens express themselves through fashion, and since many teens start earning their own money, they can buy their own clothes and choose the fashions that they want.
b. A lot of teens express themselves through fashion and since many teens start earning their own money, they can buy their own clothes and choose the fashions that they want.
c. A lot of teens express themselves through fashion, but since many teens start earning their own money, they can buy their own clothes and choose the fashions that they want.
d. A lot of teens express themselves through fashion but since many teens start earning their own money, they can buy their own clothes and choose the fashions that they want.

27. Use of formal language would be LEAST essential when addressing which of the following audiences?

a. a board of directors
b. a grammar school class
c. a gathering of college professors
d. none of the above

28. Which of the following words correctly fills in the blank in the sentence below?

The Bill of Rights protects the right to ____ arms, but one common mistake is to spell this as though the Founding Fathers were ensuring the right to go sleeveless.

a. bear
b. bare
c. barre
d. baire

Answer Key and Explanations for Test #2

Reading

1. B: The word *intermittent* suggests that something occurs at imprecise intervals, so answer choice B is the best synonym. Answer choices A and D suggest the exact opposite of the meaning indicated in the sentence. Answer choice C likely reflects another element of the woman's labor, but it has nothing to do with the meaning of the word *intermittent*.

2. C: All of these are good sources to use while developing a position on Civil Rights; nonetheless, first you must first familiarize yourself with an overview of the issue. A history textbook probably would be the most comprehensive and the least affected by personal opinion. Speeches, interviews, and blogs are great next steps in the research process, but these choices may prove too subjective to provide a necessary overview of the issue.

3. C: The correct answer is *abundance.* The sentence suggests that Kit has more zucchini than she needs, and is therefore trying to offload zucchini on anyone who might want some. The *plethora* might lead to a mild *irritation*, but the words are definitely not synonyms. (In some cases, a *plethora* is certainly not an irritation.) The word *plethora* is related to a *quantity*, but it is a specific type of quantity: an excess. Because the word *quantity* can also describe a lack of something, these words are not synonyms. Kit is obviously trying to avoid *waste*, but the words *plethora* and *waste* are not synonyms. *Waste* would also not be a natural replacement for *plethora* in the sentence.

4. C: Only the word *neglect* can fall between the guide words *needs* and *negotiate* on a dictionary page. The words *needle* and *nectar* would come before *needs*, and the word *neigh* would follow *negotiate*.

5. D: The chapter title refers to the *fictional* works of Dorothy L. Sayers, and letters generally do not fall under the category of fiction. Novels, plays, and mysteries, however, usually do.

6. C: An expository passage seeks to *expose* information by explaining or defining it in detail. As this passage focuses on describing the written works of Dorothy L. Sayers, it may safely be considered expository. The author is not necessarily telling a story, something one might expect from a strictly narrative passage. (Additionally, the author's main point, that of explaining why Sayers was such a versatile writer, represents a kind of thesis statement for shaping the overall focus of the passage. A narrative passage would focus more on simply telling the story of Sayers's life.) At no point is the author attempting to persuade the reader about anything, and there is nothing particularly technical about the passage. Rather, it is a focused look at Sayers's educational background and how she developed into a writer of many genres; this makes it solidly expository.

7. A: As indicated in the answer explanation above, the main focus of the passage is Sayers's versatility as a writer. The first paragraph notes this and then begins discussing her education, introducing the experience that would inform her later accomplishments. The second paragraph then follows this up with specifics about the types of writing she did. Answer choice B would be correct if the passage were more narrative than expository. Answer choices C and D focus on specific works for which Sayers is remembered, but both are too limited to be considered a representative summary of the entire passage.

8. B: The mention of an "unexpectedly good education" represents an opinion on the part of the author. As the author does not follow this up with an explanation about *why* such an education would be unexpectedly good, the statement is simply a moment of bias on the author's part, rather than an element within the larger argument. There is no bias in the other answer choices. Answer choices A and C are factual statements about Sayers's life and work. Answer choice D, while it might hint vaguely at disapproval on the author's part (who might, perhaps, wish to know Sayers's reasons), is not necessarily a statement containing bias. It is indeed true that Sayers turned down the doctorate of divinity, and it is also true that her reasons for doing so are unknown. Only answer choice B conveys an opinion of the author.

9. D: A search for early maps by one of the first people to study geography would certainly take Jorgen to the 900 section of the library: History, geography, and biography. For this particular study, there is no reason for Jorgen to look among books on philosophy and psychology, social sciences, or technical and applied science.

10. D: The sieve of Eratosthenes is a mathematical tool, so Jorgen should go to the science and mathematics section. While the sieve might be used in certain computer applications, there is no specific indication of this. As a result, answer choice D is a better option than answer choice A. Also, Jorgen has no reason to check the philosophy and psychology or languages sections to find out more about a mathematical topic.

11. B: Section 400 is the section on languages, so it is a good place to look for more information about the letters of the Greek alphabet. Jorgen would be unlikely to find anything useful in the sections on religion, arts and recreation, or history, geography, and biography.

12. D: Section 800 features works of literature, so that is the best place for Jorgen to begin looking for *The Iliad* and *The Odyssey*. The philosophy and psychology section will likely contain references to these works, but Jorgen would still have to go to the literature section to obtain the works themselves. The same thing can be said about the religion and arts and recreation sections.

13. C: While planning her daughter's wedding, Marci is likely to find picking out a paint color for the living room *unimportant*. Therefore, answer choice C is the most logical option. Choosing a paint color might also be meaningless at the moment, but it is not without meaning altogether. It is simply not as important. Answer choice A infers more than the sentence implies. Answer choice B could be forced into the sentence (if Marci was looking for a distraction from the stress of wedding planning, for instance), but it is not natural, and it is certainly not a synonym for *peripheral*. Answer choice D makes little sense in the context of the sentence.

14. B: The Russian population of Latvia decreased the most since 1991. The Latvian population decreased slightly, but not to the same degree. The Ukrainian population decreased by an even smaller percentage since 1991. The German population remained relatively unchanged between 1991 and 2011.

15. C: On the chart, the only ethnic group that represents approximately one percent of the population after World War II and approximately three percent by 1991 is the Ukrainian population. The Latvian and Russian populations represent much larger percentages of the total population of Latvia. The German population decreased significantly during this time period.

16. A: If Hilaire's vocabulary needs a boost, he needs a thesaurus, which provides a range of synonyms (or antonyms) for words. A dictionary is useful for word meanings, but it will not necessarily assist Hilaire in improving the words he already has in his papers. The encyclopedia is also irrelevant, particularly since the professor already approves of Hilaire's work and is not asking him to research further. The style guide will be helpful if the paper needs more attention on grammar.

17. C: As the final step indicates, the new word should end in *Y*. This immediately eliminates answer choice D. Answer choice A adds an *L* when a second one is not required, and answer choice B adds two *T*s to a word that has none. Only answer choice C follows all of the directions to spell the new word: REPLAY.

18. A: Klara's success is clearly the result of diligence, so answer choice A must be correct. It is possible that her diligence was also silent, but the sentence does not indicate this. Answer choice B, then, cannot be correct. A moderate commitment by an average student would not lead to exemplary results, so answer choice C is incorrect. Answer choice D makes no sense in the context of the sentence.

19. D: Puffed rice is a dry breakfast cereal, and therefore contains (or might contain) a dairy product. Breaded chicken parmesan contains both bread crumbs and parmesan cheese; the cheese is certainly a dairy product, and bread is on the warning list from the doctor. A sliced turkey sandwich contains deli meat and bread, both of which are discouraged by Flemming's doctor. Yogurt made from coconut milk, however, is meant to be a dairy-free alternative, so it should be a safe choice for Flemming.

20. C: Chapter III of the manual contains information about adjusting the climate within the vehicle, so it is here that Regina will find the instructions she needs to adjust the air conditioning. Chapter I would be the best choice if the manual did *not* also include Chapter III. The chapter on safety options would probably not contain information about how to operate the air conditioning, so answer choice B is incorrect. Regina should definitely adjust the air conditioning before she begins driving, but the information needed to do this is not likely to be found in Chapter IV.

21. D: An overheating vehicle is definitely an emergency, so Regina would need to consult Chapter VI. The other chapters contain useful information that Regina will need once her vehicle is back in working order, but until then she should focus on the information in the chapter about emergency situations.

22. B: As most students discover, Wikipedia is not considered a reliable source or a particularly scholarly one. The Encyclopedia Britannica is, however, as are Science.gov (which would contain officially recognized information provided by a government organization) and LexisNexis (a reputable site containing legal and educational resources).

23. B: The passage does not say that studying a foreign language will help students find jobs after high school (choice A) or gain an understanding of other cultures (choice C). The passage does say that studying a foreign language is important for college acceptance (choice D), but this point alone is not the main idea of the passage.

24. C: The passage does not claim that studying a foreign language is essential to high school graduation (choice A). Choices B and D represent claims made in the passage, but do not include all of the claims made.

25. D: Although students may find knowledge of a foreign language helpful in obtaining a job, it is an obvious exaggeration to claim that students who did not study a foreign language would be unemployable.

26. D: Choices A and C represent options that would provide information regarding the opinions of students and parents, but not actual evidence regarding the influence of studying a foreign language on future success. Choice B specifies a second language taught at home, whereas the passage focuses specifically on a foreign language taught in high school.

27. B: Choices A, C, and D do not offer a complete summary of the claims made in this passage.

28. D: Eczema is a topical condition, so Chapter 12 (section D) would be the most appropriate place to look. Eczema is not specific to either men or women, nor is it specific to adults, so Chapter 8 would not be the best place to look. Finally, eczema is neither a respiratory condition nor a digestive condition.

29. A: This question asks the reader to consider the distinction between a recognized respiratory condition (Chapter 10) and a children's condition (Chapter 7). In this case, the first and best place to check is Chapter 7, because it addresses conditions specific to children, and it describes herbs that may be useful in treating these conditions. Herbs, like pharmaceuticals, need to be used carefully, and the type of herbal remedy that would be used to treat an adult respiratory condition is not necessarily the same one that would be used to treat a respiratory condition in a child. Additionally, the dosage would certainly be different, so the chapter on children's conditions is the correct place to look. Chapters 9 and 12 (immunity and detox, respectively) would not contain useful information for this particular situation.

30. C: Chapter 5 contains information about using herbs in beverages. Since Clothilde is looking for ways to use the elderflower to make tea and wine, this chapter should be useful. Chapter 3 would not likely contain information that would be useful in this situation. Chapter 4 discusses using herbs in food, so Clothilde is unlikely to find anything in this section about beverages. Chapter 13 would certainly be the place to look in the index of herbs, but this chapter would most likely contain a listing of the herb and a summary of its properties, rather than recommendations for how to use it in tea or wine making.

31. B: Chapter 3 contains information about caring for herbs, so it is the first place Clothilde should look. The herb is clearly already planted, so Chapter 2 will not be of much use in this case. Again, Chapter 13 would certainly be the place to look in the index of herbs, but this chapter would most likely contain a listing of the herb and a summary of its properties, rather than recommendations for maintaining the plant. Chapter 14, the alphabetical listing for herbs J–O, is unlikely to contain any information either about caring for herbs in general or about the elderberry in particular.

32. C: Only Cosette fulfills all of the clearly stated requirements in the ad. She does not smoke (and is, in fact, allergic to cigarette smoke), and she needs a quiet place to study in a house that is advertised as having quiet occupants. Also implied is Cosette's need to be close to the university, since she is likely going to be studying for classes. Frances has a dog, and this is not allowed according to the ad. Adelaide is looking for a short-term lease, and the other occupants prefer a long-term renter. Felix is male, and the other occupants are looking for a female renter.

33. B: If the student's nerves are getting the better of him, it is likely that he is either very pale or very flushed. Because *flushed* is one of the options, it is the correct choice. A complexion cannot be *rambling*, so answer choice A is incorrect. Answer choice C has a hint of promise, but it makes the sentence more confusing, so it too is incorrect. It is difficult to know what is meant by the phrase "*weak* complexion," so answer choice D is too unclear to be correct.

34. B: For two pounds of each type of tea, Wholesale Tea's price would be $96, which is the best price. Tea Heaven's price would be $102. Tea by the Pound's price would be $104. Tea Express's price would be the same as Tea Heaven's price: $102.

35. B: Wholesale Tea would have the best price for these specific blends. The price for one pound of Earl Grey and two pounds of green tea would be $78. Tea Heaven's price would be $87. Tea by the Pound's price would be $83. Tea Express's price would be $88.

36. B: Answer choice B is the most logical conclusion. The passage states that, "Primary sources are the more direct type of information. They are accounts of an event that are produced by individuals who were actually present." Therefore, it is reasonable to assume that an account prepared by someone who was present would be more accurate than one prepared by somebody decades later who had to rely on the accounts of others.

37. D: Ten nations received independence in the first thirty years of the nineteenth century. Choice A is incorrect because the American Revolution was fought during the latter 1770s and early 1780s. This was decades before the independence movements in South America. In fact, the American Revolution inspired some of the movements. France did not have many possessions in South America. So, choice B is wrong. Nations on the west coast were among the last to gain independence. So, that makes choice C incorrect.

38. C: The only logical conclusion that can be made based on the announcement is that the library has applied a fee to Internet usage beyond 30 minutes to discourage patrons from spending too long on the computers. There is nothing in the announcement to suggest that the library plans to add more computers. The announcement mentions a limited number of computers, but there is no indication that there are plans to change this fact. The announcement makes no mention of the library's budget, so it is impossible to infer that the library is facing budget cuts or that the library is compensating for budget cuts with the fee. Similarly, the announcement says nothing about the library's Internet costs, so it is impossible to conclude logically that the library is attempting to offset its own Internet fees.

39. C: Raoul will need the computer for a total of 90 minutes. The first 30 minutes are free, so Raoul will need to be prepared to pay for 60 minutes. This is equal to four intervals of 15 minutes. Each 15-minute interval costs $3, so Raoul will need to pay $12 for his Internet usage at the library.

40. A: The author says that victims of Marah's disease "appear" to be comfortable but "beneath it all" are in pain. He says that they are "inaccurately" diagnosed as low on the pain scale. This shows that the pain scale is not an accurate way to measure Marah's disease.

41. B: The topic sentence is placed at the beginning of each supporting paragraph. Supporting evidence is presented after the topic sentence in each supporting paragraph. The passage states "Next come the supporting paragraphs. Each paragraph contains a topic sentence, supporting evidence, and finally a type of mini-conclusion that restates the point of the paragraph."

42. B: Answer choices A, C, and D are all mentioned in the passage, but they are part of the overall purpose, which is to give an overview of how leeches have been used throughout history.

43. C: Although it never specifically addresses the babysitter, the directions are clearly instructions for how to take care of a little girl. A mother or father would not need this information written down in such detail, but a babysitter might. You can infer the answer in this case.

44. D: You cannot assume gender, and the note never indicates whether the writer is male or female. You can tell that the writer is the main caretaker of the child in question, so "parent" is the best choice in this case. A teacher or nurse might be able to write such a note, but parent is probably more likely, making it the best choice.

45. B: The information in the passage lets you know that only the serving team can score. This rule is different in different leagues, so it is important to read the passage instead of going by what you know from your own life.

46. D: Although any number of people could play in a volleyball game, the passage mentions that the entire class could participate in a game. Do all of them have to participate? No. But that wasn't the question.

47. C: The author does not make predictions of a radically rejuvenated planet (choice A) or the complete annihilation of life as we know it (choice B). The author is also not accusatory in his descriptions (choice D). Instead, the author states what he believes to be the current state of the planet's environment, and makes practical suggestions for making better use of its resources in the future.

48. B: As the passage states: "Locally grown food and other products manufactured within your community are the best choices. The fewer miles a product traveled to reach you, the fewer resources it required."

49. C: The author does not mention running out of resources in a specific time period (choice A), the cost of water and energy (choice B), or the possibility of hardship for local farmers (choice D).

50. D: As the passage states: "You should try to be aware of your consumption of water and energy. Turn off the water when you brush your teeth, and limit your showers to five minutes. Turn off the lights, and don't leave appliances or chargers plugged in when not in use." The contexts of these sentences indicate that consumption means the depletion of goods (e.g., water and energy).

51. C: Of the choices available, this is the only sentence that offers specific ideas for carrying out the author's suggestion to the reader of limiting consumption of energy.

52. D: B and C are only briefly mentioned, allowing them to be eliminated as possibilities. Although the passage does discuss what could happen to two balls released at the top of a mountain, that is not the purpose of the passage, so A can be eliminated. The purpose is to show how small differences (in this case two inches between two rubber balls) can have large effects. This is essentially what the butterfly effect is, and the purpose of the passage is to give an example to demonstrate this principle.

53. B: This is the correct answer because the birthdates show that the youngest children are on the right and their older siblings are on the left side of the family tree. Choice A is incorrect because Queen Victoria and Prince Albert are the oldest generation, and they are at the top of the family tree. Choice C is incorrect because the youngest children are on the left, not the right (the reader can see this by looking at the birthdates). Choice D is partially correct because Queen Victoria and Prince Albert are at the top of the family tree, but the family tree does not show great-grandchildren. Although it looks like there are more than three layers, the middle layers all show Queen Victoria and Prince Albert's children.

Mathematics

1. C: According to the problem statement, 60% of the class wanted to work with the elderly. Therefore, convert 60% to a fraction by using the following steps:

$$60\% = \frac{60}{100}$$

Now simplify the above fraction using a greatest common factor of 20.

$$\frac{60}{100} = \frac{3}{5}$$

2. B: Since 35% of the staff will take vacation days, only 100% – 35% = 65% of the staff is available to work. Of the remaining 65%, only 20% are certified to work in the neonatal unit. Therefore multiply 65% by 20% using these steps:

Convert 65% and 20% into decimals by dividing both numbers by 100.

$$\frac{65}{100} = 0.65 \text{ and } \frac{20}{100} = 0.20$$

Now multiply 0.65 by 0.20 to get

$$(0.65)(0.20) = 0.13$$

Now convert 0.13 to a percentage by multiplying by 100.

$$(0.13)(100) = 13\%$$

3. B: The patient's dosage must decrease by 30%. So calculate 30% of 340:

$$(0.30)(340 \text{ mg}) = 102 \text{ mg}$$

Now subtract the 30% decrease from the original dosage.

$$340 \text{ mg} - 102 \text{ mg} = 238 \text{ mg}$$

4. C: Since 70% of the patients in the study were women, 30% of the patients were men. Calculate the number of male patients by multiplying 100 by 0.30.

$$(100)(0.30) = 30$$

Of the 30 male patients in the study, 10% were overweight as children. So 90% were not overweight. Multiply 30 by 0.90 to get the final answer.

$$(30)(0.90) = 27$$

5. C: If the incoming class has 100 students, then $\frac{3}{4}$ of those students will major in nursing.

$$(100)\left(\frac{3}{4}\right) = 75$$

So 75 students will major in nursing but only $\frac{1}{5}$ of that 75 will complete the nursing program.

$$(75)\left(\frac{1}{5}\right) = 15$$

Therefore, 15 students will complete the program.

6. A: The first midwife contributes $2000 per month, and she uses $\frac{2}{5}$ of that amount for rent and utilities.

$$(\$2000)\left(\frac{2}{5}\right) = \$800$$

So the midwife pays $800 for rent and utilities, which leaves her with

$$\$2000 - \$800 = \$1200$$

The midwife divides the remaining $1200 in half.

$$\frac{\$1200}{2} = \$600$$

The midwife saves $600 and buys medical supplies with the remaining $600.

7. A: The second midwife allocates $\frac{1}{2}$ of her funds for an office administrator plus another $\frac{1}{10}$ for office supplies. So add $\frac{1}{2}$ and $\frac{1}{10}$ by first finding a common denominator.

$$\frac{1}{2} = \frac{5}{10}$$

$$\frac{5}{10} + \frac{1}{10} = \frac{6}{10}$$

Now simplify $\frac{6}{10}$ by using the greatest common factor of 6 and 10, which is 2.

$$6 \div 2 = 3 \text{ and } 10 \div 2 = 5$$

Therefore, $\frac{6}{10} = \frac{3}{5}$.

8. C: The following proportion can be written $\frac{4}{2} = \frac{x}{18}$. Solving for x gives $x = 36$. Thus, there are 36 data analysis problems on the test.

9. A: The flat rate of $65 represents the y-intercept, and the charge of $0.12 per roaming minute used represents the slope. Therefore, the expression representing his monthly phone bill is $65 + 0.12x$.

10. B: First, determine how many miles can be driven on one tank of gas by multiplying the numbers of gallons in a tank by the miles per gallon:

12 gallons/tank × 30 miles/gallon = 360 miles

Next, divide the total miles for the trip by the number of miles driven per tank of gas to determine how many total tanks of gas Robert will need:

1,800 miles ÷ 360 miles/tank = 5 tanks

11. C: To obtain the new dosage, subtract 1/5th of 310 mg from the original dosage of 310 mg, then subtract 20 mg.

$$310 \text{ mg} - \left(310 \times \frac{1}{5}\right) \text{mg} - 20 \text{ mg} = 228 \text{ mg}$$

12. C: Find $\frac{1}{7}$ of 100 by multiplying

$$(100)\left(\frac{1}{7}\right) = \frac{100}{7} = 14.2857$$

$\frac{100}{7}$ is an improper fraction. Convert the fraction to a decimal and round to the nearest hundredth to get 14.29.

13. B: A single straight line can be drawn that is close to many of the points. The slope of that line would be negative, so the points have a negative, linear association.

14. D: In order to determine the number of questions Joshua must answer correctly, consider the number of points he must earn. Joshua will receive 4 points for each question he answers correctly, and x represents the number of questions. Therefore, Joshua will receive a total of 4x points for all the questions he answers correctly. Joshua must earn more than 92 points. Therefore, to determine the number of questions he must answer correctly, solve the inequality $4x > 92$.

15. D: To determine the total cost of Susan's outfit, add all her purchases.

$$\$69.99 + \$39.99 + \$34.76 = \$144.65$$

16. C: Group B is negatively skewed since there are more high scores. With more high scores, the mean for Group B will be higher.

17. A: Apply the order of operations to solve this problem. Multiplication and division are computed first from left to right. Then addition and subtraction are computed next from left to right.

$$2 + (2)(2) - 2 \div 2 =$$
$$2 + 4 - 2 \div 2 =$$
$$2 + 4 - 1 =$$
$$6 - 1 =$$
$$5$$

18. A: The numbers listed for Choice A can all be converted to decimal form for comparison. The given sequence can be written as $-2, -0.75, -0.45, 0.03, 0.36$. The negative integers are the least values, with the negative integer with the greatest absolute value, serving as the least integer. The percentage, 3%, is written as 0.03, and is less than 0.36.

19. B: Compare and order the rational numbers by finding a common denominator for all three fractions. The least common denominator for 3, 5, and 15 is 15. Now convert the fractions with different denominators into fractions with a common denominator.

$$\frac{4}{15} = \frac{4}{15}$$

$$\frac{2}{5} = \frac{6}{15}$$

$$\frac{1}{3} = \frac{5}{15}$$

Now that all three fractions have the same denominator, order them from smallest to largest by comparing the numerators.

$$\frac{4}{15} < \frac{5}{15} < \frac{6}{15}$$

Since $\frac{4}{15}$ of the patients are in Group Alpha, this group has the smallest number of patients. The next largest group has $\frac{5}{15}$ of the patients, which is Group Gamma. The largest group has $\frac{6}{15}$ of the patients, which is Group Beta.

20. A: Solve the equation for x.

$$2x + 6 = 14$$

$$2x = 14 - 6$$

$$2x = 8$$

$$x = \frac{8}{2}$$

$$x = 4$$

21. C: To determine the mean time for this event, add up all 8 event times (181.42) and then divide that value by 8: $\frac{181.42}{8} = 22.6775 \approx 22.68$ sec. Answer A is the mode value of the event times. Answer B is the median value of the event times. In Answer D, the mean was incorrectly calculated by only adding the first and last times ($22.33 + 23.22$) and then dividing that value by 2.

22. A: During week 1, Nurse Cameron worked 5 shifts.

$$\text{shifts for week 1} = 5$$

During week 2, she worked twice as many shifts as she did during week 1.

$$\text{shifts for week 2} = (2)(5)$$

During week 3, she added 4 shifts to the number of shifts she worked during week 2.

$$\text{shifts for week 3} = (2)(5) + 4$$

23. A: Use the order of operations to solve this problem.

$$(3)(-4) + (3)(4) - 1$$

$$-12 + (3)(4) - 1 =$$

$$-12 + 12 - 1 =$$

$$0 - 1 =$$

$$-1$$

24. A: The volume formula for a rectangular solid is $V = lwh$. Plugging in values then evaluating will yield the final answer.

$$V = (30 \ in)(10 \ in)(12 \ in)$$
$$V = 3600 \text{ cubic inches}$$

25. B: If a line-of-fit is drawn through the points, the slope will be $-\frac{1}{5}$ so the snow melts 5 centimeters every day.

26. D: The variables are the objects the graph measures. In this case, the graph measures the Hospital Staff and the Average hours worked per week. The dependent variable changes with the independent variable. Here, the average hours worked per week depends on the particular type of hospital staff. Therefore, the dependent variable is Average hours worked per week and the independent variable is Hospital Staff.

27. D: The prefix, milli-, means 1000th. In this case,

$$1 \text{ g} = 1000 \text{ mg}$$

Therefore,

$$(5)(1 \text{ g}) = (5)(1000 \text{ mg})$$

$$5 \text{ g} = (5)(1000 \text{ mg})$$

$$5 \text{ g} = 5000 \text{ mg}$$

28. B: The number of people who voted for the proposition is 9.5% of 51,623. If we only require an approximation, we can round 9.5% to 10%, and 51,623 to 50,000. Then 9.5% of 51,623 is about 10% of 50,000, or $(0.1)(50,000) = 5,000$.

29. D: To calculate the total time taken, divide the distance driven by the speed it was driven at:

$$305 \text{ mi} \div 65 \text{ mph} = 305 \text{ miles} \times \frac{1 \text{ hour}}{65 \text{ miles}} = 4.69 \text{ hours}$$

$$162 \text{ mi} \div 80 \text{ mph} = 162 \text{ miles} \times \frac{1 \text{ hour}}{80 \text{ miles}} = 2.03 \text{ hours}$$

Convert the minutes spent at the gas station to hours: $15 \text{ min} \times \frac{1 \text{ hour}}{60 \text{ minutes}} = 0.25 \text{ hours}$

Find the total time taken on the trip by summing all the times: $4.69 + 2.03 + 0.25 = 6.97 \text{ hours}$

30. C: Use the formula $Volume = length \times width \times height$:

$$200 = 5 \times 5 \times h$$

$$25h = 200$$

31. D: Integers include all positive and negative whole numbers and the number zero. The product of three integers must be an integer, so you can eliminate any answer choice that is not a whole number: choices (A) and (C). The product of two even integers is even. The product of even and odd integers is even. The only even choice is 24.

32. C: Divide the mg the child should receive by the number of mg in 0.8 mL to determine how many 0.8 mL doses the child should receive: $\frac{240}{80} = 3$. Multiply the number of doses by 0.8 to determine how many mL the child should receive: $3 \times 0.8 = 2.4$ mL

33. B: The chart indicates that each x value must be tripled to equal the corresponding y value, so $y = 3x$. One way you can determine this is by plugging corresponding pairs of x and y into the answer choices.

34. D: Use the following proportion: $\frac{1\ in}{45\ miles} = \frac{3.2\ in}{x\ miles}$

Cross multiply: $x = (45)(3.2) = 144$ miles

35. A: The amount of money he has already saved represents the y-intercept. The amount of money he intends to save per month represents the slope. Thus, his savings can be represented by the equation, $y = 28x + 15$, also written as $y = 15 + 28x$.

36. B: The number of trees planted by the Juniors is skewed left, with more higher numbers of trees planted. The number of trees planted by the Seniors is skewed right, with more lower numbers of trees planted.

Science

1. C: The circulatory system consists of the heart, blood vessels, lymph, lymph nodes, and blood. It circulates materials throughout the entire body, providing tissues and organs with nutrients and oxygen. It is also responsible for transporting hormones and removing waste. The nervous system is responsible for transmitting nerve impulses that originate in the brain and coordinate action in the rest of the body.

2. B: The digestive system helps the body process food. The stomach, mouth, and esophagus all participate in food digestion. Common diseases infecting the digestive system include Crohn's disease, ulcerative colitis, and diverticulosis. Diabetes is a disease of the endocrine system, that impacts the release of insulin from the pancreas.

3. A: The nervous system is the body's communication center. The body uses the respiratory system to breathe, and blood is transported by the circulatory system. The digestive system breaks down food for the body.

4. A: The respiratory system uses the lungs, diaphragm, trachea, alveoli and bronchi to help the body distribute oxygen and remove carbon dioxide. While the ribs contain and protect many of these elements, the ribs are part of the musculoskeletal system, which is responsible for providing structure, stability and protection to the internal organs.

5. A: The immune system helps protect the body from bacteria, viruses, infections, and other elements that could cause illness. Depending on the foreign element that enters the body, different cells respond to attack the foreign element. Cells that contribute to this protection and response include leukocytes, or white blood cells (eosinophils, basophils, natural killer (NK) cells, and mast cells), and phagocytic cells (dendritic cells, macrophages and neutrophils) in addition to cells of adaptive immunity (B cells and T cells) which are produced in the bone marrow. A neuron is a nerve cell that is central to the nervous system and transmits nerve impulses.

6. A: The human body has five types of bones: long bones, short bones, irregular bones, flat bones, and sesamoid bones. While bones may be dense, this is not a major category of bones in the body.

7. B: Sesamoid bones are embedded in tendons. Vertical bones, is not a major bone type. Long bones contain a long shaft, and flat bones are thin and curved.

8. A: A triple beam balance would be used to measure the mass (in grams) of the gum in this experiment. An anemometer is used to measure wind speed. A hot plate is used to heat liquids. A microscope is used to magnify microscopic particles or organisms.

9. C: In respiration, the human inhales air, consisting of oxygen, and then produces energy (ATP) and exhales nitrogen, carbon dioxide, and water (in the form of vapor). While oxygen is a main component of the respiratory system's process, it is not produced by the respiratory system. Rather, it is utilized and distributed throughout the body, and then what is not absorbed, is exhaled back into the environment.

10. C: The pulmonary artery carries oxygen-depleted blood from the heart to the lungs, where CO_2 is released and the supply of oxygen is replenished. This blood then returns to the heart through the pulmonary vein, and is carried through the aorta and a series of branching arteries to the capillaries, where the bulk of gas exchange with the tissues occurs. Oxygen-depleted blood returns to the heart through branching veins (the femoral veins bring it from the legs) into the vena cava, which carries it again to the heart. Since the pulmonary artery is the last step before replenishment of the blood's oxygen content, it contains the blood which is the most oxygen depleted.

11. D: The myocardium is the layer of the heart that contains the muscle fibers responsible for contraction (Hint: myo- is the prefix for muscle). The endocardium and epicardium are the inner and outer layers of the heart wall, respectively. The pericardium is the sac in which the heart sits inside the chest cavity.

12. A: While generally speaking, veins carry deoxygenated blood and arteries carry oxygenated blood, in this case, the pulmonary veins carry oxygenated blood from the lungs to the left side of the heart and the pulmonary arteries carry deoxygenated blood from the right side of the heart to the lungs. The aorta, takes oxygenated away from the left side of the heart and distributes it throughout the body. The superior vena cava returns unoxygenated blood back to the right side of the heart, to then be distributed through the lungs and reoxygenated.

13. C: The independent variable is the variable that is changed in the experiment in order to determine its effect on the dependent variable or the outcome of the experiment. The dependent variable results from the experimenter making only one change to an experiment that can be repeated with the same results. Mrs. Jones's class was comparing the effects of sugar and artificial sweetener on the overall color of cookies once they are baked; thus, the one thing that should be changed in the experiment is the sugar and artificial sweetener in the recipe. All of the other ingredients stay the same. For the experiment to be valid and not influenced by any other variables, the students should keep the temperature and baking time the same, as these could affect the color of the cookies as well.

14. C: Mitochondria are often called the power house of the cell because they provide energy for the cell to function. The nucleus is the control center for the cell. The cell membrane surrounds the cell and separates the cell from its environment. Cytoplasm is the thick fluid within the cell membrane that surrounds the nucleus and contains organelles.

15. B: Ribosomes are organelles that help synthesize proteins within the cell. Cilia and flagella are responsible for cell movement. The cell membrane helps the cell maintain its shape and protects it from the environment. Lysosomes have digestive enzymes.

16. B: Cells differentiate so that simple, less specialized cells can become highly specialized cells. For example, humans are multicellular organisms who undergo cell differentiation numerous times. Cells begin as simple zygotes after fertilization and then differentiate to form a myriad of complex tissues and systems before birth.

17. C: Both meiosis and mitosis occur in humans, animals, and plants. Mitosis produces cells that are genetically identical, and meiosis produces cells that are genetically different. Only mitosis occurs asexually.

18. B: A decrease in a natural predator, such as a wolves, coyotes, bobcat, or wild dogs, would allow the population to become out of control. In a population of deer that has increased, there would be a natural decrease in a food source for the nutritional needs for the animals in surrounding areas. Although deer have been known to share a human's developed habitat, it is often forced by reduced territory and food sources. An increase in hunting licenses would be used by local officials to try to control the population, helping to decrease the number of adults of breeding age.

19. B: DNA is the primary carrier of genetic information in most cells. RNA serves as a messenger that transmits genetic information from DNA to the cytoplasm of the cell.

20. C: Food enters the digestive system through the mouth and proceeds down to the stomach after mastication by the teeth. Once in the stomach, enzymes are secreted that begin to digest the specific substances in the food (proteins, carbohydrates, etc.). Next, the food passes through to the small intestine where the nutrients are absorbed and then into the large intestine where extra water is absorbed.

21. C: After cell division, the daughter cells should be exact copies of the parent cells. Therefore, the DNA should replicate, or make an exact copy of itself, so that each daughter cell will have the full amount of DNA.

22. A: Genes are the molecular units that enable parents to pass hereditary traits on to their offspring. The blood, organs, cells and hair all contain the genes that makeup the offspring, but these are not basic molecular units.

23. A: Both DNA and RNA are made up of 4 nucleotide bases. Both DNA and RNA contain cytosine, guanine, and adenine. However, DNA contains thymine and RNA contains uracil. Choice B is incorrect because DNA and RNA do not have the same 4 nucleotides, and choices C and D are incorrect because neither DNA nor RNA contains 6 nucleotides. Furthermore, DNA has a double helix structure, and RNA has a single helix structure.

24. B: The genotype describes a person's genetic makeup. The phenotype describes a person's observable characteristics. Among the choices, the CFTR gene refers to genetic makeup while the other choices all describe traits that are observable.

25. B: The complete Punnett square is shown below.

	B	**b**
B	BB	Bb
b	Bb	bb

Because male pattern baldness is a recessive gene, the offspring would need the *bb* gene combination in order to inherit this trait. Possibility 4 corresponds to the *bb* gene combination.

26. C: Because male pattern baldness is recessive, the offspring would need the *bb* gene combination in order to inherit this trait. Therefore, any offspring with the *B* gene will have a full head of hair. Possibilities 1, 2, and 3 all have the *B* gene.

27. B: Interstitial fluid is found in the tissues around the cells; intracellular fluid is found within the cells. Fluid in the ventricles of the brain and down into the spinal cord is called cerebrospinal fluid. Cerebrospinal fluid bathes these sensitive tissues in a fluid that helps to protect them. Blood and lymph are the fluids that carry nutrients, oxygen, waste, and lymph material throughout the body.

28. D: *Plasma* cells secrete antibodies. These cells, also known as plasmacytes, are located in lymphoid tissue. Antibodies are only secreted in response to a particular stimulus, usually the detection of an antigen in the body. Antigens include bacteria, viruses, and parasites. Once released, antibodies bind to the antigen and neutralize it. When faced with a new antigen, the body may require some time to develop appropriate antibodies. Once the body has been exposed to an antigen, however, it does not forget how to produce the correct antibodies.

29. A: A catalyst increases the rate of a chemical reaction without becoming part of the net reaction. Therefore, chemical C increases the rate of the reaction between A and B. The catalyst does not change the chemicals within the reaction or initiate the reaction itself.

30. B: Enzymes are protein molecules produced by living organisms. Enzymes serve as catalysts for certain biological reactions.

31. A: The hypothalamus controls the hormones secreted by the pituitary gland. This part of the brain maintains the body temperature and helps to control metabolism. The adrenal glands, which lie above the kidneys, secrete steroidal hormones, epinephrine, and norepinephrine. The testes are the male reproductive glands, responsible for the production of sperm and testosterone. The pancreas secretes insulin and a fluid that aids in digestion.

32. A: Gas exchange occurs in the *alveoli*, the minute air sacs on the interior of the lungs. The *bronchi* are large cartilage-based tubes of air; they extend from the end of the trachea into the lungs, where they branch apart. The *larynx*, which houses the vocal cords, is positioned between the trachea and the pharynx; it is involved in swallowing, breathing, and speaking. The *pharynx* extends from the nose to the uppermost portions of the trachea and esophagus. In order to enter these two structures, air and other matter must pass through the pharynx.

33. C: The esophagus is the only structure that is not part of the respiratory system, it is part of the digestive system. The larynx houses the voice box; it also acts as a passageway for air to travel into the lungs. The trachea connects the larynx to the lungs. The trachea splits into the right and left bronchi, which divide into smaller passageways called the bronchioles.

34. C: In order to have accurate measurements, the use of a graduated cylinder would be the best measurement equipment for a liquid solution. A triple beam balance measures the weight of an object in grams. A flask and a test tube are used to contain a liquid while being heated or stored.

35. C: The atom is negatively charged. Neutrons have no charge. Protons have positive charge and electrons have negative charge equal in magnitude to the positive charge of the proton. Because the atom has more electrons than protons, the atom has a negative charge.

36. C: The genitourinary system is responsible for removing waste from the body through urine. Components include two kidneys, two ureters that drain the urine from the kidney to the bladder, and the urethra that drains urine from the bladder out of the body. The rectum is the last section of the large intestine, and part of the digestive system.

37. C: The neurovascular structure found under each rib in descending order is the vein, artery, and nerve. When a procedure such as a thoracocentesis or chest tube needs to be performed, the medical professional should aim for directly over the rib in order to avoid damaging to these structures.

38. D: The atomic number equals the number of protons and the number of electrons in an atom. Since Be has an atomic number of 4, it has 4 protons and 4 electrons. H has the fewest protons and electrons, as denoted by its atomic number of 1.

39. B: The spleen's job is to filter the blood by removing dead or dying red blood cells as well as microorganisms. In humans it is found in the left upper quadrant of the abdomen lateral to the liver.

40. C: Vaporization is the process of changing from a liquid to a gas. For instance, water vaporizes when boiled to create steam. Freezing is the process of changing from a liquid to a solid. Condensation describes changing from a gas to a liquid, and sublimation is the process of changing from a solid to a gas.

41. C: The nurse wants to investigate her patients' body temperatures. A thermometer is the only tool in the list that will help measure the temperature of a person's body.

42. A: The researcher should use statistical analysis to understand trends in the data. Different statistics tools can help manage and examine large data sets. The researcher would probably miss important correlations by looking at the individual data points, and eliminating most of the data would defeat the purpose of conducting the study. Simply staring at the data would not be helpful.

43. B: Based on the evidence, the most likely explanation for fly larvae in the spoiled food is that flies laid their eggs in the food. When the food was left out in the open, the flies had access to it and laid their eggs. However, when the food was in a sealed container, the flies could not lay their eggs in the food. Hence, the spoiled food in the sealed container had no fly larvae.

44. D: Longer life expectancy could be explained by any or all of the alternatives presented. Advances in medical technology, basic cleanliness, and vaccines could all help people live longer in the 21st century.

45. C: A scientific argument should be based on measurable and observable facts such as the patient's current symptoms and health history. Discussing the patient's appearance or the doctor's feelings does not communicate a scientific argument. While insurance may be a factor in most healthcare systems, the status of the patient's insurance does not communicate a scientific argument that justifies the need for the test.

46. C: Interferons are members of a larger class of proteins called cytokines. Cytokines are specialized proteins that carry signals between cells. Interferons are proteins that are produced by cells infected by pathogens such as viruses. They signal neighboring cells to produce antiviral proteins which help prevent the spread of infection.

47. D: Humans have three layers of skin called the epidermis, the dermis, and subcutaneous fat. Epidermis is the top layer of the skin, the dermis is the second layer, and subcutaneous makes up the bottom layer. The epidermis does not contain blood vessels.

48. A: The hypothalamus is a tiny gland at the base of the brain. It helps regulate temperature, sleep, emotions, sexual function and behavior. During puberty it secretes hormones that stimulate the gonads which initiate sexual development.

49. D: Of the given structures, veins have the lowest blood pressure. *Veins* carry oxygen-poor blood from the outlying parts of the body to the heart. An *artery* carries oxygen-rich blood from the heart to the peripheral parts of the body. An *arteriole* extends from an artery to a capillary. A *venule* is a tiny vein that extends from a capillary to a larger vein.

50. C: Of the four heart chambers, the left ventricle is the most muscular. When it contracts, it pushes blood out to the organs and extremities of the body. The right ventricle pushes blood into the lungs. The atria, on the other hand, receive blood from the outlying parts of the body and transport it into the ventricles. The basic process works as follows: Oxygen-poor blood fills the right atrium and is pumped into the right ventricle, from which it is pumped into the pulmonary artery and on to the lungs. In the lungs, this blood is oxygenated. The blood then reenters the heart at the left atrium, which when full pumps into the left ventricle. When the left ventricle is full, blood is pushed into the aorta and on to the organs and extremities of the body.

51. A: The *cerebrum* is the part of the brain that interprets sensory information. It is the largest part of the brain. The cerebrum is divided into two hemispheres, connected by a thin band of tissue called the corpus callosum. The *cerebellum* is positioned at the back of the head, between the brain stem and the cerebrum. It controls both voluntary and involuntary movements. The *medulla oblongata* forms the base of the brain. This part of the brain is responsible for blood flow and breathing, among other things.

52. C: A vaccination is a way of acquiring active artificial immunity, where an antigen is deliberately introduced into an individual to stimulate the immune system. Vaccines contain dead or dying pathogens which are not enough to cause an infection, but allow the immune system to "remember" the pathogen and become immune to it.

53. C: The *parasympathetic nervous system* is responsible for lowering the heart rate. It slows down the heart rate, dilates the blood vessels, and increases the secretions of the digestive system. The *central nervous system* is composed of the brain and the spinal cord. The *sympathetic nervous system* is a part of the autonomic nervous system; its role is to oppose the actions taken by the parasympathetic nervous system. So, the sympathetic nervous system accelerates the heart, contracts the blood vessels, and decreases the secretions of the digestive system.

English and Language Usage

1. A: Semicolons are used to separate items in a series when those items contain internal commas, such as in a listing of cities and states. Answer choice A correctly demonstrates this. Answer choice B places the semicolon between the city and its state, instead of between *each* listing of the city and its state, and this is incorrect. A comma is always used to separate a single instance of a city and a state. Answer choice C separate the items in the series with commas, but this creates confusion for the reader, since there are already commas between each city and its state. Answer choice D places commas between each item in the series, but fails to include the necessary comma between each city and its state.

2. B: This sentence best conveys the information without using too many words (choice D) or having an awkward construction (choices A and C).

3. D: Research papers are formal exercises that should not include several types of speech used in informal spoken settings. Colloquialisms are non-standard forms of language, such as "ain't," or slang, like "dude." Contractions represent the words as they sound in speech, so "do not" is formal whereas "don't" is informal. Relative pronouns are necessary in grammar. In the phrase "The boy who I met…," "who" is a relative pronoun.

4. C: When a plural word is made possessive, the standard rule is to place the apostrophe after the final *s*, as in *jurors'*. Answer choice C correctly demonstrates this. Answer choices A and D place the possessive apostrophe within *meals* (*meal's* and *meals'*), and these forms of the word do not make sense within the context of the sentence. Answer choice B places the possessive apostrophe before the final *s*, as in *juror's*, which indicates only a single juror. This form is incorrect in the context of the sentence.

5. B: A complex sentence contains a single independent clause in addition to a dependent clause. Answer choice B opens with the dependent clause *Before Ernestine purchases a book* and ends with the independent clause *she always checks to see if the library has it*. Answer choice A is a simple sentence, as it has no dependent clause. Answer choice C is a compound sentence, because it has two independent clauses. Answer choice D is also a simple sentence, although it has a compound subject.

6. D: In the context of the sentence, it appears that Finlay's parents are attempting to *coax* him by promising a trip to his favorite toy store. Answer choice A makes little sense, as the sentence indicates Finlay's parents want him to participate in the recital. Answer choice B might work, but the promise of a trip to the toy store seems more like a reward than a punishment. Answer choice C makes no sense when added to the sentence in place of the word *cajole*.

7. C: The correct plural form of *tempo* is *tempi*. This word has an Italian root, and thus follows the pattern of other, similar words that end in *-i* in their plural form. Note also that *tempo*, meaning time, is simply the Italian form of the Latin *tempus*. (Recall the Latin expression *tempus fugit*, or "time flies.") Other Latin-based nouns ending in *-us* also take the *-i* ending when made plural: *octopus > octopi, syllabus > syllabi*, etc.

8. A: In answer choice A, *aunt Jo* is correctly capitalized, because although *aunt* identifies a specific person, the word her makes *aunt* into an adjective rather than being part of her name. Titles such as uncle or aunt are only to be capitalized if they are at the beginning of a sentence or are used as part of the proper noun. Answer choice B fails to capitalize *Brother Mark*, as *Brother* is part of the full proper noun. In answer choice C, cousin should remain lower case as it is used to describe who Martha is, but is not used as part of her name. Answer choice D incorrectly capitalizes *Fall*. Seasons are not to be capitalized. *Chicago* is correctly capitalized as it is the name of a city, which is a proper noun.

9. C: *Acrimonious* means "bitter" or "vitriolic," and is very similar in meaning to *rancorous*.

10. B: Answer choice B demonstrates a comma splice, which is the use of a comma to join two independent clauses. Note that *however* is not a conjunction, and cannot join two sentences like other coordinating conjunctions (e.g., *and*, *but*, *or*, etc.) can. Answer choice A correctly uses a semicolon between the independent clauses. Answer choice C correctly uses a period between the independent clauses. Answer choice D correctly uses a comma and the coordinating conjunction *but* to join the independent clauses.

11. B: Answer choice B combines the sentences in the best way. The sentences are combined into a single sentence, and all of the details are still included. Answer choices A and D do a good job of combining the sentences, but still consist of more than one sentence. Answer choice C combines the sentences, but leaves out the part about how she "tried to find a way to attend both." There is no clear reason to leave this out, so answer choice C is not the best choice.

12. D: The context of the sentence indicates that Mara would feel great happiness.

13. D: If the root *meare* means "to pass," and the word *permeate* means "to penetrate or pervade," the most likely meaning of the prefix *per-* is "through." This would yield a literal word meaning of "to pass through," which is similar in meaning to the original: "to penetrate or pervade." The phrase "to pass across" does not match the original Latin origins. Similarly, "to pass by" and "to pass with" are not consistent with the meaning of "passing through."

14. B: Anthropology is the study of human culture. Cosmetology is the study of cosmetic techniques. Etymology is the study of word meanings. Genealogy is the study of family history. All of these words would indicate that the suffix *-logy* refers to the study of something. It cannot refer to a record, since that indicates something in the past, and the words in question describe activities that are ongoing. An affinity for something is not the same as a committed study of it, and each item in the question represents its own dedicated field. The suffix for "fear" is *-phobia*.

15. D: An adverb modifies a verb, and in the sentence, the word *well* modifies the verb *did* by indicating *how* Jacob did with his speech. The word *worried* is a verb. The word *about* is a preposition. The word *but* is a conjunction.

16. A: This answer provides an example of a formal speech, lays out the steps to a solution in a concise manner, and utilizes the correct transition words.

17. C: It is correct to pair a plural verb with a collective noun when that noun indicates a plural context. In answer choice C, it is clear that the faculty members are acting individually in their disagreement, so the plural verb makes sense. In answer choice A, the pronoun *neither* is singular, so the verb that accompanies it should also be singular. In answer choice B, the pronoun *all* is plural, so the accompanying verb should be plural. Similarly, in answer choice D, the pronoun *both* is plural, so the verb that accompanies it should also be plural.

18. D: The sentence suggests that the scholar was very *knowledgeable* about his subject matter; it is just that his presentation went over the students' heads. The word *authentic* suggests an external guarantee of correctness, which makes little sense in the context of the sentence. The word *arrogant* might be accurate, except that there is nothing in the sentence to suggest the guest speaker deliberately spoke over the students' heads. It is simply that his knowledge was not presented effectively given the audience. Finally, there is nothing in the sentence to suggest that the guest speaker was *faulty* in any way. Rather, he knew so much that he failed to connect with an audience that was less knowledgeable.

19. C: The word *sacrilegious* indicates a violation of sacred expectations, and wearing white to a funeral would be something that would violate the sacred expectations of many. The other answer choices are spelled incorrectly, particularly *sacreligious*, which spells the word with the correct spelling of *religious*. This is not correct, as the spelling is adjusted when joined to the other root.

20. D: A comma and the conjunction *and* are required to combine the sentences. *And* is a better choice than *but* because the second sentence is a continuation of the first rather than a contradiction. Choices A and B are incorrect because the conjunction *but* doesn't fit the meaning of the sentences. Choice A is also missing the required comma. Choice C uses the correct conjunction, *and*, but is missing the comma.

21. D: Answer choice D has a plural subject, but is still a simple sentence. Answer choice A is a compound sentence, as it is composed of two independent clauses. Answer choice B consists of two independent sentences that are joined by a semicolon. (The punctuation is correct, and creates two simple sentences, not one.) Answer choice C contains a dependent clause, so it is a complex sentence.

22. D: Answer choice D is a pronoun: the subjective case *I*. Answer choice A is a helping verb. Answer choice B is an adjective. Answer choice C is an adverb.

23. B: Answer choice B is the clearest and the most concise. Answer choices A and C include more than one independent clause. As the statement can function as a single independent clause, this is unnecessary. Answer choice D works, but it is not the best option in terms of style, clarity, and concision. The coordinating conjunction with the added independent clause makes the sentence more unwieldy than answer choice B.

24. B: The context of the sentence suggests that Mrs. Vanderbroek would not be delighted about any changes to her routine. Thus, answer choice B makes the most sense. Answer choice A has promise, but it does not exactly fit the meaning of the sentence. It is not that Mrs. Vanderbroek would be incapable of accepting change, but rather that she would not welcome it. Answer choices C and D indicate Mrs. Vanderbroek's overall response to changes, but they do not work as synonyms for the word *amenable*.

25. D: The words *quick*, *available*, and *little* are all adjectives in the sentence. *Quick* modifies *review*; *available* modifies *housing options*; *little* modifies *choice*. The word *rent* is part of the infinitive (i.e. verbal) phrase *to rent*.

26. A: Choice A uses correct punctuation and a logical conjunction. The conjunction *and* connects two independent clauses (meaning that they can stand on their own as sentences), there must be a comma before the conjunction. Therefore, choices B and D are incorrect because they are missing this comma. While choice C does have a comma before the conjunction, it uses the conjunction *but* rather than *and*. *But* implies that the two clauses contradict each other. *And* is a better choice because the two clauses are connected and support each other.

27. B: Young people will respond to and better comprehend informal, friendly speech. However, you would not want to be too informal when addressing an educated gathering of college professors or a professional board of directors. Informal speech likely would weaken addresses made before such audiences.

28. A: The form *bear* is correct in this context, because it suggests the right to carry or own arms. The form *bare* indicates an uncovered limb. The word *barre* is the French form of *bar*, and is typically used to describe a ballet barre where dancers train. The word *baire* is an alternative colloquial form that refers to a mosquito net in some parts of the United States.

TEAS Practice Test #3 (Online Interactive)

Special feature: In addition to the two full-length practice tests included in this section, you also have access to an **online interactive practice test!** Just follow the link below on your computer or mobile device to get started.

> **Online Interactive Practice Test**
> Visit mometrix.com/university/teas-bonus-practice-test

Image Credits

Fertilization: "Fertilization Sequence" by Wikimedia user Chippolito
(https://commons.wikimedia.org/wiki/File:Acrosomal_reaction_of_fertilization.PNG)

Fertilization: "Fertilization Sequence part two" by Wikimedia user Chippolito
(https://commons.wikimedia.org/wiki/File:Cortical_reaction_of_fertilization.PNG)

Respiratory System: "Respiratory System Diagram" by Wikimedia user BruceBlaus
(https://commons.wikimedia.org/wiki/File:Blausen_0770_RespiratorySystem_02.png)

Respiratory Zone: "Respiratory Zone Diagram" by Wikimedia user OpenStax College
(https://commons.wikimedia.org/wiki/File:2309_The_Respiratory_Zone_esp.jpg)

Thoracic Cavity: "Inspiration and Expiration" by OpenStax CNX user OpenStax College
(https://cnx.org/contents/14fb4ad7-39a1-4eee-ab6e-3ef2482e3e22@6.27)

Human Heart: "Diagram" by Wikimedia user Wapcaplet
(https://commons.wikimedia.org/wiki/File:Diagram_of_the_human_heart_(cropped).svg)

Pancreas: "Pancreas biliary" by Wikimedia user Boumphreyfr
(https://commons.wikimedia.org/wiki/File:Pancrease_biliary1.png)

Nervous System: "Diagram of Nervous System" by Fuzzform at English Wikipedia
(https://commons.wikimedia.org/wiki/File:NSdiagram.png)

Spinal Cross Sections: "Role of Spinal Cord" by Wikimedia user Polarlys
(https://commons.wikimedia.org/wiki/File:Medulla_spinalis_-_Section_-_English.svg)

Neurons: "Types of Neurons" by Wikimedia user Jonathan Haas
(https://commons.wikimedia.org/wiki/File:Neurons_uni_bi_multi_pseudouni.svg)

Neuroglia: "Types of Neuroglia" by Wikimedia user BruceBlaus
(https://commons.wikimedia.org/wiki/File:Blausen_0870_TypesofNeuroglia.png)

Capillary: "Fenestrated Capillary" by OpenStax CNX user OpenStax College
(https://cnx.org/contents/FPtK1zmh@6.27:zMTtFGyH@4/Introduction)

Blood: "Centrifuge Blood Sample" by KnuteKnudsen at English Wikipedia
(https://commons.wikimedia.org/wiki/File:Blood-centrifugation-scheme.png)

Lymphatic System: "Anatomy of the Lymphatic System" by OpenStax CNX user OpenStax College
(https://cnx.org/contents/FPtK1zmh@6.27:zMTtFGyH@4/Introduction)

Gastric Gland: "Diagram" by Wikimedia user Boumphreyfr
(https://commons.wikimedia.org/wiki/File:Gastric_gland.png)

Small Intestine: "Small Intestine Anatomy" by Wikimedia user BruceBlaus
(https://commons.wikimedia.org/wiki/File:Blausen_0817_SmallIntestine_Anatomy.png)

Large Intestine: "Large Intestine Anatomy" by Wikimedia user BruceBlaus
(https://commons.wikimedia.org/wiki/File:Blausen_0603_LargeIntestine_Anatomy.png)

Kidney and Nephron: "Kidney and Nephron Structures" by Wikimedia users Madhero88 and PioM
(https://commons.wikimedia.org/wiki/File:KidneyAndNephron-v4_Antares42.svg)

Loop of Henle CounterCurrent Multiplier System: "Diagram" by OpenStax CNX user OpenStax College (https://cnx.org/contents/FPtK1zmh@6.27:zMTtFGyH@4/Introduction)

Male Anatomy: "Diagram" by Wikimedia user Stephanie~commonswiki (https://commons.wikimedia.org/wiki/File:Male_anatomy.png)

Female Anatomy: "Diagram" by Wikimedia user CFCF (https://commons.wikimedia.org/wiki/File:Female_Reproductive_Anterior.JPG)

Skeletal Muscle: "Vein Pump" by OpenStax CNX author OpenStax College (https://cnx.org/contents/FPtK1zmh@6.27:zMTtFGyH@4/Introduction)

Cartilage: "Types of Cartilage" by OpenStax CNX user OpenStax College (https://cnx.org/contents/FPtK1zmh@6.27:zMTtFGyH@4/Introduction)

Epidermis: "Epidermis Structure" by Wikimedia user BruceBlaus (https://commons.wikimedia.org/wiki/File:Blausen_0353_Epidermis.png)

LICENSED UNDER CC BY 2.5 (CREATIVECOMMONS.ORG/LICENSES/BY/2.5/DEED.EN)

Stomach: "Stomach Diagram" by Wikimedia user Olek Remesz (https://commons.wikimedia.org/wiki/File:Ventriculus.svg)

Uterus and Mullerian Ducts: "Diagram" by StemBook authors J. Teixeira, B.R. Rueda, and J.K. Pru (https://commons.wikimedia.org/wiki/File:The_uterus_differentiates_from_the_fetal_M%C3%BCllerian_ducts..jpg)

Bone: "Composition of Bone" by Wikimedia user BDB (https://commons.wikimedia.org/wiki/File:Composition_of_bone.png)

How to Overcome Test Anxiety

Just the thought of taking a test is enough to make most people a little nervous. A test is an important event that can have a long-term impact on your future, so it's important to take it seriously and it's natural to feel anxious about performing well. But just because anxiety is normal, that doesn't mean that it's helpful in test taking, or that you should simply accept it as part of your life. Anxiety can have a variety of effects. These effects can be mild, like making you feel slightly nervous, or severe, like blocking your ability to focus or remember even a simple detail.

If you experience test anxiety—whether severe or mild—it's important to know how to beat it. To discover this, first you need to understand what causes test anxiety.

Causes of Test Anxiety

While we often think of anxiety as an uncontrollable emotional state, it can actually be caused by simple, practical things. One of the most common causes of test anxiety is that a person does not feel adequately prepared for their test. This feeling can be the result of many different issues such as poor study habits or lack of organization, but the most common culprit is time management. Starting to study too late, failing to organize your study time to cover all of the material, or being distracted while you study will mean that you're not well prepared for the test. This may lead to cramming the night before, which will cause you to be physically and mentally exhausted for the test. Poor time management also contributes to feelings of stress, fear, and hopelessness as you realize you are not well prepared but don't know what to do about it.

Other times, test anxiety is not related to your preparation for the test but comes from unresolved fear. This may be a past failure on a test, or poor performance on tests in general. It may come from comparing yourself to others who seem to be performing better or from the stress of living up to expectations. Anxiety may be driven by fears of the future—how failure on this test would affect your educational and career goals. These fears are often completely irrational, but they can still negatively impact your test performance.

> **Review Video: <u>3 Reasons You Have Test Anxiety</u>**
> Visit mometrix.com/academy and enter code: 428468

Elements of Test Anxiety

As mentioned earlier, test anxiety is considered to be an emotional state, but it has physical and mental components as well. Sometimes you may not even realize that you are suffering from test anxiety until you notice the physical symptoms. These can include trembling hands, rapid heartbeat, sweating, nausea, and tense muscles. Extreme anxiety may lead to fainting or vomiting. Obviously, any of these symptoms can have a negative impact on testing. It is important to recognize them as soon as they begin to occur so that you can address the problem before it damages your performance.

Review Video: 3 Ways to Tell You Have Test Anxiety
Visit mometrix.com/academy and enter code: 927847

The mental components of test anxiety include trouble focusing and inability to remember learned information. During a test, your mind is on high alert, which can help you recall information and stay focused for an extended period of time. However, anxiety interferes with your mind's natural processes, causing you to blank out, even on the questions you know well. The strain of testing during anxiety makes it difficult to stay focused, especially on a test that may take several hours. Extreme anxiety can take a huge mental toll, making it difficult not only to recall test information but even to understand the test questions or pull your thoughts together.

Review Video: How Test Anxiety Affects Memory
Visit mometrix.com/academy and enter code: 609003

Effects of Test Anxiety

Test anxiety is like a disease—if left untreated, it will get progressively worse. Anxiety leads to poor performance, and this reinforces the feelings of fear and failure, which in turn lead to poor performances on subsequent tests. It can grow from a mild nervousness to a crippling condition. If allowed to progress, test anxiety can have a big impact on your schooling, and consequently on your future.

Test anxiety can spread to other parts of your life. Anxiety on tests can become anxiety in any stressful situation, and blanking on a test can turn into panicking in a job situation. But fortunately, you don't have to let anxiety rule your testing and determine your grades. There are a number of relatively simple steps you can take to move past anxiety and function normally on a test and in the rest of life.

Review Video: How Test Anxiety Impacts Your Grades
Visit mometrix.com/academy and enter code: 939819

Physical Steps for Beating Test Anxiety

While test anxiety is a serious problem, the good news is that it can be overcome. It doesn't have to control your ability to think and remember information. While it may take time, you can begin taking steps today to beat anxiety.

Just as your first hint that you may be struggling with anxiety comes from the physical symptoms, the first step to treating it is also physical. Rest is crucial for having a clear, strong mind. If you are tired, it is much easier to give in to anxiety. But if you establish good sleep habits, your body and mind will be ready to perform optimally, without the strain of exhaustion. Additionally, sleeping well helps you to retain information better, so you're more likely to recall the answers when you see the test questions.

Getting good sleep means more than going to bed on time. It's important to allow your brain time to relax. Take study breaks from time to time so it doesn't get overworked, and don't study right before bed. Take time to rest your mind before trying to rest your body, or you may find it difficult to fall asleep.

Review Video: <u>The Importance of Sleep for Your Brain</u>
Visit mometrix.com/academy and enter code: 319338

Along with sleep, other aspects of physical health are important in preparing for a test. Good nutrition is vital for good brain function. Sugary foods and drinks may give a burst of energy but this burst is followed by a crash, both physically and emotionally. Instead, fuel your body with protein and vitamin-rich foods.

Also, drink plenty of water. Dehydration can lead to headaches and exhaustion, especially if your brain is already under stress from the rigors of the test. Particularly if your test is a long one, drink water during the breaks. And if possible, take an energy-boosting snack to eat between sections.

Review Video: <u>How Diet Can Affect your Mood</u>
Visit mometrix.com/academy and enter code: 624317

Along with sleep and diet, a third important part of physical health is exercise. Maintaining a steady workout schedule is helpful, but even taking 5-minute study breaks to walk can help get your blood pumping faster and clear your head. Exercise also releases endorphins, which contribute to a positive feeling and can help combat test anxiety.

When you nurture your physical health, you are also contributing to your mental health. If your body is healthy, your mind is much more likely to be healthy as well. So take time to rest, nourish your body with healthy food and water, and get moving as much as possible. Taking these physical steps will make you stronger and more able to take the mental steps necessary to overcome test anxiety.

Review Video: <u>How to Stay Healthy and Prevent Test Anxiety</u>
Visit mometrix.com/academy and enter code: 877894

Mental Steps for Beating Test Anxiety

Working on the mental side of test anxiety can be more challenging, but as with the physical side, there are clear steps you can take to overcome it. As mentioned earlier, test anxiety often stems from lack of preparation, so the obvious solution is to prepare for the test. Effective studying may be the most important weapon you have for beating test anxiety, but you can and should employ several other mental tools to combat fear.

First, boost your confidence by reminding yourself of past success—tests or projects that you aced. If you're putting as much effort into preparing for this test as you did for those, there's no reason you should expect to fail here. Work hard to prepare; then trust your preparation.

Second, surround yourself with encouraging people. It can be helpful to find a study group, but be sure that the people you're around will encourage a positive attitude. If you spend time with others who are anxious or cynical, this will only contribute to your own anxiety. Look for others who are motivated to study hard from a desire to succeed, not from a fear of failure.

Third, reward yourself. A test is physically and mentally tiring, even without anxiety, and it can be helpful to have something to look forward to. Plan an activity following the test, regardless of the outcome, such as going to a movie or getting ice cream.

When you are taking the test, if you find yourself beginning to feel anxious, remind yourself that you know the material. Visualize successfully completing the test. Then take a few deep, relaxing breaths and return to it. Work through the questions carefully but with confidence, knowing that you are capable of succeeding.

Developing a healthy mental approach to test taking will also aid in other areas of life. Test anxiety affects more than just the actual test—it can be damaging to your mental health and even contribute to depression. It's important to beat test anxiety before it becomes a problem for more than testing.

Review Video: Test Anxiety and Depression
Visit mometrix.com/academy and enter code: 904704

Study Strategy

Being prepared for the test is necessary to combat anxiety, but what does being prepared look like? You may study for hours on end and still not feel prepared. What you need is a strategy for test prep. The next few pages outline our recommended steps to help you plan out and conquer the challenge of preparation.

STEP 1: SCOPE OUT THE TEST

Learn everything you can about the format (multiple choice, essay, etc.) and what will be on the test. Gather any study materials, course outlines, or sample exams that may be available. Not only will this help you to prepare, but knowing what to expect can help to alleviate test anxiety.

STEP 2: MAP OUT THE MATERIAL

Look through the textbook or study guide and make note of how many chapters or sections it has. Then divide these over the time you have. For example, if a book has 15 chapters and you have five days to study, you need to cover three chapters each day. Even better, if you have the time, leave an extra day at the end for overall review after you have gone through the material in depth.

If time is limited, you may need to prioritize the material. Look through it and make note of which sections you think you already have a good grasp on, and which need review. While you are studying, skim quickly through the familiar sections and take more time on the challenging parts. Write out your plan so you don't get lost as you go. Having a written plan also helps you feel more in control of the study, so anxiety is less likely to arise from feeling overwhelmed at the amount to cover.

STEP 3: GATHER YOUR TOOLS

Decide what study method works best for you. Do you prefer to highlight in the book as you study and then go back over the highlighted portions? Or do you type out notes of the important information? Or is it helpful to make flashcards that you can carry with you? Assemble the pens, index cards, highlighters, post-it notes, and any other materials you may need so you won't be distracted by getting up to find things while you study.

If you're having a hard time retaining the information or organizing your notes, experiment with different methods. For example, try color-coding by subject with colored pens, highlighters, or post-it notes. If you learn better by hearing, try recording yourself reading your notes so you can listen while in the car, working out, or simply sitting at your desk. Ask a friend to quiz you from your flashcards, or try teaching someone the material to solidify it in your mind.

STEP 4: CREATE YOUR ENVIRONMENT

It's important to avoid distractions while you study. This includes both the obvious distractions like visitors and the subtle distractions like an uncomfortable chair (or a too-comfortable couch that makes you want to fall asleep). Set up the best study environment possible: good lighting and a comfortable work area. If background music helps you focus, you may want to turn it on, but otherwise keep the room quiet. If you are using a computer to take notes, be sure you don't have any other windows open, especially applications like social media, games, or anything else that could distract you. Silence your phone and turn off notifications. Be sure to keep water close by so you stay hydrated while you study (but avoid unhealthy drinks and snacks).

Also, take into account the best time of day to study. Are you freshest first thing in the morning? Try to set aside some time then to work through the material. Is your mind clearer in the afternoon or evening? Schedule your study session then. Another method is to study at the same time of day that you will take the test, so that your brain gets used to working on the material at that time and will be ready to focus at test time.

STEP 5: STUDY!

Once you have done all the study preparation, it's time to settle into the actual studying. Sit down, take a few moments to settle your mind so you can focus, and begin to follow your study plan. Don't give in to distractions or let yourself procrastinate. This is your time to prepare so you'll be ready to fearlessly approach the test. Make the most of the time and stay focused.

Of course, you don't want to burn out. If you study too long you may find that you're not retaining the information very well. Take regular study breaks. For example, taking five minutes out of every hour to walk briskly, breathing deeply and swinging your arms, can help your mind stay fresh.

As you get to the end of each chapter or section, it's a good idea to do a quick review. Remind yourself of what you learned and work on any difficult parts. When you feel that you've mastered the material, move on to the next part. At the end of your study session, briefly skim through your notes again.

But while review is helpful, cramming last minute is NOT. If at all possible, work ahead so that you won't need to fit all your study into the last day. Cramming overloads your brain with more information than it can process and retain, and your tired mind may struggle to recall even previously learned information when it is overwhelmed with last-minute study. Also, the urgent nature of cramming and the stress placed on your brain contribute to anxiety. You'll be more likely to go to the test feeling unprepared and having trouble thinking clearly.

So don't cram, and don't stay up late before the test, even just to review your notes at a leisurely pace. Your brain needs rest more than it needs to go over the information again. In fact, plan to finish your studies by noon or early afternoon the day before the test. Give your brain the rest of the day to relax or focus on other things, and get a good night's sleep. Then you will be fresh for the test and better able to recall what you've studied.

STEP 6: TAKE A PRACTICE TEST

Many courses offer sample tests, either online or in the study materials. This is an excellent resource to check whether you have mastered the material, as well as to prepare for the test format and environment.

Check the test format ahead of time: the number of questions, the type (multiple choice, free response, etc.), and the time limit. Then create a plan for working through them. For example, if you have 30 minutes to take a 60-question test, your limit is 30 seconds per question. Spend less time on the questions you know well so that you can take more time on the difficult ones.

If you have time to take several practice tests, take the first one open book, with no time limit. Work through the questions at your own pace and make sure you fully understand them. Gradually work up to taking a test under test conditions: sit at a desk with all study materials put away and set a timer. Pace yourself to make sure you finish the test with time to spare and go back to check your answers if you have time.

After each test, check your answers. On the questions you missed, be sure you understand why you missed them. Did you misread the question (tests can use tricky wording)? Did you forget the information? Or was it something you hadn't learned? Go back and study any shaky areas that the practice tests reveal.

Taking these tests not only helps with your grade, but also aids in combating test anxiety. If you're already used to the test conditions, you're less likely to worry about it, and working through tests until you're scoring well gives you a confidence boost. Go through the practice tests until you feel comfortable, and then you can go into the test knowing that you're ready for it.

Test Tips

On test day, you should be confident, knowing that you've prepared well and are ready to answer the questions. But aside from preparation, there are several test day strategies you can employ to maximize your performance.

First, as stated before, get a good night's sleep the night before the test (and for several nights before that, if possible). Go into the test with a fresh, alert mind rather than staying up late to study.

Try not to change too much about your normal routine on the day of the test. It's important to eat a nutritious breakfast, but if you normally don't eat breakfast at all, consider eating just a protein bar. If you're a coffee drinker, go ahead and have your normal coffee. Just make sure you time it so that the caffeine doesn't wear off right in the middle of your test. Avoid sugary beverages, and drink enough water to stay hydrated but not so much that you need a restroom break 10 minutes into the test. If your test isn't first thing in the morning, consider going for a walk or doing a light workout before the test to get your blood flowing.

Allow yourself enough time to get ready, and leave for the test with plenty of time to spare so you won't have the anxiety of scrambling to arrive in time. Another reason to be early is to select a good seat. It's helpful to sit away from doors and windows, which can be distracting. Find a good seat, get out your supplies, and settle your mind before the test begins.

When the test begins, start by going over the instructions carefully, even if you already know what to expect. Make sure you avoid any careless mistakes by following the directions.

Then begin working through the questions, pacing yourself as you've practiced. If you're not sure on an answer, don't spend too much time on it, and don't let it shake your confidence. Either skip it and come back later, or eliminate as many wrong answers as possible and guess among the remaining ones. Don't dwell on these questions as you continue—put them out of your mind and focus on what lies ahead.

Be sure to read all of the answer choices, even if you're sure the first one is the right answer. Sometimes you'll find a better one if you keep reading. But don't second-guess yourself if you do immediately know the answer. Your gut instinct is usually right. Don't let test anxiety rob you of the information you know.

If you have time at the end of the test (and if the test format allows), go back and review your answers. Be cautious about changing any, since your first instinct tends to be correct, but make sure you didn't misread any of the questions or accidentally mark the wrong answer choice. Look over any you skipped and make an educated guess.

At the end, leave the test feeling confident. You've done your best, so don't waste time worrying about your performance or wishing you could change anything. Instead, celebrate the successful completion of this test. And finally, use this test to learn how to deal with anxiety even better next time.

Review Video: 5 Tips to Beat Test Anxiety
Visit mometrix.com/academy and enter code: 570656

Important Qualification

Not all anxiety is created equal. If your test anxiety is causing major issues in your life beyond the classroom or testing center, or if you are experiencing troubling physical symptoms related to your anxiety, it may be a sign of a serious physiological or psychological condition. If this sounds like your situation, we strongly encourage you to seek professional help.

Thank You

We at Mometrix would like to extend our heartfelt thanks to you, our friend and patron, for allowing us to play a part in your journey. It is a privilege to serve people from all walks of life who are unified in their commitment to building the best future they can for themselves.

The preparation you devote to these important testing milestones may be the most valuable educational opportunity you have for making a real difference in your life. We encourage you to put your heart into it—that feeling of succeeding, overcoming, and yes, conquering will be well worth the hours you've invested.

We want to hear your story, your struggles and your successes, and if you see any opportunities for us to improve our materials so we can help others even more effectively in the future, please share that with us as well. **The team at Mometrix would be absolutely thrilled to hear from you!** So please, send us an email (support@mometrix.com) and let's stay in touch.

> **If you'd like some additional help, check out these other resources we offer for your exam:**
> **http://MometrixFlashcards.com/TEAS**

Additional Bonus Material

Due to our efforts to try to keep this book to a manageable length, we've created a link that will give you access to all of your additional bonus material.

Please visit https://www.mometrix.com/bonus948/teas6 to access the information.